Fitness in Special Populations

Roy J. Shephard, MD
University of Toronto, Ontario, Canada

Human Kinetics Books
Champaign, Illinois

Library of Congress Cataloging-in-Publication Data

Shephard, Roy J.
  Fitness in special populations / Roy J. Shephard.
    p. cm.
  Includes bibliographical references.
  ISBN 0-87322-270-9
  1. Physical fitness for the physically handicapped. 2. Physical
fitness--Testing. 3. Physical education for handicapped persons.
I. Title.
  GV482.7.S54 1990
  613.7'087--dc20   89-27879
                                                       CIP

ISBN: 0-87322-270-9

Copyright © 1990 by Roy J. Shephard

Figures 2.1 through 2.9 and Figure 7.2 appear courtesy of Dr. Robert Jackson. Figures
4.1 and 4.2 appear courtesy of M. Luc Noreau. Figure 7.3 appears courtesy of the Athletic
Information Bureau.

Developmental Editors: Kathy Kane and Joanne Fetzner
Production Director: Ernie Noa
Copyeditor: Julie Anderson
Assistant Editors: Robert King and Timothy Ryan
Proofreader: Laurie McGee
Typesetter: Brad Colson
Text Design: Keith Blomberg
Text Layout: Jill Wikgren
Cover Design: Hunter Graphics
Printer: Braun-Brumfield

Printed in the United States of America

10 9 8 7 6 5 4 3 2 1

Human Kinetics Books
A Division of Human Kinetics Publishers, Inc.
Box 5076, Champaign, IL 61825-5076
1-800-747-4HKP

Contents

Preface

"We can no longer tolerate the invisibility of the handicapped in America."
Senator Hubert Humphrey (1972), Congressional Record **118**, p. 525.

At one time the disabled were an invisible minority, kept in the supposed security of homes and institutions (where they quickly died of infection or of despair). The medical miracles of the late 20th century have unfortunately failed to reduce the size of the disabled population; indeed, the proportion of those with certain types of lesions has actually increased. Technological advances, including widespread use of the automobile and the continuing horrors of modern warfare, have served to augment the incidence of spinal cord injuries; moreover, the use of antibiotics and modern techniques of rehabilitation have greatly enhanced the survival prospects of individuals with paraplegia, thus increasing the overall proportion of such people in the community. In similar fashion, the improved medical treatment of other disabling conditions has extended the average period of survival and thus the representation of the disabled in our world of the late 20th century.

Nevertheless, much of the apparent increase in the numbers of disabled individuals is due to their greater visibility, as they have taken their rightful place in the mainstream of society. In the United States, this trend has been helped by the fight of the late President Franklin D. Roosevelt against poliomyelitis and the support of the Kennedy family for the mentally retarded. In Canada, feats such as the completion of a wheelchair marathon in under two hours, Rick Hanson's world wheelchair tour, and transcontinental walks by amputees such as Steve Fonyo have shown that the disabled are not a group of "cripples" to be locked away with minimal support until they die. Given an adequate program of rehabilitation, the great majority of the disabled are neither diseased nor unhealthy. If granted appropriate consideration by the able-bodied, they are capable of playing a vital role in our society and can stir our emotions through challenging performances in both solo activities and team sports.

Over the past decade, physical educators and physiotherapists have become increasingly aware of the exciting potential of disabled competitors. Sports that began merely as a pleasant form of rehabilitation or psychotherapy have developed to extremely high levels of competitive performance. They offer not only a means of self-actualization for the disabled individual, but also a clear demonstration to both the critical and the over-sympathetic of the potential contribution special populations can make to society.

Professional recognition of the social and economic potential of the successfully rehabilitated disabled person has led to the introduction of an increasing number of university courses and programs in adapted physical activity at both undergraduate and graduate levels of instruction. Graduates from such programs have sought to help the disabled to develop personal fitness (thus countering some of the medical hazards of a sedentary lifestyle), to move with greater efficiency (thus making better use of their restricted physiological potential), and to find pleasure in active recreation (thus addressing some of the adverse psychological effects of disability).

A series of six international conferences on adapted physical activity have been organized, the most recent in Berlin (June, 1989), and selected papers from these events have subsequently been published. There have also been several books offering detailed suggestions on exercise programming for the disabled. However, to date, there has been no attempt to provide a clear, synthetic account of the current fitness status of the disabled and their responses to vigorous, competitive physical activity. The present volume is designed to address this need. It provides detailed information on the performance of individuals with conditions recognized by national and international sports organizations—spinal cord injury, amputations, blindness, deafness, cerebral palsy, muscular dystrophies and multiple sclerosis, scoliosis, and mental retardation. No discussion of emotional disturbances or other health impairments is attempted, although it should be noted that these are official U.S. Department of Education categories of disability. The material that is offered should appeal to senior undergraduate and graduate students in physical education and physiotherapy, together with a variety of health professionals who offer exercise prescriptions or advice on training to the active disabled person who wishes to participate in competition.

Inevitably, I have encountered some difficulty in presenting the known facts about the various types of disability, physical and mental, in a way that would not stereotype the affected individual. I recognize that agencies ministering to the disabled have objected to the indiscriminate use of such words and phrases as handicap, victim, wheelchair athlete, wheelchair bound, or "confined" to a wheelchair, and that opinions differ on an optimum, non-pejorative terminology. I certainly remain open to alternative suggestions of language for any future edition of this book but, nevertheless, I also recognize that the physiological status of a person who spends all of his or her waking hours in a wheelchair is different from that of the person who has the good fortune to expend a similar amount of energy in walking and running. Such terms as disability, handicap, wheelchair confined, and mentally retarded are retained in order to allow clear descriptions of the different types of disability, but I would stress at the outset that this in no way denies the right of such individuals to be treated as equal members of society.

The text has been organized into 10 chapters. These cover in turn normal human responses to exercise and training, historical aspects of exercise for the disabled, current issues in disability classification, methods of fitness assessment, current functional status of various categories of the disabled, training programs, bio-mechanical issues (including an analysis of movement patterns and mechanical efficiency, practical considerations in the design of equipment such as racing wheelchairs, and the prevention of injuries), psycho–social aspects (current patterns of lifestyle adopted by the disabled, the impact of disability upon attitudes and personality, methods of motivation to increased physical activity, and the impact of such activity upon mood and lifestyle), practical issues in program design (particularly the design of effective training regimens that will enhance physical condition while improving the mental health of the individual), and comparative international issues (particularly differences in legislation, programs, and patterns of treatment in various world cultures). A comprehensive bibliography provides convenient access to recent literature in this rapidly growing area of scientific investigation, and a glossary provides simple definitions of medical terms that may be unfamiliar to the more general reader.

As has commonly been the case in my writings, I have drawn heavily upon both personal experience and research investigations, which have been shared with a number of gifted colleagues and graduate students. In the present context, I may make special mention of Dr. R.W. Jackson and Dr. J. Crawford of the Toronto Hospital, Professors Graham Ward and Gaston Godin (both formerly with our graduate program in exercise sciences), the late Professor Mavis Berridge (who for many years taught our school's undergraduate courses in adapted physical activity), Mary Bluechardt, Glen Davis, Peggy Kofsky-Singer, Luc Noveau, Mary Lee, Marion Fraser, Heather Hattin, and Josie diNatale. All of these individuals have in their own special way enriched the contents of this book through their insights, their research, and a real personal dedication to the cause of the disabled. A special word of gratitude must also be expressed to our disabled subjects themselves; I particularly appreciate how cheefully they faced the practical problems of repeated travel in a large city in order to contribute to our controlled laboratory studies of exercise training. It is my hope that all of these wonderful people will find some recompense for their efforts in the appearance of this book.

Roy J. Shephard

Chapter 1

Normal Human Responses to Exercise and Training

Before proceeding to a discussion of exercise and training responses in various forms of physical disability, we will briefly review general concepts of exercise, fitness, and training. For a detailed treatment of the subject, including full references and a discussion of differences in response encountered in children and older adults, see Shephard (1982a, 1982b, 1987).

Some Basic Definitions of Exercise and Fitness

Caspersen, Powell, and Christenson (1985) reviewed the terminology of exercise and fitness, drawing clear distinctions between the physical demands of employment, deliberate structured leisure activity designed to improve or maintain some component of fitness (i.e., exercise), and habitual physical activity (which encompasses the physical demands of employment, exercise, normal ambulation, and domestic chores). In this schema, physical fitness was regarded as a set of attributes that influence one's ability to perform physical activity, itself being augmented by repeated physical activity, whether undertaken at work, at leisure, or at home.

The World Health Organization (WHO) earlier reviewed physical fitness in the context of cardiovascular health (Shephard, 1968), defining it as "the ability to perform muscular work satisfactorily." This definition also reflects the ability of the individual to undertake demanding physical activity wherever it is encountered—at work, at home, or on the sports field. Such a concept seems appropriate to the disabled person, who may face a severe physical challenge several times during a normal day. The level of fitness thus defined is influenced by the basic exercise responses of the person (an expression of constitutional endowment and any chronic pathology), the extent to which these basic responses are optimized by vigorous habitual activity, the efficiency with which the individual applies the available physiological capacity to the performance of a given mechanical task, and the motivation to succeed as effort approaches the limits of physiological capacity.

Other authors, particularly those interested in high-performance sport, have taken a more task-specific approach to fitness, asking "fitness for what?" Thus, an individual may be very well prepared for an event such as wheelchair weight lifting but in very poor physical condition to undertake a wheelchair marathon race. Fitness for athletic events depends heavily upon body build and muscle fiber type; thus the weight lifter has a high percentage of fast twitch muscle fibers in the arm and shoulder muscles, whereas a successful distance wheelchair competitor has a high percentage of slow twitch fibers in the same muscle groups. Such sport-specific fitness is largely inherited rather than induced by deliberate habitual activity, and although it is important to those selecting national teams of gold medalists, it has less relevance to the health professional who is attempting to improve the physical condition of the average disabled individual.

The Biochemical Basis of Work Performance

Any type of physical activity requires the performance of physical work as the mass of the individual's body, a wheelchair, or other objects are displaced against the resisting forces of gravity, inertia, and wind. Additional amounts of energy must be expended internally in stabilizing the body and meeting the demands of increased ventilation and cardiac pump function.

The immediate source of power for the performance of both external and internal work is the muscle fiber. Here, a chemical combination of the muscle proteins actin and myosin induces a shortening of the muscle filaments. In skeletal muscle this allows a force to be applied through the tendon to related bones and external objects, whereas in the heart tension is sustained in the ventricular wall and effort is applied to the expulsion of blood against the impedance offered by the arterial blood pressure.

Chemical energy for the actin/myosin combination is supplied by two high-energy phosphate compounds—adenosine triphosphate (ATP) and creatine phosphate. Both are stored within the active muscle fibers. Unfortunately, the local reserve of these "phosphagens" is extremely limited (a total of 15-25 mmol/kg wet weight), and depots are thus exhausted within a few seconds of beginning all-out muscular activity. Thereafter, energy derived from ingested foods must be used to resynthesize adenosine triphosphate and creatine phosphate if muscle contraction is to continue. The principal metabolic options are a breakdown of glycogen (previously stored within the active muscle fibers) or of free fatty acids (transported via the bloodstream from adipose tissue depots). The metabolism of free fatty acids occurs only within the muscle mitochondria, and oxygen is essential for this process (aerobic metabolism). If oxygen is freely available, glycogen is oxidized to carbon dioxide and water, but if the local oxygen supply is inadequate, a partial breakdown to pyruvate is also possible within the muscle cytoplasm (anaerobic metabolism). An important by-product of the anaerobic reaction is lactic acid. Conversion of accumulating pyruvate to lactic acid quickly raises the acidity of the muscle fiber to a critical level, inhibiting key enzymes involved in the breakdown of glycogen (particularly phosphorylase and phospho-fructokinase). Thus, all-out anaerobic exercise is self-limiting, being halted by a build-up of lactic acid within 30 to 40 seconds. At exhaustion the arterial pH of a well-trained athlete may drop as low as 6.80 (Kindermann, Keul, & Lehmann, 1975), corresponding to an intramuscular pH of about 6.60, but sedentary subjects commonly stop exercising at a blood pH of around 7.20.

Thereafter, the continuation of vigorous physical activity depends on a steady supply of oxygen to the working tissues; each 21 kJ (5 kcal) of energy usage requires about 1 L of oxygen. Delivery should thus match metabolic demand during endurance exercise. This is possible if the intensity of effort remains moderate. However, if a certain threshold is passed (often 60-70% of peak oxygen intake for a given task), the quantity of oxygen supplied by the circulation becomes inadequate to meet the needs of some of the muscle fibers (the so-called anaerobic threshold). At higher intensities of exercise lactic acid is produced faster than it can be removed, and there is a progressive intramuscular and intravascular accumulation of this substance. A limiting point of fatigue is thus reached similar to that which would have been encountered with a brief bout of all-out effort.

The preferred fuel of the skeletal muscles is glycogen. However, intramuscular reserves of this substance become exhausted over about 100 minutes of vigorous rhythmic exercise (longer if special high-carbohydrate diets have been adopted to boost local glycogen stores). Thereafter, the only source of carbohydrate is gluconeogenesis (the formation of glucose by the liver from hepatic glycogen stores, glycerol metabolism, conversion of circulating lactate or pyruvate, and amino acid breakdown). Under anaerobic conditions, physical work becomes virtually impossible after glycogen depletion because of local muscle weakness and fatigue. For example, a person who has been operating a wheelchair continuously for some hours will have exhausted arm and shoulder glycogen stores. He or she may continue to function moderately well while wheeling on a level road but will find it impossible to climb a slight rise because the resultant increase of muscle tension restricts blood flow to the working muscles, preventing aerobic metabolism of fat. If oxygen is available to glycogen-depleted muscles, effort can continue, but aerobic performance becomes limited by the rate at which depot fat can be mobilized and transported to the muscle mitochondria.

Types of Muscular Activity

Two main types of muscular activity are distinguished—rhythmic or isotonic movements and static or isometric muscle contractions. During an isotonic movement, the tension within the muscle remains constant (typically at a low level) so that a major part of the available chemical energy can be applied to the process of muscle shortening. In contrast, during an isometric contraction the muscle is not allowed to shorten; instead, tension is developed against an internal or an external resistance.

Although researchers can devise relatively pure forms of both isotonic and isometric effort in the laboratory, most of the activities encountered in ordinary daily life demand varying proportions of both isometric and isotonic effort. For example, propulsion of a wheelchair across a smooth and level surface involves mainly isotonic activity, but isometric effort is also required to maintain body posture within the wheelchair. In contrast, weight lifting demands the development of a large tension in the active muscles, but it also requires some shortening as the weights are lifted to their final position. Eccentric contraction is a third type of activity in which the muscles contract as their fibers are lengthened by an external force (e.g., the braking of a wheelchair by applying tension to the push rim when descending a steep slope). A final variant, commonly applied to the testing of muscle function, is an isokinetic contraction; here, a constant-speed motor allows a major joint such as the elbow to be rotated at a predetermined slow or rapid speed, and the maximum isokinetic force of the individual is recorded throughout the arc of rotation.

Blood flow to the working muscles is strongly influenced by the local intramuscular tension (Kay & Shephard, 1969; Royce, 1959). Flow restriction begins when 15 to 20% of maximum voluntary force is exerted, and occlusion of the intramuscular blood vessels becomes complete at about 70% of maximum voluntary force. Isometric (postural) and eccentric (braking) contractions are much more fatiguing than isotonic movements; not only is the intramuscular tension high during an isometric contraction, but there is a relaxation phase when the local circulation is restored.

Types of Isotonic Activity

Isotonic activities can be classified in terms of their duration; categories of performance include explosive power, anaerobic power, anaerobic capacity, aerobic power, and very prolonged work.

Explosive Power

Occasional throwing and jumping feats call for a single explosive movement, typically documented as a maximum instantaneous rate of power production. In the able-bodied person, a simple measure of this performance is provided by the jump-and-reach test, power being calculated from body mass and the height of jump; the force plate allows a more accurate measurement of such an impulse in the laboratory. Analogous tests can be applied in a wheelchair, for example, the distance the chair is propelled up a ramp by a single movement.

Anaerobic Power

A sprint-type activity (whether for individual competition or for the sudden bursts of speed demanded by a team sport) involves anaerobic power, the maximum rate at which external work can be performed in the absence of oxygen. Simple field tests can be based on track performance over short distances. In the laboratory, researchers can test the able-bodied with a timed staircase sprint or all-out cycle ergometry. Parallel ergometer tests can be devised for the wheelchair disabled. Performance is usually expressed as a peak power output measured over a brief interval (5 s in the Wingate test; Bar-Or, 1981), although an equivalent steady-state oxygen delivery is sometimes calculated. The latter depends upon mechanical efficiency. Some authors assume that a maximum of 25% of food energy is converted to useful work, but the efficiency may be rather higher during a very brief effort, as ATP is not necessarily resynthesized.

Anaerobic Capacity

Somewhat more protracted exercise (10 s to 2 min duration, as in a 400-m track event) is limited primarily by the individual's tolerance of accumulating lactic acid, the so-called anaerobic capacity. An individual's performance may be expressed as the maximum power output developed over an arbitrary period (e.g., 30 s of all-out cycle ergometry in the Wingate test; Bar-Or, 1981), or an equivalent oxygen transport may again be calculated.

Aerobic Power

If activity continues steadily for more than 1 to 2 minutes (e.g., a 1,500- or 5,000-m track or road race), the dominant factor influencing performance becomes the aerobic power, the steady-state transport of oxygen to the working muscles. Once more, the status of an individual may be documented as a maximum power output, in this case determined during progressive ergometer exercise sufficient to exhaust the subject within perhaps 10 minutes. Alternatively, the peak oxygen transport may be determined in the final 30 seconds prior to exhaustion of the subject. The able-bodied person is best tested by uphill treadmill running, but in those with spinal injuries analogous testing can be undertaken using a wheelchair or an arm ergometer. The recorded maximum oxygen intake values relate to body mass and even more closely to lean body mass; thus, data are often expressed as a relative oxygen transport (ml/kg • min) rather than as the absolute value (L/min). Controversy continues as to whether peak oxygen transport is determined simply by central cardiorespiratory factors or whether there is a significant influence from the volume of active muscle in the working limbs. During uphill treadmill running, the observed peak of oxygen intake is not substantially modified by adding arm work. On the other hand, the peak oxygen intake that an able-bodied person can develop when using the arms is only about 70% of that developed when using the legs. A limitation of ostensibly aerobic performance by the volume of active muscle rather than by cardiac output seems particularly likely in individuals whose major muscle groups are no longer functional.

Very Prolonged Exercise

In very prolonged competitions, considerations other than oxygen transport influence performance. We have noted the possibility that intramuscular glycogen reserves will become exhausted; at present, no simple tests of muscle glycogen exist other than biopsy and histochemical examination. In adverse environments (extremes of heat or cold), fluid depletion and an increase or decrease of core temperature can reach dangerous levels. A rising core temperature, depletion of blood volume, and a switch from carbohydrate to fat metabolism may cause an upward drift of heart rate as exercise is prolonged. Finally, if prolonged bouts

of exercise are repeated over many days, as in the transcontinental events undertaken by some disabled athletes, the extent of fat and protein stores and the strength
of the bones and joints can become factors limiting performance.

Determinants of Muscular Performance

Peak Isometric Force

Isometric force is measured by a dynamometer (preferably of the strain gauge
type) or a cable tensiometer. In general, the peak isometric force that can be
developed by a given group of muscles is proportional to the cross section of
the muscle (Ikai & Fukunaga, 1968; Maughan, Watson, & Weir, 1983), although
scores also depend on coordination, synchronization of effort, and motivation.
The external forces that are recorded by the measuring device further depend
on the point of insertion of the muscle into bone and the resultant lever arm about
the moving joint. Interindividual variations in peak isometric force per unit of
muscle cross section reflect the influence of neural factors such as central inhibition of peak effort (the strength of an isometric effort can sometimes be boosted
10-15% if inhibition is lessened by hypnosis or encouragement), the extent of
relaxation of antagonist muscles, and the subject's ability to initiate a simultaneous burst of activity in a large proportion of the relevant motor units. A further
factor in tasks that are accompanied by body movement is the mass of the part
to be displaced; indeed, some authors express peak isometric muscle force in
newtons (the SI unit of force) per kilogram of body mass.

Isometric Endurance

The endurance of isometric effort is tested by having the subject develop a predetermined fraction of the peak dynamometer or tensiometer score for as long
as possible. Results depend in part on the predominant muscle fiber type. Slow
twitch fibers are more tolerant than fast twitch fibers with respect to the local
accumulation of lactic acid and resultant fatigue. A second important variable
is again the motivation of the individual. Scores reflect his or her willingness
to continue effort through the recruitment of less favorably positioned accessory
muscles in the face of pain and exhaustion.

Isotonic Power Output

Leverage, and thus tension in the muscles, varies as a joint rotates, so that there
are no true isotonic tasks. However, a lightly loaded ergometer provides an
approximation to light isotonic work, and the lifting of weights in a metal frame
provides a heavier but predominantly isotonic task.

   The external power that is generated by these various forms of isotonic contraction depends upon the external loading. If a suboptimal load is selected the muscle
contracts very rapidly, and a substantial part of the available force is dissipated
as internal friction occurs between the individual muscle filaments. However,
if the loading is too heavy muscle tension rises, intramuscular blood vessels are
occluded, and after a few repetitions the effort is halted by local lack of oxygen

within the working tissues. Study of the operation of machines such as bicycles shows us that the optimum transfer of useful work from muscle to machine occurs when the force applied to the pedals demands 25 to 35% of the maximum voluntary force of the muscle group concerned (Hoes, Binkhorst, Smeeks-Kuyl, & Vissurs, 1968). Internal frictional losses at any given velocity of muscle contraction depend in part on viscosity of the tissue. A preliminary warm-up of the limb reduces viscosity and thus improves performance.

Isotonic Endurance

Isotonic endurance is commonly reported as the number of repetitions of a task that can be made at a fixed fraction of maximum effort (e.g., the number of lifts achieved at 50% of the maximum load that a person can lift once through the same distance). Performance depends on the individual's tolerance of a local accumulation of lactic acid within the working muscles. As with isometric effort, the end point is influenced quite markedly by fiber type, motivation, and willingness to use accessory muscles to complete a given task. Other variables are (a) the local perfusion of the active limbs (an expression of the health of the peripheral blood vessels and muscle capillaries), (b) the ability of the cardiac pump to increase perfusion of the available vascular bed by an increase of systemic blood pressure, (c) the percentage of maximum voluntary muscle force that is being exerted (and thus the pressure compressing blood vessels within the body of the muscle), (d) the buffering of acid in the working tissues (this factor being influenced favorably by anaerobic training), and (e) the rate of diffusion of hydrogen ions into the bloodstream.

Eccentric Force and Endurance

Researchers do not commonly make formal measurements of eccentric force and endurance. However, it is well established that the forces generated during eccentric effort are greater than those associated with a peak isometric effort, since the normal strength of the active muscle is supplemented by external forces. In consequence, muscle ischemia is very likely during eccentric activity. A prolonged bout of eccentric exercise will probably be followed by muscle soreness, leakage of intramuscular enzymes into the bloodstream, and other signs of subclinical damage to the active part.

Isokinetic Force and Endurance

Isokinetic force and endurance are usually measured by a commercial dynamometer such as the Cybex II. During an isokinetic contraction, the peak force developed by a muscle depends on the speed of rotation of the joint at which it acts. Slow movements (e.g., rotation at an angular velocity of 18°/s) reflect mainly the activity of slow twitch fibers, whereas rapid movements (e.g., an angular velocity of 360°/s) reflect mainly the force that is developed by fast twitch fibers. Performance of the individual may be expressed as either the peak isokinetic force that is observed or the average force developed over the entire arc of rotation. Endurance is commonly assessed from the decrease in these two measurements over 50 repetitions of a maximal isokinetic contraction.

Determinants of Anaerobic and Aerobic Performance

Anaerobic Power

The observed anaerobic power of an individual depends largely upon the mass of muscle that can be brought to bear upon the required task. Thus scores are much greater for a leg ergometer than for an arm-cranking device, unless the latter is arranged to allow a substantial contribution of the shoulder and back muscles to the cranking process. The predominant type of muscle fiber in the active limbs (fast or slow twitch) is also an important consideration, and because the common means of assessment (Bar-Or's cycle ergometer test) has a total duration of only 5 seconds, scores are heavily influenced by the individual's knowledge of an appropriate pace to achieve exhaustion within the 5-second test period. The individual's motivation and coordination are also exceedingly important determinants of how much work can be accomplished within the specified time limit; this is true even in laboratory ergometry but becomes much more obvious in field tests such as a 50-m sprint.

Anaerobic Capacity

The reported anaerobic capacity also depends largely on the muscle mass activated by the required task. In essence, the amount of work that can be performed before the intramuscular acidity reaches its ceiling depends on (a) the local buffering capacity, (b) the tissue volume in which accumulating lactic acid is dispersed, (c) the ability of the person to metabolize lactate in other, better perfused parts of the working muscle, and (d) the speed of diffusion of hydrogen ions from the muscle into the bloodstream (Brooks & Fahey, 1984). Other important determinants of performance include an optimum loading of the system (and thus an optimum speed of muscle shortening), the motivation of the subject, coordination, and knowledge of a pace of movement that will produce total exhaustion of the active limbs within the specified time of 30 seconds.

Aerobic Power

Maximum oxygen intake, or its synonym aerobic power, may be defined as the maximum steady-state oxygen consumption observed after 9 to 11 minutes of all-out effort involving the major muscle groups of the body. Ideally, each person reaches a plateau of oxygen consumption (an increase of less than 2 ml/kg • min in response to a substantial increase of work rate). If a plateau is not demonstrated, an attempt may be made to infer maximum effort from heart rate, respiratory gas exchange ratio, lactate accumulation, and ratings of perceived effort.

In a large-muscle task such as uphill treadmill running or the propulsion of a racing bicycle with toe stirrups and drop handlebars, sustained performance normally depends on the ability of the individual's cardiorespiratory system to pump oxygen from the atmosphere to the working muscles. Nevertheless, a detailed analysis of the process (Shephard, 1977) suggests that in disease any one of a number of closely linked variables can limit oxygen transport. Critical factors include the unpleasant sensation associated with a high level of external ventilation, an enlargement of the anatomical dead space of the conducting airways, a poor distribution of alveolar ventilation in relationship to perfusion of the lung, consumption of an excessive fraction of the available oxygen by the respiratory muscles, limitation of gas exchange across the alveolar membrane, poor maximum cardiac output, reduced oxygen carrying capacity of the blood, failure to direct the available circulation to the working muscles, and poor arterial or capillary blood supply within the working muscles. However, in the normal individual the main factor limiting any type of large muscle exercise is the cardiovascular transport of oxygen from the lungs to the working tissues.

As the volume of active muscle is reduced, either by design of the ergometer or by disability of the individual, the balance between central (cardiovascular) and peripheral (muscular) determinants of performance changes (Shephard, Vandewalle, Bouhlel, & Monod, 1988). Thus, in the usual design of arm crank the total volume of active muscle is relatively small, and effort is made at a high percentage of maximal force for the muscles concerned. Intramuscular pressure becomes very high, and despite a substantial rise of systemic blood pressure, the heart becomes unable to perfuse the working muscles. It thus fails to reach the full potential maximal output that would be observed if there were a large muscle bed to perfuse. The small volume of active muscle also pumps less blood back to the heart, leaving the vascular beds of inactive or paralyzed muscle filled with blood. The resultant reduction of venous return and of "preloading" of the left ventricle further hampers cardiac performance. A combination of these several peripheral factors thus sets a ceiling to small-muscle endurance effort.

Respiration and Performance

Ventilation and Breathlessness

Respiration is important to physical performance in terms of both gas transport (oxygen and carbon dioxide) and modifications of acid/base balance associated with a change in body CO_2 stores. Ventilation increases linearly with oxygen consumption until the anaerobic threshold is reached; thereafter, the accumulation of lactic acid leads to a disproportionate hyperventilation. Older people frequently stop exercising not because they have reached a ceiling of cardiovascular performance but rather because they perceive that breathlessness has reached an intolerable level (the sensation of dyspnea). The determinants of breathlessness include the fraction of the vital capacity used, the rate of breathing, and any unusual resistance to airflow encountered at the mouth or within the airways. Typically, the subject complains when the tidal volume exceeds 50 to 60% of his or her vital capacity; dyspnea is particularly likely if the anaerobic threshold is surpassed, as ventilation then becomes disproportionate to metabolism.

The effective vital capacity may be reduced through postural deformities or fixation of the chest; the latter occurs when the arms begin to perform external work. If only small or weakened muscles are available to develop a given power output, the tendency to accumulation of lactic acid in the blood increases correspondingly, and thus the respiratory minute volume becomes larger for any given rate of oxygen consumption. Furthermore, the sensations perceived by the respiratory muscles depend in part upon the percentage of maximal force that they must exert. The percentage is inevitably increased if the chest muscles are weakened by disability, and the margin to the onset of dyspnea shows a corresponding reduction.

Dead-Space Ventilation

A proportion of the respiratory minute volume is "wasted" in ventilating the anatomical dead space of the conducting airways and the physiological dead space attributable to poorly perfused parts of the lung.

During exercise, dead space accounts for perhaps 25 to 30% of total ventilation in a young adult, but the percentage of "wasted ventilation" tends to increase as a person becomes older. Deformities of the thoracic cage and weakness of muscles in the lower part of the thorax and abdomen also exaggerate unequal distribution of ventilation at any age.

Oxygen Cost of Breathing

During all-out effort, the oxygen cost of breathing accounts for 5 to 10% of the total maximum oxygen intake in a young adult (Shephard, 1966). If the peak oxygen intake of an individual is reduced because work is restricted to the relatively small muscles of the arms and shoulder girdle, an unchanged oxygen cost of breathing can account for a larger percentage of total oxygen transport. The proportion of transported oxygen used by the respiratory muscles may be further increased by the mechanical problems associated with either deformities of the chest or a deliberate, voluntary fixation of the rib cage in order to allow arm work.

Pulmonary Diffusion

Equilibration of oxygen between the alveolar spaces and the pulmonary capillaries is normally fairly complete, although very well-trained subjects with an exceptionally large maximum cardiac output may experience a residual gradient of oxygen pressure as blood leaves the lungs (Dempsey, 1987). A poor matching of ventilation and perfusion in the lungs can lead to an appreciable shunting of reduced venous blood into the pulmonary veins; this increases the alveolar–arterial oxygen pressure gradient in affected individuals.

The Cardiovascular System and Performance

Oxygen transport from the pulmonary capillaries to the working tissues ($\dot{V}O_2$) depends on peak cardiac output ($\dot{Q}$, the product of peak heart rate and peak stroke volume), hemoglobin concentration, oxygenation of arterial blood, oxygenation of mixed venous blood, and distribution of the available cardiac output between muscles, skin, and viscera. The overall process can be summarized by Fick's principle:

$$\dot{V}O_2 = \dot{Q} \, (Cao_2 - C\bar{v}o_2)$$

where Cao_2 is the oxygen content of arterial blood, and $C\bar{v}o_2$ is the oxygen content of mixed venous blood.

Peak Cardiac Output

The resting heart rate commonly averages 70 to 80 beats/min in a sedentary person, but it is much lower in a well-trained athlete. The peak exercise heart rate is normally about 210 beats/min in a young child and 195 beats/min in a young adult, dropping to 160 to 170 beats/min in a person aged 65 years. Training decreases the heart rate at a given submaximum power output, but it has little effect on the maximum heart rate.

When sitting or standing, the resting stroke volume of a young adult is about 80 ml/beat, values varying roughly in proportion to body mass. During vigorous exercise, output increases to 110 to 120 ml/beats (in part by an increase of end-diastolic volume, but mainly by a more complete emptying of the ventricle and thus a decrease of end-systolic volume). A healthy, older person may experience some increase of stroke volume during vigorous work to compensate for the decrease of maximum heart rate. Endurance training also commonly increases the maximal stroke volume of the heart.

In a normal adult, the various acute exercise responses are brought about progressively over 2 to 4 minutes through three main mechanisms:

1. a direct action of sympathetic nerve endings upon the heart (including both a "chronotropic" increase of heart rate and an "inotropic" increase in the force of ventricular contraction for a given end-diastolic volume),

2. an increase of venous return due to activation of the muscle pump, an increase of ventilation, and a sympathetically mediated augmentation of venous tone. These three factors together cause a weak stimulation of heart rate and a more substantial increase of stroke volume, the latter being due to the increase of end-diastolic volume, and

3. an increase in the level of circulating catecholamines. Blood levels of epinephrine and norepinephrine rise over several minutes in response to vigorous effort; these hormones also induce both chronotropic and inotropic responses.

Some forms of disability interfere with the normal sympathetic outflow from the spinal cord (thus limiting the normal exercise-induced increase of heart rate and myocardial contractility). Weakened muscles may also impair venous return, thus reducing preloading of the ventricles. Any exercise-induced increase of cardiac output may be left to the rather tardy chronotropic and inotropic impact of circulating catecholamines. Moreover, if disability restricts the volume of active muscle, the high intramuscular pressure presents a severe impedance to ventricular out-flow, limiting the increase of stroke volume that occurs in response to a given catecholamine release (the condition of "increased afterload"). If these various constraints cause a sluggish cardiac response to exercise, the result will be a proportionately larger accumulation of anaerobic metabolites such as lactic acid in the early stages of physical activity.

Arteriovenous Oxygen Difference

The quantity of oxygen transported by each liter of blood depends on the difference in oxygen content between arterial and venous blood. We have already noted the possibility that a small decrease in arterial oxygen saturation may arise from a poor matching of pulmonary ventilation and perfusion. The oxygen content of mixed venous blood reflects its hemoglobin content and the relative proportions of the venous return that are derived from the active muscles (where a large part of the available oxygen has been extracted) and from the skin and viscera (where oxygen extraction is quite limited). If a given exercise task is performed by small arm muscles rather than by the much larger muscles of the leg, then the propor-tion of the total venous return contributed by parts of the body where oxygen extraction is fairly complete will drop, and mixed venous oxygen content will increase correspondingly. This means in turn that less oxygen will be transported from the lungs for any given cardiac output.

The hemoglobin content of the blood is the second main determinant of oxygen transport per unit of cardiac output. An average sedentary person may not neces-sarily have an abnormal hemoglobin concentration, but the hemoglobin reading is of sufficient importance to an individual's competitive performance that it is worth checking in any endurance athlete.

Distribution of Cardiac Output

At the beginning of vigorous exercise, the sympathetic nervous system normally experiences intense activity. This serves to redirect blood flow from the viscera and inactive muscles to the working tissues, including skeletal and respiratory muscles, the heart, and (particularly in a hot environment) the skin. Diastolic blood pressure remains relatively unchanged, but systolic blood pressure rises sharply. The latter response seems a reflection of local oxygen lack in the muscles; the pressure rise is particularly marked if the exercise is performed by small muscles or has a substantial isometric component.

If the sympathetic outflow is interrupted (e.g., by a spinal cord injury), the process of redirection of blood flow at the beginning of exercise is disturbed. Blood pressure fails to show the anticipated rise, and there is a corresponding difficulty in perfusing muscles that are contracting vigorously.

Cellular Factors and Physical Performance

Cellular factors normally have little influence upon aerobic performance. Recent studies suggest that the muscle cells have a substantial reserve of enzyme activity and a further increase in the activity of specific enzymes does not have any great influence upon peripheral oxygen extraction, which in any event is relatively complete. However, there is a very substantial hypertrophy of the arm and shoulder muscles in some forms of lower-limb disability, and because the local oxygen pressure within a given muscle fiber is inversely related to the square of the diffusion distance from the supplying capillaries, we may need to consider a possible peripheral limitation of endurance effort in such cases.

The patterns of enzyme activity differ substantially between individuals with predominantly fast twitch fibers and those with mainly slow twitch fibers. The main consequence of this metabolic differentiation seems a diversion of metabolic pathways, so that fat rather than carbohydrate provides the fuel for the slow twitch fibers. Such an arrangement favors conservation of available glycogen stores over a distance event.

Other Aspects of Fitness and Health

Although the main focus of fitness testing is upon cardiovascular and muscular function, a full examination of fitness and health should also include determination of the amount of body fat, the flexibility of the major joints, and the nature of electrocardiographic responses to exercise.

Body Fat

The body fat content may be assessed quite simply from the relationship of body mass to height. Excess mass relative to actuarial standards and various height/mass ratios are widely used in large-scale surveys, although abnormalities of lean muscle mass influence such indices as well. Skinfold determinations of subcutaneous fat provide a more direct measure of adiposity, but differences in the relative proportions of deep and superficial fat affect estimates of total body fat. The determination of body density by underwater weighing is often said to provide a very reliable estimate of body fatness, but in practice the simplistic lean and fat tissue model can give erroneous results if there are substantial changes in bone density or the relative proportions of muscle and bone.

An excessive accumulation of body fat has important implications for future health, as excess fat is commonly associated with hypertension and atherosclerotic disease of the major blood vessels (Keys et al., 1972). The impact of prognosis is particularly marked if the fat has a "masculine" distribution (i.e., chest and abdomen rather than hips and thighs; Krotkiewski, Björntorp, Sjöstrom, & Smith, 1983). From the practical point of view, an excessive reserve of body fat also constitutes an additional mass that must be carried and accelerated against gravity, with corresponding negative effects upon both the anaerobic and the aerobic performance of the person concerned. Finally, in a hot environment, a thick layer of subcutaneous fat impedes the elimination of body heat, increasing the proportion of the total cardiac output that must be diverted to the skin circulation during vigorous exercise.

Flexibility

Flexibility unfortunately varies substantially from one joint to another, and no single, simple, overall test of flexibility exists. The sit-and-reach test provides a quantitative measure of flexion in the lower back and hips, whereas a goniometer can be used to assess the range of motion at other major joints.

Flexibility is of considerable importance to top performance in many sports—for example, the shoulder mobility of a world-class swimmer is much greater than that of an average person. Flexibility has relatively little impact upon the perceived fitness of an ordinary young adult, but as age advances, loss of flexibility in key joints eventually restricts the activities of daily living. Such losses of flexibility develop more rapidly and the consequences are more severe if there are associated joint deformities, contractures, or weaknesses of major muscle groups.

Electrocardiogram and Blood Pressure

During exercise, the electrocardiogram is conveniently recorded from a series of unipolar chest leads, corresponding to the resting V-2, V-4, and V-6 lead placements. If leg work is to be performed, the second exploring electrode is placed over the manubrium sterni, and the neutral lead is attached to the nape of the neck. However, such placements are less suited to arm exercise; if arm work is to be performed, it may be necessary to place the second exploring and neutral electrodes over the left and right iliac crests, respectively.

Exercise electrocardiography should be carried to at least 85% of peak effort, with recording during both exercise and the first 5 minutes of recovery. Simultaneous recording of the systemic blood pressure during a progressive stress test may show static or decreasing readings despite an increase of work rate; this reflects deteriorating left ventricular function and is an urgent indication to halt an exercise test.

In a healthy young adult the electrocardiogram shows no abnormalities even during vigorous exercise, but a substantial proportion of individuals over the age of 40 years show some evidence of "silent ischemia" of the myocardium, typically a horizontal or downward depression of the ST segment or the appearance of frequent early and polyfocal premature ventricular contractions. A disability that causes a person to become extremely inactive enhances the risk of atherosclerosis; as the condition progresses, ECG abnormalities appear at an earlier age or at a lower work rate. Unfortunately, stress-induced ECG changes are harbingers of an increased risk of death during vigorous exercise.

Mechanical Efficiency

Biomechanical Fundamentals

The maximum amount of physical work that a person can accomplish over a given time interval depends partly upon the relevant physiological ability (anaerobic power, anaerobic capacity, or aerobic power) and partly upon the efficiency with which the chemical energy expended in the muscle can be converted to useful external work.

A ceiling of mechanical efficiency is generally set by the nature of the biochemical processes involved. During aerobic exercise, a maximum of about 25%

of available food energy can be applied to muscular shortening, the remaining 75% appearing as heat. During anaerobic effort the mechanical efficiency is much lower, initially 1 to 2% but rising to 13% as accumulating lactate is metabolized. Interindividual differences of mechanical efficiency reflect the person's skill in performing a particular task. For instance, when walking individuals vary in the extent of pelvic tilt, the amplitude of limb movements, and the extent of vertical displacement of the body's center of mass. In our present context, additional energy costs are incurred through unwanted muscle spasms, moving against spasm, and using poorly placed muscles as substitutes for the normal prime movers. Usually, training decreases the cost of a given activity; the individual learns better techniques and strengthened prime movers no longer need assistance from less well-positioned muscles.

Even the able-bodied display quite low mechanical efficiencies during the performance of many daily tasks. This is partly because the loading of the individual muscles has not been optimized and partly because much of the observed energy expenditure is directed to stabilizing the body rather than to accomplishing the desired movement. A conceptual problem also arises in the calculation of mechanical efficiency when the body is displaced on level ground (e.g., in running or in wheelchair propulsion). No net performance of external work exists, since neither the subject nor the chair are displaced with respect to gravity. Nevertheless, energy is expended during both level running and wheelchair ambulation. Losses are incurred due to acceleration and deceleration of body parts, friction between the ground and the shoes or the driving wheels of a chair, friction in the wheel bearings of a chair, the viscous air resistance encountered by a subject or chair (this resistance increasing as the third power of the speed of forward movement), and any opposing wind.

Estimation of Mechanical Efficiency

Human mechanical efficiency has traditionally been calculated as the ratio of the energy consumed to the external work that is performed. In theory, energy consumption could be calculated from the energy yield of the food that is eaten, but in practice a steady state in which energy intake matches energy output is not reached for a week or more. Energy consumption is thus estimated indirectly from the fairly constant relationship between metabolism and oxygen consumption. On a normal mixed diet, 1 L of oxygen consumption is associated with an energy expenditure of about 21 kJ (5 kcal). Work may be performed against some type of ergometer (a cycle, arm, or wheelchair ergometer), in which case the loss of energy in the crank bearings and chains (8-10% of the total external work) is usually neglected. Alternatively, if the subject climbs a step, ramp, or upward-sloping treadmill, work may be estimated as the product of the mass of the body plus any wheelchair multiplied by the vertical displacement of the center of mass. In this type of calculation, energy expenditures associated with forward or downward movement of the body and acceleration/deceleration of individual body parts are commonly neglected. Recent developments of infrared technology now allow a sophisticated three-dimensional analysis of movement patterns for each of the body segments (Waterloo Spatial Motion Analysis and Recording Technique

[WATSMART], Northern Digital Inc., Waterloo, Ontario, Canada), and future calculations of efficiency may take account of the energy expended in relative displacement of the various body parts.

Mechanical efficiency calculation is divided into several categories (see chapter 6). Gross efficiency relates the total consumption of food energy to the performance of external mechanical work. Net efficiency notes the increased consumption of energy as activity increases above the basal or the resting state, and delta efficiency looks at the slope of the relationship between work output and energy consumption.

Responses of the Body to Physical Training

Appropriate forms of physical training can increase an individual's muscular strength, aerobic power, and flexibility and can reduce the amount of body fat and the likelihood of electrocardiographic abnormalities at any given rate of working. Training may also improve mechanical efficiency as muscles become stronger and the subject learns the skills associated with a particular task.

Anthropometric data show a decrease of body fat and an increase in the dimensions of the active muscles as training progresses. Repeated weight-bearing exercise may also increase bone density in the active body parts. During submaximal exercise, there is a lesser increase of heart rate and a lesser secretion of various hormones including the catecholamines.

Determinants of Training Response

The primary determinant of the response to physical training is the intensity of the prescribed exercise relative to the initial physical condition of the subject (Shephard, 1969b). For development of either cardiovascular or muscular performance, any given person has a potential ceiling of ability that is genetically determined, and the response to a given dose of training becomes progressively smaller as the person approaches this ceiling. Furthermore, some evidence implies that individuals show genetically determined differences in their susceptibility to training. With aging, a person normally commences a training program further from the potential response ceiling, but that person also displays an age-related decrease of trainability. The response to a conditioning regimen may thus remain unchanged in terms of the percentage gain over baseline values, but in absolute units the response is much smaller in an older person.

Optimum Training Regimen

Whether the subject seeks to develop muscular or cardiovascular performance, the general principle of a successful training program is that of moderate overload. In biochemical terms, it is probable that the tension developed in the muscle fibers during each bout of conditioning causes a sustained increase in the rate of protein synthesis. At the same time, the overload required to initiate a satisfactory training response is close to the tolerance limit of the muscles concerned. Thus, unless due care is taken, signs of an excessive overload may develop, including delayed muscle soreness and the escape of intramuscular enzymes into the bloodstream.

Two specific examples illustrate the enormous variety of possible training programs. If the objective is to develop isotonic muscular strength, the trainer first determines the maximum isotonic load; the subject is then asked to perform at each training session a total of three sets of 10 repeated contractions (repetitions), individual efforts corresponding to 50% of the maximum tolerated load for the muscle group concerned. The subject repeats the conditioning stimulus on alternate days, with an increase in loading as the muscle group becomes stronger.

Likewise, if the objective is to develop cardiorespiratory endurance, a sedentary subject may be given an initial exercise prescription that includes in each session 20 minutes of large-muscle exercise such as running, swimming, or cross-country skiing at a heart rate corresponding to 60% of the individual's maximum oxygen intake. The endurance component of the prescription is repeated 4 times per week, and when the subject is performing the task comfortably, he or she gradually progresses to longer and more arduous exercise sessions (perhaps demanding 30-40 min at 70-80% of the current maximum oxygen intake). A period of gentle stretching and warm-up exercises should precede the definitive components of both muscular and cardiovascular bouts, not only to improve the individual's peak performance but also to minimize the risk of musculoskeletal injuries or abnormalities of heart rhythm. A gentle cool-down should follow each bout of cardiovascular exercise, as a sudden venous pooling at the end of a training session may precipitate a transient loss of consciousness and cardiac emergencies.

The choice between a personally programmed exercise such as jogging and participation in a team sport or a gymnasium class depends very much on the personality of the individual concerned. Programmed exercise can be adjusted to the current capacity of the individual and is well received by an introverted person (Massie & Shephard, 1971). Team sport and gymnasium programs have more motivational appeal, particularly to the gregarious type of individual; however, a participant in group activity may receive either an inadequate bout of exercise (because the other class participants are unfit) or may be challenged beyond his or her capacity (because other members of the group are younger or in better physical condition).

Specificity of Response

Training responses show a substantial specificity (Clausen, 1977). It is fairly obvious that training the arm muscles has little effect upon the condition of the legs, unless the muscles in the latter region are used to stabilize the body or to walk to the gymnasium. However, there is also a specificity with respect to the type of muscle training that occurs. Isometric training, for example, has little influence upon subsequent isotonic performance, and indeed an individual isometric program is relatively specific to the joint angle at which contractions have been developed during training.

Likewise, although a course of cycle ergometer training leads to some improvement in subsequent arm-cranking performance, repeated bouts of training upon an arm-crank ergometer have little influence upon an individual's subsequent ability to undertake leg exercise. There are corresponding specificities of cellular responses. Thus, running induces hypertrophy of the myocardium and slow twitch muscle fibers in the legs, whereas isometric training has little effect on the heart but favors fast twitch fiber hypertrophy in the exercised skeletal muscles (Henriksson, 1980).

Key Ideas

1. We must draw a distinction between the physical activity required for work, for deliberate leisure activity (exercise), and for habitual activity (the sum of work, leisure, and domestic chores).

2. Physical fitness is the ability to undertake these various forms of activity. Fitness is itself increased by regular and vigorous physical activity.

3. The ability to undertake very brief activity (anaerobic power) depends upon the application of locally stored phosphagen energy (adenosine triphosphate and creatine phosphate) to the bonding of actin and myosin molecules within the muscle fibers. Activity lasting from 10 seconds to 2 minutes is sustained largely by the breakdown of intramuscular glycogen to pyruvate (glycolysis) with an associated accumulation of lactic acid; the anaerobic capacity reflects the ability to undertake this type of activity. Endurance activity depends upon a steady oxygen supply that matches metabolic needs (the aerobic power of the individual). In very prolonged effort, performance can be limited by problems of fluid balance and temperature regulation, the exhaustion of glycogen and fat stores, or an inadequate strength of joints and bones.

4. The primary categories of muscular contraction are isometric (constant tension) and isotonic (constant length). In daily life, most activities demand changes in both the length and tension of the active muscles. Other categories of muscle activity include eccentric contraction (lengthening of the muscle as it contracts) and isokinetic contraction (development of maximal force while a joint is rotated at a predetermined and constant angular speed).

5. The anaerobic power and capacity of the individual are determined largely by the dimensions of the active muscles relative to body mass.

6. Any of the links in the chain transporting oxygen from the environment to the working muscles can influence aerobic power. Critical respiratory variables include the sensation of breathlessness, the extent of dead-space ventilation, the oxygen cost of breathing, and possible limitations of pulmonary diffusion. Cardiovascular factors influencing peak oxygen transport include peak cardiac output (the product of maximum stroke volume and maximum heart rate), the proportion of the total blood flow reaching the working muscles, and the arteriovenous oxygen difference. In the healthy adult, performance of large-muscle endurance exercise is normally limited by the individual's maximum cardiac output.

7. Tissue enzyme levels apparently have more influence upon the type of fuel that is consumed during activity (glycogen vs. fat) than upon the peak level of performance.

8. A full assessment of fitness must examine not only muscular and cardiovascular performance but also body fat distribution, the flexibility of major joints, and electrocardiographic responses to maximal exercise.

9. Performance is determined not only by current physiological status but also by the mechanical efficiency with which energy is translated into the performance of external work.

10. An appropriate training regimen can improve physiological responses to a bout of exercise. When developing an appropriate exercise prescription, an individual must consider the intensity of activity in relation to his or her initial condition. The exerciser must apply a moderate overload but avoid overtraining. The extent of the training response depends also upon the gap between current physical condition and genetic potential. The gains induced by training are specific with respect to the part of the body that has been exercised (arms vs. legs) and the type of training that has been undertaken (muscular vs. cardiovascular, isometric vs. isotonic).

Practical Applications

1. If you were attempting to determine the physical condition of a substantial group of adults, would you embark upon a survey of habitual activity patterns or would you prefer to test the physical fitness of a representative sample of the population?

2. Why does the net mechanical efficiency of exercise rarely rise above 25%? What might be the explanation in a few cases in which figures as high as 40 to 45% have been reported?

3. Which of the various types of physical fitness discussed in this chapter would be most important to the performance of a person propelling a wheelchair?

4. If a person is able to sustain a power output of 150 watts throughout a 10-minute ergometer test, what would be his or her likely power output during 10 seconds of all-out exercise? What figure might be observed with 3 hours of sustained exercise?

5. What elements would you include when developing an exercise prescription for a healthy young adult? How would you modify your advice if the person were 65 years old?

Chapter 2

An Historical View

This chapter first examines the scope of physical performance studies in the disabled, discussing the prevalence of various types of disability and exploring the particular health problems of the paraplegic. A second section then discusses possible forms of increased activity and traces the concept of a handicapped competition from its early English origins to present-day disabled sports. A final section considers the current organization of sports for the disabled and future prospects for this area of enquiry.

Scope of Physical Performance Studies

The broad theme of this book is the scientific study of physical performance in the disabled, including current fitness status and gains of physical condition whether realized by habitual activity or sports participation. Both the amount and the intensity of the daily physical activity undertaken currently varies widely from one disabled individual to another. At one extreme, we find very inactive people who badly need a modest amount of physical conditioning to reduce the risk of degenerative diseases and minimize the limitations imposed by life in a wheelchair (Arheim & Sinclair, 1985; Auxter & Pyfer, 1985; Dendy, 1978; Jochheim & Strohkendl, 1973; Sherrill, 1986c; Weiss & Beck, 1973). At the other extreme, an increasing number of the disabled now elect a pursuit of athletic excellence, undertaking the intensive and rigorous training necessary to participate in suitably adapted international contests (Adams, Daniel, McCubbin, & Rullman, 1982; Buell, 1987; Croucher, 1976, 1978; Guttmann, 1946, 1973, 1976a, 1976b; Huberman, 1971, 1976; Hullemann, List, Matthes, Wiese, & Zika, 1975; Jackson & Frederickson, 1979; Jokl, 1958; Price, 1986; Shephard, 1978b; Sherrill, 1986a, 1986c; Steadward & Walsh, 1986; Stewart, 1986; Van Hal, Rarick, & Vermeer, 1984; Weiss, 1971).

Merits of Exercise Prescription

The very idea of prescribing a deliberate increase of physical activity for the disabled is of quite recent origin. Traditionally, people were prepared to accept the dictum of Victorians such as Herbert Spence, who viewed active recreation as the irresponsible waste of a limited energy store (Bedbrook, 1974). In response to such reasoning, the disabled were confined to institutions where physical activity was held to a minimum. At best, the inmates of such centers were offered occasional promenades in adapted buses or battery-driven wheelchairs.

However, we now generally recognize that a carefully graded increase of physical activity can make an important contribution to the immediate health, life satisfaction, and life expectancy of the disabled (N. Stewart, 1981). Among the potential benefits of involvement in a program of vigorous activity, Bedbrook (1974) noted an improvement of psychomotor skills, a stimulation of motivation for other tasks, a reestablishment of contact with the normal human environment, a reduction of emotional tensions with a release of natural anger and aggression, and an increase of relaxation. Other, more recent authors (Bar-Or, 1983; Davis, Shephard, & Jackson, 1981; Sherrill, 1986c) noted similar benefits, while frequent articles in such journals as *Palaestra* and *Sports 'N Spokes* attest to the intense involvement of disabled people in a multitude of sports. Weiss and Beck (1973) concluded that during the critical period immediately following spinal trauma, sports training resulted in a 100% faster increase of upper body strength than that seen with more traditional forms of bedside treatment. Moreover, the early introduction of sports and active games reduced depression scores and increased motivation to restoration of function.

Because the performance of ordinary activities is harder for a disabled person than for an average subject, the disabled inevitably have an enhanced need for physical fitness in order to meet the demands of daily life. Moreover, even after successful rehabilitation, many disabled individuals remain severely restricted compared to their able-bodied peers in such areas as personal relationships, travel, and cultural experiences (Yale, 1982). Thus disabled people have an increased need for the pleasurable relaxation, interest, and relief of monotony that regular, barrier-free physical activity can provide. Finally, the disabled segment of the population is by no means immune to such long-term consequences of an inactive lifestyle as obesity, hypertension, and ischemic heart disease; however, participation in a regular program of endurance exercise offers the prospect of protection against such problems.

Prevalence and Incidence Statistics

Epidemiologists distinguish the prevalence of a condition from its incidence. Prevalence statistics describe the proportion of individuals affected by a given condition as found by a carefully conducted survey of a population, whereas incidence statistics indicate the proportion of individuals from the same population who will present themselves for treatment of the condition over a specified period, usually 1 year. Much of the information on disabled individuals describes the prevalence rather than the incidence of the various types of disorder.

Types of Disability

A wide variety of conditions can handicap physical performance. The glossary contains brief definitions of the various types of disability. Some forms of disability date from birth—the deformed limbs resulting from intrauterine thalidomide poisoning (Pascoe, 1971), several types of spastic paralysis (Corcoran, Jebsen,

Brengelmann, & Simons, 1970), many types of deafness and blindness (Cartmel & Banister, 1968; Cumming, Goulding, & Baggley, 1971; Hattin, Fraser, Ward, & Shephard, 1986; Lee, Ward, & Shephard, 1985), and the majority of instances of mental retardation (Grossman, 1984; Hayden, 1962).

Other types of disability are incurred in young adulthood. Until recently, persistent muscle wasting was an all-too-common sequel of paralytic poliomyelitis. Paraplegia and quadriplegia remain consequences of spinal injuries sustained in war, industrial accidents, motor vehicle accidents, and contact sports. Amputations may be needed following trauma to the limbs, and eye injuries lead to acquired blindness.

Further problems may arise in later life. Paralysis may be caused by multiple sclerosis or the various manifestations of cerebral atherosclerosis, whereas spasticity and tremor may be due to Parkinsonian degeneration. Amputations may be made necessary by diabetes or (less frequently) by gangrene secondary to arteriosclerosis obliterans or Buerger's disease (Najenson & Levy, 1971). Although only a part of the cardiovascular "epidemic," the incidence of amputations for ischemic vascular disease has apparently increased fivefold over the last quarter of a century (Grundy & Silver, 1983).

Prevalence of Disability

The prevalence of the various classes of disability is important background information for those organizing athletic meetings, particularly if they wish to assure a reasonable number of contestants in each category of competition. A convenient source of information for the school-aged handicapped population in the United States is the Department of Education Annual PL 94-142 Report to Congress. Free copies are obtainable from U.S. Dept. of Education, Office of Special Education and Rehabilitation Services, 400 Maryland Avenue, S.W., Washington, DC 20202. Although the proportion of handicapped individuals is quite large in most developed countries (see Tables 2.1 and 2.2), the extent of participation in competitions is generally no more frequent than among the able-bodied.[1] Thus, if we take account of both the prevalence of disability and the likely participation rate, we see that the potential pool of athletes is small enough to significantly impact the structuring of competitions.

Statistics on the prevalence of disability are nevertheless hard to interpret. First, different groups define disability from differing perspectives—legal, medical, or educational. For many clinical conditions, a continuum ranges from those with mild to those with very severe lesions. Moreover, disability does not necessarily parallel clinical severity, and some individuals are affected by multiple disorders. Quite small physical and mental disabilities can impair the processes of training and athletic competition; moderate deafness, for example, can impair the ability of a rower to hear a coach's instructions bellowed from the towpath or the whistle of the referee in an ice hockey match (Lagerstom, 1980). The overall proportion of the population with complete or partial disability is thus very large.

---

[1]Young adults with accidental spinal injuries show a relatively high participation rate in wheelchair sports. This probably reflects a preexisting adventurous lifestyle.

Table 2.1   Prevalence of Disability Among Children in West Germany in 1962/63

Type of disability	Prevalence (per 1,000)
Blindness	0.13
Deafness	0.9
Weak vision	1.0
Weak hearing	2.5
Malfunction of lower limbs	5.0
Mental retardation	5.0
Physical handicaps	5.0
Problems of speech	15.0
Problems of behavior	20.0
Slow learners	60.0

Note. Based on data from "Physical Education of the Mentally Retarded" by K.A. Jochheim in *Sports as a Means of Rehabilitation*, edited by U. Simri, 1971, Natanya, Israel: Wingate Institute.

Table 2.2   Prevalence of Disability Among United States School-Age Children

Type of disability	Prevalence (per 1,000)	
	Crowe et al., 1981	Sherrill, 1986c
Deaf and blind and other multihandicapped	0.6	1.54
Visually handicapped	1.0	0.70
Deafness	0.75	1.70
Hard of hearing	5.0	1.70
Orthopedically impaired and other health impaired	5.0	1.30 + 1.1
Mental retardation	23.0	17.6
Speech impaired	35.0	25.1
Emotionally disturbed	20.0	8.0
Learning disabled	30.0	39.4

Note. Based on data from *Adapted Physical Education and Recreation* by C. Sherrill, 1986, Dubuque: W.C. Brown and *Adapted Physical Education and Recreation*, 4th ed. by W.C. Crowe, D. Auxter, and J. Pyfer, 1981, St. Louis: Mosby.

Verbeek (1984) and Hoeberigs (1985) discussed some recent data for the Netherlands. In 1968, the prevalence of locomotor disorders among Dutch boys was 10.7 per 1,000 (orthopedic 3.7, cerebral palsy 3.4, other neurological disorders, 2.7, and sequelae of poliomyelitis 1.1). The survey of Verbeek (1984), which covers a wider age range, shows a lower prevalence of these various conditions. In vaccinated areas, poliomyelitis is now a disappearing problem, although the number of patients with residual symptoms is still 0.32 to 0.36 per 1,000.

The prevalence of cerebral palsy remains difficult to assess, because there is a continuum from mild to severe spasticity; a third of patients show a hemiplegia and a further third a diplegia, but in the remaining third, manifestations of the disorder are much less clear-cut. The total prevalence of cerebral palsy in Holland is about 1.50 per 1,000 in children of school age and 0.12 per 1,000 in adults; even if 20% of this group were to become interested in athletics, the total pool of Dutch male competitors with cerebral palsy could not exceed 2,500. The annual incidence of accidental paraplegia is 150 to 200 cases, giving a prevalence rate of 0.22 per 1,000 in people aged 15 to 50 years; again, the numbers available for competitions are relatively limited. Finally, amputations of the leg and the arm have respective prevalence rates of 0.25 and 0.20 per 1,000 over the same age span. Some 87 per 1,000 of the overall Dutch population is handicapped in some fashion, with a disability prevalence rate of 40 per 1,000 between the ages of 15 and 50 years. Locomotor dysfunction substantially outweighs disorders affecting the arms and hands, particularly in the older age groups.

In the United States, about 12% of the school-age population is handicapped. Some 100,000 citizens (about 0.44 per 1,000, mostly older adults of employable age) receive federal aid for economic blindness, and 500,000 others (2.2 per 1,000) are rated as "totally disabled" or legally blind, with a vision of less than 20/200 after correction of refractive errors.[2] In children, the numbers are much lower (0.7-1.0 per 1,000 with visual impairment). People in this group are unable to read even the large E on the Snellen test chart, although they may retain a useful appreciation of form and color. A further 5% of the population have lost sight in one eye. Unfortunately, many of both unilateral and bilateral visual handicaps are due to preventable conditions such as injuries, diabetes, and glaucoma. Young's study (cited in Cowell, Squires, & Raven, 1986) showed that in 1982 there were also 94,000 paraplegics (about 0.4 per 1,000 of the U.S. population), and this number is increasing by some 3,700 new cases per year, due largely to motor vehicle accidents and other types of trauma.

The U.S. Office of Special Education distinguishes a broad category of orthopedic impairment in children; this includes congenital lesions (club foot, congenital dislocation of the hip, spina bifida, and cleft palate) and acquired conditions (trauma, infections such as poliomyelitis and osteomyelitis, and the osteochondroses), with a total prevalence of about 1.3 per 1,000 according to recent statistics. Cerebral palsy reflects damage to the motor areas of the brain before or during birth; often there is associated mental retardation. The prevalence among U.S. children is about 3.5 per 1,000. The disabled group classes as "les autres"

---

[2]The ability to see at 20 feet what a normal eye could distinguish at 200 feet.

includes individuals with arthritis (20 per 1,000), muscular dystrophy (0.03 per 1,000), multiple sclerosis (0.06 per 1,000), and other rare conditions. Hearing impairment affects about 1.7 children per 1,000, but in the total population about 32 per 1,000 are hard of hearing and a further 8.7 per 1,000 are deaf. In addition to these various physical problems, some 7 million U.S. citizens (30 per 1,000 in adults, 18-23 per 1,000 in children) have some degree of mental handicap (Sherrill, 1986c; Zasueta & Kasch, 1973).

In the United Kingdom, a special register is kept of 650,000 persons (about 12 per 1,000) who are substantially handicapped in obtaining or holding employment on account of injury, disease, or congenital deformity. All companies employing more than 20 personnel are required to accept a standard percentage of employees from this register, and in certain industries well suited to the employment of the handicapped, a special quota is imposed. In the school system, about 0.45% are classed as severely educationally subnormal (McLeish, 1983).

Australian investigators estimate that 90 per 1,000 of their population have chronic disorders sufficient to cause some restriction in moving to and from work, making business contacts, or enjoying sports and social activities (M.J. Fox, 1974). The limitation is judged as severe in 50 cases per 1,000 of the population (Yeo, 1974). Statistics are less readily available for developing countries, but given the lesser availability of medical care one might anticipate an even larger proportion of disabled people in such regions of the world.

Health Problems of the Disabled

Health problems may sometimes arise from an extension of the disease itself, for example, in those with ischemic vascular lesions or multiple sclerosis. The general lifestyle of many disabled people is also poor, the adverse health effects of inadequate physical activity being compounded by obesity, smoking, and an excessive consumption of alcohol (see chapter 8). However, spinal paralysis is the category of disability with the greatest direct implications for general health; historically, it has been associated with early death.

Historical Trends

Classical Hippocratic writings referred to "the retention of urine and feces, the loss of strength and torpor of the lower limbs, the cold skin and the fatal termination" of those sustaining a vertebral injury (Breithaupt, Jousse, & Wynne-Jones, 1961, p. 73). Early medical statistics apparently confirmed a very unfavorable prognosis for this type of disorder. Gurlt (1864/1889) recorded a mortality as high as 80% for 272 paraplegic and tetraplegic[3] patients over a 1-year period of follow-up. Likewise, Burrell (cited in Breithaupt, Jousse, & Wynne-Jones, 1961) found a 72% 1-year mortality rate among 244 patients who had been treated

---

[3]The word paraplegia infers a paralysis of the lower limbs, whereas the terms tetraplegia and quadriplegia are used synonymously in this book for paralytic problems affecting the function of all four limbs. Depending on the level of the lesion, those with spinal injuries are paraplegic or quadriplegic. However, many of those with cerebral palsy and other types of lesion are also paraplegic.

between 1864 and 1903. Among those with cervical lesions, only 10% had survived for 3 years, 87% of deaths occurring in the 1st month following injury.

In the period before World War II, figures for the spinally paralyzed continued to be almost as discouraging (Riches, 1943; Gutteman, Riches, Whitteridge, & Jonason, 1947; Nesbit & Lapides cited by Breithaupt et al., 1961). Frazier and Allan (1918) found that prior to 1911, 68% of patients died in the first 90 days following a traumatic injury of the spinal cord, but between 1911 and 1915 the early mortality rate decreased to 27% of cases. Nevertheless, the long-term prognosis remained very poor, with mortality rates of 90% in 1 year (V.A. Technical Bulletin on Spinal Injuries, 1948), 81% over two years (E.N. Cook, 1942), and 60% (Nesbit & Lapides cited by Breithaupt et al., 1961) or 80% (Guttmann, Whitteridge, & Jonason, 1947; Riches, 1943) over unspecified periods of long-term follow-up.

A combination of the availability of antibiotics and the adoption of more vigorous physical therapy contributed to a drastic improvement in these statistics immediately after World War II. Thus, by 1954 Guttmann reported a 10-year mortality rate of only 8.3% among 1,000 patients who had been treated at Stoke Mandeville Hospital, and in Toronto, Breithaupt et al. (1961) noted a 13-year survival of 84.3% (12.1% mortality per decade) in 599 patients who had been followed from 1945 to 1958. Nevertheless, for the group as a whole (partial and complete spinal paralysis), the Toronto experience remained 3 times poorer than actuarial norms; for those with complete spinal paralysis, the prognostic disadvantage was fivefold relative to able-bodied norms, and for those with tetraplegia it was 12-fold. Further studies of the Toronto group (Geisler, Jousse, & Wynne-Jones, 1977; Jousse, Wynne-Jones, & Breithaupt, 1968) were complicated by the inclusion of additional patients in the analysis. This led to wide variations in the average follow-up period; cumulative death rates of 21% and 29% were reported for the expanded samples.

Causes of Worsening Disability and Death

The main causes of worsening disability and delayed death among the spinally paralyzed who were treated during the war and in the immediate postwar period were renal failure (43%), gastrointestinal complications (11%), cardiovascular disease (10%), and respiratory infections (9%) (Breithaupt et al., 1961; Riches, 1943). Respiratory complications (including a progressive paralysis of the respiratory muscles, pulmonary consolidation or collapse, and pulmonary edema) were particularly likely hazards in those with high level lesions (Cheshire & Coats, 1966).

Perhaps in part because many patients had survived to middle and old age, the main change seen in two subsequent studies of the Toronto population of disabled individuals (Geisler et al., 1977; Jousse et al., 1968) was an increase in the percentage of deaths from cardiovascular disease (to 16% and 20% of the total sample, respectively). The trend to a high incidence of cardiovascular disease among those with lower-limb disabilities was confirmed in the epidemiological study of Wilcox, Stauffer, and Nickel (1968).

In a substantial sample of 739 paraplegics, Young and associates (cited by Cowell, Squires, & Raven, 1986) found that although 72% were affected by renal disease or dysfunction, as many as 39% had cardiovascular disease, 44% had pulmonary disease or dysfunction, and 10% had osteoporosis. Blocker, Merrill, Krebs, Cardus, & Ostermann (1983) reported that hypertension was the commonest form of cardiovascular disease among the spinally injured. Among possible etiological factors, the researchers suggested spinal shock, excessive release of norepinephrine by the heart muscle, vascular effects of disrupted autonomic function (see chapter 5), and emotional distress.

Amputees are also very vulnerable to cardiovascular disease. This is partly because of the causal lesion (often peripheral vascular disease) and partly because physical activity is subsequently restricted. If the amputee has a combination of vascular disease and diabetes, he or she may have great difficulty in maintaining health of the amputated limb stump. Hrubec and Ryder (1980) found that as many as 48% of proximal and 43% of distal amputees subsequently died of cardiovascular disease. Kavanagh and Shephard (1973) also observed that 48% of amputees had significant cardiovascular disease, whereas Sawka, Glaser, Laubach, Al-Samkari, and Surprayasad (1981) noted a 56% incidence of cardiovascular disorders in this type of population. Goals of therapeutic exercise should be to increase the range of joint movement, to prevent or correct contractions, to minimize the risk of subsequent musculoskeletal problems by encouraging a correct alignment of the body, to toughen the stump and develop its circulation, and to avoid atrophy of affected muscles. Pulmonary disease is a likely complication in any type of disability in which movement is restricted, the chest muscles are weakened or spastic, or the thoracic cage is deformed.

Any condition leading to weakness or paralysis of muscles can progress to contractures and deformities, with poor posture and movement patterns, leading ultimately to muscle atrophy and osteoarthritic problems. In muscular dystrophies, the cardiac muscle may also be affected, and coordination and balance are usually impaired, with an increased risk of injury. The blind and the deaf are also at increased risk of injury, as are individuals liable to seizures (for example, some forms of cerebral palsy).

Osteoporosis is a general response of the skeleton to the immobilization that follows spinal trauma and other forms of muscle weakness or paralysis. It affects particularly the paralyzed limbs (Claus-Walker & Halstead, 1982). In some patients, the bones become so weakened that there is a danger they will be fractured during muscle spasm, minor movements, or even stretching exercises. Additional problems arise from increased local levels of glycosaminoglycans in the ground substance; the presence of these polysaccharides impedes recalcification of the demineralized bone (Naftchi, Vian, Sell, & Lowmann, 1980; Nilsson, Staff, & Pruett, 1975; Pilonchery, Minaire, Milan, & Revol, 1983). At the same time, there may be enhanced collagen formation in various tissues, with a risk that the calcium liberated from the bone may be deposited in the extracellular spaces (Claus-Walker & Halstead, 1982) making deformities more permanent and giving rise to urinary calculi (Kaplan, Gandhavadi, Richards, & Goldschmidt, 1978; Nilsson et al., 1975). Many disabled individuals suffer renal infections secondary to calculus formation.

Choice of Activity

Chapter 9 discusses program options for an improvement of physical condition. The choice of increased activity for a disabled person lies between formal remedial exercises in a hospital setting, unsupervised recreational activity, individual supervised training sessions with weights or ergometers, and participation in some sort of adapted sport. Although the disabled can relatively easily accept the effort necessary to increase physical activity within the regimented framework of a hospital rehabilitation program, they need considerable self-discipline to persist with any of the possible exercise modalities after returning home (Cowell et al., 1986).

Various authors such as Lipton (1970), Huberman (1971), Weiss (1971), Rosen (1973), Weiss and Beck (1973), Guttmann (1976a), and Jackson and Frederickson (1979) cite the advantages of participation in vigorous sport programs that restore strength, coordination, and endurance. Others maintain that the psychological trauma due to the disability itself is such that it is unfair to expose a paraplegic to the normal type of athletic competition, with the associated possibility of further defeat (Lorenzen, 1961). One practical expression of the latter type of reasoning was seen at the 1963 International Games for the Disabled, which were held in Linz; here, participants all performed a pentathlon-type event, in which they competed only against a stopwatch and a tape measure. Likewise, in Canada, Red Foster (founder of the Canadian Special Olympics) has argued that every child participant should be allowed to attend the national meet, regardless of the physical standards that he or she may demonstrate in local contests.

Proponents of the more usual type of athletic competition maintain that a disability such as paraplegia does not change the basic characteristics of human nature; the wheelchair athlete has the same desire to move faster or to throw farther that can be found in an able-bodied competitor, and this desire can best be satisfied by allowing a real contest, albeit appropriately handicapped (Huberman, 1971).

One important potential bonus of the public type of contest relative to individual or unsupervised activity programs is that it may provide an opportunity for the disabled athlete to become integrated into normal society (see chapter 8). This is helpful not only to the participant but also to the spectators, who gain fresh insights into both the problems and the potential of disabled individuals. However, a danger remains that disabled contests can in themselves become a kind of ghetto for participants, officials, and spectators alike.

The Concept of a Handicap

The term *handicap* is used as a close synonym of *disability*, but it refers also to an appropriate adjustment of competitive conditions between participants of differing ability. The latter concept can be traced to an ancient English game of chance known as ''hand-i-cap.'' A player would challenge an opponent to some form of athletic feat, offering as a stake a prized personal possession. If the challenge were entertained, the opponent would also stake a personal possession, and an umpire would be appointed to decide the difference in value between the two articles that had been wagered. At this stage, all three parties would deposit forfeit money in a cap. The umpire would next indicate the "boot" to be added to the inferior article, and the two contestants would then draw out full or empty hands, thereby signifying their acceptance or rejection of the terms of competition. If the contestants agreed on the proposed terms, the entire sum that had been deposited in the cap would be passed to the umpire, but if the two players disagreed, the forfeit money would be claimed by the person who was willing that the contest should stand as determined by the umpire.

Handicapping of Sports

The term handicap was gradually extended from the equating of wagers to the matching of horses and of people, as umpires or judges awarded advantages or penalties that would permit fair and well-matched competition between differently endowed contestants. As such, it has particular relevance to athletic events involving participants who differ in the nature and severity of their disability.

Whereas a score may be modified or a race distance adjusted to match the ability of an individual (particularly if the total number of contestants is small), many competitions for the disabled now attract sufficient entrants that a reasonable level of equality can be assured by an appropriate classification of disability levels (see chapter 3) rather than by an adjustment of scores or race distances for the individual competitor. In essence, classification has taken the place of a handicap.

Development of Disabled Sports

Recreation for the disabled can be traced back at least to 1908, when the Playground Association of America set "play in institutions" as one of its objectives (Nesbitt, 1983); Sherrill (1986c) provides a detailed chronology. Sport for the deaf has perhaps the longest history, but more recently fast-moving sports such as wheelchair basketball have gained a higher profile.

Range of Sports

Traditional interests of the disabled such as fencing (see Figure 2.1; Jokl, 1958), equitation (Bicknell, 1972; Bieber, 1986; Davies, 1976; V.M. Fox, Lawlor, & Luttges, 1984; Hoskin, Erdman, Bream, & MacAvay, 1974; Reichenbach, 1973; Rosenzweig, 1987; Scott, 1974), basketball, swimming, archery, and javelin throwing (see Figures 2.2 and 2.3) have now been augmented by wheelchair rugby, football, volleyball, tennis, waterskiing (Wilkinson, 1982), sailing (Brabant, 1982; Roeren, 1987), canoeing (Lais & Schurke, 1982; Ware, 1982), and rowing (Cahill, 1982; Shasby & Lyttle, 1981).

Competitions for the blind, amputees, and cerebral palsied also include jumping events (high jump, long jump, and triple jump). Amputees play a form of standing volleyball. Goalball and judo (Loetze, 1981) are popular with the blind (Morisbak, 1980).

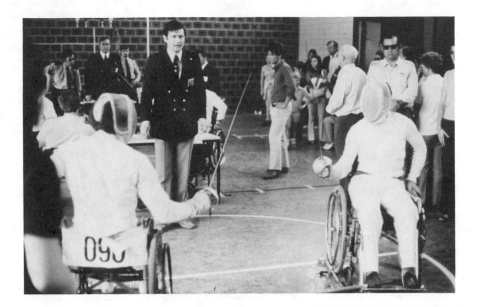

Figure 2.1. Fencing was introduced to paraplegics at an early stage in the development of wheelchair sports.

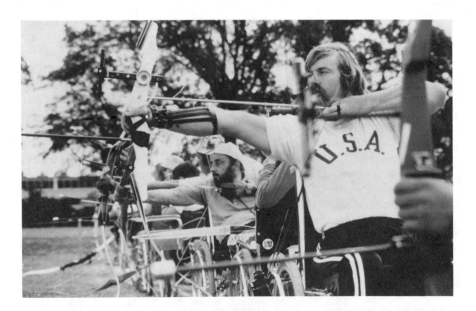

Figure 2.2. Archery has long been a popular sport for the wheelchair disabled. In some cases an orthotic is used to facilitate grasping of the bow.

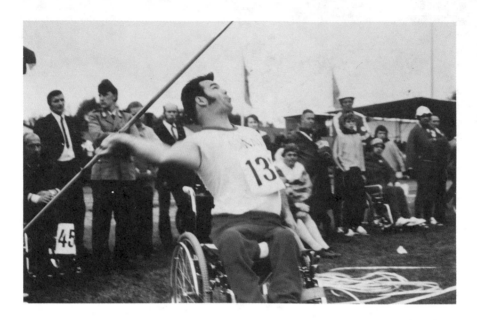

Figure 2.3.   Javelin competitions exploit the well-developed shoulder muscles of the paraplegic.

Winter sports began with ampute downhill skiers, individuals who performed three-track skiing (one regular ski and two smaller outrigger skis attached to poles) while navigating a slalom course (Kabsch, 1973). As other types and degrees of disability have been included in competitions, variants have included four-track (two regular skis plus two outriggers), one-track (a single ski with normal poles), and two-track skiing (two skis with or without poles used, for example, by below-knee amputees). More recently, blind amputees have also competed (using a guide; McCormick, 1984), and paraplegics have been able to enjoy downhill contests sitting in a sled or *pulk* (see Figures 2.4 and 2.5) or using a mono-ski (a seat and leg supporting device mounted on a single ski; Hottinger, 1980; Benedick, 1985). Cross-country skiing and speed-skating are also part of the Winter Olympic Games for the blind. Ice hockey, using small sleds, has proven quite popular with paraplegic athletes (Rappoport, 1982).

The growth of competitive events has, moreover, been matched by an increased recreational interest of the disabled in many of these same pursuits. In addition, suitably adapted forms of adventure sports such as gliding, rock climbing, canoeing, and parachute jumping (over water) now reach special segments of the disabled population (Croucher, 1976, 1978).

Wheelchair Sports

The idea of wheelchair sports was promoted by Stafford (1939) in the context of corrective physical education; such sport became popular during World War II, when a need was recognized to provide exercise and encouragement for the many

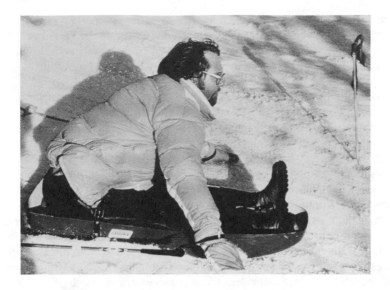

Figure 2.4.   Competitive winter sports are a relatively recent pleasure for the physically disabled.

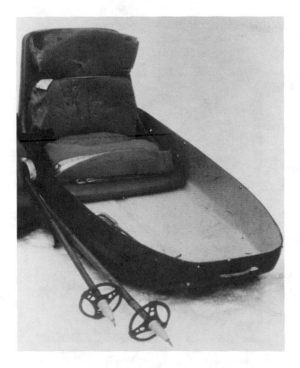

Figure 2.5.   A suitably padded toboggan with appropriate back support allows the paraplegic to enjoy many of the thrills of downhill skiing.

service personnel with severe spinal injuries. Independent initiatives were started at Veterans Administration hospitals in the United States, at British Army hospitals in Egypt, and at the Stoke Mandeville Hospital near Aylesbury in England. In each case, competitions were arranged on the basis of a disability-weighted handicap.

The concept of a wheelchair sports meet became established on an international basis through the efforts of Sir Ludwig Guttmann (see Figure 2.6), founder of the British National Unit for Paraplegics at Stoke Mandeville (Jokl, 1980; Scruton, 1979). Daily contact with spinally injured veterans convinced Sir Ludwig of the frequency with which a paralyzed person developed an inferiority complex, becoming anxious, self-pitying, and antisocial, with a lack of self-confidence. Sport was seen as a "rediscovery of the sensation and command of the body," according to Von Hallinger (cited by A.N. Witt, 1973, p. 257). Sport played a vital and immediate psychotherapeutic role, bringing the spinally injured person to terms with the anatomical defect, renewing his or her contact with the able-bodied world, providing the companionship and encouragement of other disabled persons, and restoring self-respect and self-discipline (Guttmann, 1973). Guttmann emphasized the unity of chair and rider: "The paraplegic and his chair have become one, in the same way as a first class horseman and his mount" p. 257; thus, all competitions were to be played from a wheelchair, irrespective of the level of disability in the individual contestant. This philosophy has led to some disagreement with organizations catering to the cerebral palsied and amputees, where competition is permitted from a standing position.

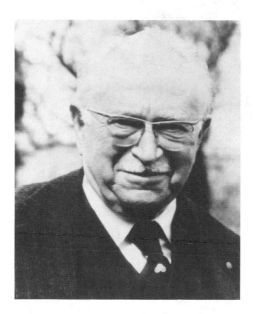

Figure 2.6. Sir Ludwig Guttman is credited with developing the International Stoke Mandeville Games immediately following World War II.

Development of International Wheelchair Competition

Initial competitions involved wheelchair patients in such activities as archery, table tennis, bowling, punchball, darts, and snooker (a type of billiards played in Great Britain; see Figure 2.7). Emphasis was next placed on events involving use of the wheelchair (100-m races and slalom competitions), as ability to maneuver a wheelchair was seen as important to daily living. These initiatives were quickly followed by the introduction of more vigorous sports, including wheelchair polo, badminton, and basketball (see Figure 2.8). The last of these activities provided spinally injured patients with a real challenge, in that they had to master both the chair and the ball while maintaining a correct orientation toward both opponents and fellow team members.

The first formal wheelchair games were held at the Stoke Mandeville Paraplegic Unit in 1948, with a mere 14 male and 2 female participants, all former military personnel (Guttmann, 1973; Steadward & Walsh, 1986). By chance, the competition coincided with the opening of the Olympic Games in London. Four years later, in 1952, the organization initiated by Sir Ludwig had already become the International Stoke Mandeville Games Federation (ISMGF). It soon affiliated with more than 50 national organizations, and its leaders began planning quadrennial contests in the same countries that hosted the Olympic Games for the able-bodied.

The first Olympic contest for the disabled (Paralympics, Rome, 1960) attracted 400 wheelchair competitors, and an almost equal number (390) visited Tokyo in 1964. The 1968 Games were not held in Mexico City, partly for organizational reasons and partly because it was thought that the added altitude would present too great a stress for the disabled competitors. This decision effectively broke

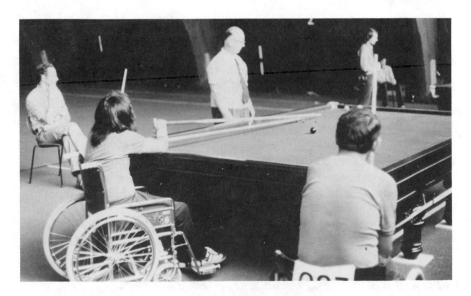

Figure 2.7. Quite severely disabled paraplegics can participate in billiards competitions.

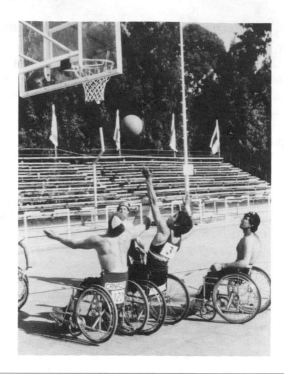

Figure 2.8. Basketball is regarded by many as one of the most exciting of wheelchair sports.

the linkage between the disabled and the able-bodied Olympics. Subsequent international competitions for the disabled have thus been held in Tel Aviv (1968), Heidelberg (1972), Toronto (1976), and Arnhem (1980).

Blind and amputee athletes were first allowed to participate in the Toronto olympiad of 1976. This event attracted not only participants from 38 countries but also more than 100,000 paying spectators (Jackson & Frederickson, 1979). Those with cerebral palsy were also allowed to participate in the games held at Arnhem in 1980. At the request of the International Olympic Committee, the term "Olympics" was dropped from the 1984 contests; the ISMGF met at Stoke Mandeville with an attendance of about 1,000 competitors, and about 3,000 from other groups such as the International Sports Organization for the Disabled (ISOD), the International Blind Sports Association (IBSA), and the Cerebral Palsy International Sports and Recreation Association (CP-ISRA) met in New York. Happily, in 1988 these various groups reunited in Seoul at the International Games for the Disabled (IGD).

Regional and National Events

Various regional events now supplement the quadrennial international competitions for the disabled. A quadrennial Commonwealth Paraplegic Games was initiated in Perth, Australia, in 1962. It has generally been hosted by the country organizing the Commonwealth Games for able-bodied individuals (e.g., the host cities were Kingston, Jamaica, in 1966, Edinburgh, Scotland, in 1970, and Dunedin, New Zealand, in 1974). Other wheelchair events have been organized in parallel with the Pan-American Games, commencing in 1967.

The U.S. National Wheelchair Basketball Association (NWBA) was founded in 1949, and the U.S. National Wheelchair Athletic Association (NWAA) had its debut in 1956. Initially, wheelchair sports were open to all contestants with significant and permanent disability of the lower limbs (whether due to spinal cord injury, spina bifida, poliomyelitis, amputation, orthopedic defects, or muscular weakness). The NWBA still accepts this view, now classifying competitors on functional ability (see chapter 3), but the NWAA excludes individuals with cerebral palsy and those (les autres) with other motor disabilities such as muscular dystrophy and multiple sclerosis.

Range of Contests

The range of competitions permitted at the wheelchair games has progressively extended as the ability of the contestants has become more widely recognized. Wheelchair track events over distances of more than 100 m were first introduced at the olympiad of 1976, and times for endurance races of this type have since improved rapidly (see Figure 2.9). Since 1980, ISMGF disability Classes II and III (see chapter 3) have been allowed to compete distances of over 400 m, and

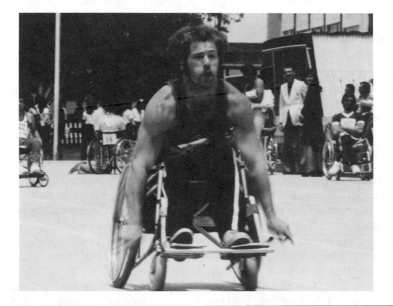

Figure 2.9. The body is held low in track events to minimize air resistance. Notice also the camber of the racing wheels and the need for wide lanes on the track.

since 1981 quadriplegics have also contested distances of more than 200 m. By 1983, six wheelchair athletes with spinal lesions graded as ISMFG Classes II to V (see chapter 3) completed the Toronto 1500-m event in less than 4 minutes. Wheelchair marathons were first attempted informally in 1975, and in 1977 the first U.S. National Wheelchair Marathon was held in conjunction with the Boston Marathon; a number of paraplegic athletes have completed the 42.2 km distance in under 2 hours. Some authors (Cowin, O'Riain, Sibille, & Layeux, 1987; Sherrill, 1986c) currently include motorized wheelchair games in their definition of disabled sport.

Sports for Amputees

Many amputees participate in wheelchair sports organizations, including the NWBA and open NWAA competitions (track, field, swimming, table tennis, and archery). The U.S. Amputee Athletic Association (USAAA) was founded in 1981, governing lesion-specific summer sports for amputees and those with major burn injuries. International competition is through ISOD.

Winter sports participation was introduced to the United States from Germany and Austria, gaining a major impetus from the need to rehabilitate casualties sustained in the Vietnam war (Benedick, 1985). Competitions in the United States have been coordinated by the National Handicapped Sports and Recreation Association since 1967; the first national handicapped ski championships at Winter Park, Colorado, attracted 50 competitors, and by the 1981-1982 competition numbers were such that regional qualifying events were added; by the 1984-1985 event, some 1,000 racers attempted to qualify for national competition.

Sports for the Blind

The U.S. Association of Blind Athletes (USABA) was founded in 1976, and 27 members of the association competed at the Toronto Paralympics in the same year. National competitions were initiated in 1977 and are now held annually, covering such events as weight lifting, wrestling, swimming, track, and cross-country and downhill skiing (Buell, 1979).

Sports for the Deaf

Many deaf people are excellent athletes and could compete readily in integrated events, but because of communication problems, they prefer to associate with others having a similar disability. The international organization dealing with deaf competitors, the Comité International des Sports Silencieux (CISS), can claim quite a long history, hosting a World Games for the Deaf in Paris in 1924 (Ammons, 1986). Events are restricted to those with a pure-tone hearing loss of 55 decibels or more in the better of the two ears.

With the exception of a 10-year hiatus due to World War II, the World Summer Games for the Deaf have been held every 4 years since 1924, usually 1 year following the able-bodied Olympics. The Los Angeles event of 1985 attracted 2,500 deaf competitors from 42 nations; sports included cycling, wrestling, swimming, track and field, tennis, table tennis, badminton, shooting, soccer, water polo, handball, volleyball, and basketball.

A quadrennial World Winter Games for the Deaf began in Austria in 1949; events include speed skating and cross-country and downhill skiing. The American Athletic Association for the Deaf (AAAD) was founded in 1945, and the U.S. Deaf Skiers Association had its debut in 1968. The AAAD now has 20,000 members; it organizes basketball and softball tournaments and prepares national competitors for the World Games. A Pan-American Games for the Deaf was also initiated in 1958.

Sports for the Cerebral Palsied

The first international games for the cerebral palsied were hosted by France in 1968, but CP-ISRA was not founded until 1978. The National Association of Sports for Cerebral Palsy (NASCP), a national organization for the United States, was established in the same year; membership is restricted to those with average or above-average intelligence.

The two team sports recommended for the cerebral palsied are soccer (played standing or from a wheelchair, according to the level of disability) and boccie. Most cerebral palsied persons perform better in individual sports; popular contests include archery, bowling, cycling, tricycling, horseback riding, shooting, swimming, slalom events with hand-propelled or motorized wheelchairs, table tennis, track and field, and weight lifting (Jones, 1984).

Sports for Les Autres

Les autres comprise individuals with a variety of locomotor disabilities such as muscular dystrophy, multiple sclerosis, Friedrich's ataxia, arthrogryposis, and osteogenesis imperfecta who are not eligible to compete in wheelchair events organized by the NWAA or cerebral palsy events sponsored by the NASCP.

International competition for les autres is regulated by ISOD, founded in 1976 (Lindstrom, 1984). The athletic potential of this group was highlighted by the 1984 ISOD competitions in New York, where les autres competitors from 20 nations participated in rifle and pistol shooting, archery, bowling, swimming, table tennis, track, volleyball, and weight lifting. Within the United States, the first national Les Autres Games was hosted at Detroit in 1985 in conjunction with the 5th National Cerebral Palsy Games. Les autres also compete in NWBA events.

Sports for the Mentally Retarded

Day camps involving informal sport and physical activities for the mentally retarded were initiated by Eunice Kennedy Shriver in 1963. Five years later, the Kennedy Foundation organized the first International Special Olympics in Chicago; some 1,000 mentally retarded competitors attended (Shriver, 1983). Despite the designation "international," this particular organization has retained a strong American influence; at the Baton Rouge meet of 1983, more than 80% of the 4,393 participants were still drawn from the United States. A rival organization is the Federation for Sports for Persons with Mental Handicap (INHS-FMH).

Although the Special Olympics does involve some competition, its prime goals are year-round activity and events in which the first eight participants can be winners. It is hoped that such recognition will boost self-esteem. Activities include aquatics, basketball, bowling, floor hockey, gymnastics, figure and speed skating, cross-country and downhill skiing, soccer, softball, track and field, and volleyball (Songster, 1986). The first Winter Special Olympics was hosted in 1977, and by 1985 the winter event attracted more than 800 participants. In both summer and winter events competitors are usually classified according to disability, but this decision is made by the meet director rather than by use of national norms.

Disabled Sports: Present and Future

Unfortunately, the organization of events for the disabled has at times been marked more by intergroup rivalry than by cooperation, as various associations have each pleaded the cause of their selected type of disability. Nevertheless, each of the organizations has seen vigorous growth over the past decade, and particularly in North America most categories of disabled sport are extremely viable.

ISOD was founded in 1976 as the blind and amputees were admitted to what had begun as a wheelchair Olympic competition. Although ISOD was at first intended as an umbrella organization for all disabled athletes, in practice it has developed as the representative of amputees, disabled skiers, and les autres.

A second International Coordinating Committee (ICC) was established in 1983 (McCann, 1987), with representatives from ISMGF, CP-ISRA, IBSA, and ISOD. Specific responsibilities of the ICC include (a) the avoidance of calendar conflicts between athletic events sponsored by member organizations, (b) the hosting of events involving multiple types of disability, and (c) the development of structures that allow cooperation rather than competition between the individual international sports organizations for the disabled.

Unfortunately, the group with the longest history of organizing contests for the disabled, CISS, initially prided itself on lack of participation in the ICC. Three recent events apparently presage greater cooperation in the future. In September 1986, CISS and INHS-FMH decided to join the ICC. However, they agreed that CISS– and INHS-FMH–affiliated athletes would still not participate in the Paralympics and World Championships organized by the ICC. A meeting of representatives from the six federations in 39 nations met in Arnhem in March 1987 to affirm that there would in future be one international sports organization for the disabled (McCann, 1987). Even more significantly, the Seoul Games of 1988 saw a reunion of the ISMGF and ISOD competitors, who had separated in 1984.

Research Efforts

The first of a series of international symposia discussing research on adapted physical activity was held in Quebec City in 1977. Subsequent meetings have been hosted in Brussels (1979), New Orleans (1981), London (1983), Toronto (1985),

Brisbane, Australia (1987), and West Berlin (1989). The first World Congress of Research on Sport and Exercise for the Physically Disabled was hosted in Banff, Alberta, in 1986.

An International Association for the Research of Sport and Exercise for the Disabled (IARSED) was founded in 1984 at the Olympic Scientific Congress in Eugene, Oregon, with Dr. Robert Steadward (of Edmonton, Alberta) as its first president. The same year, a research journal (*The Adapted Physical Activity Quarterly*) began publication, under the editorship of Dr. Geoffrey Broadhead. Other useful journals are *Palaestra* and *Sports 'N Spokes*. In some sports such as wheelchair basketball, techniques have now advanced to the point that methods of developing and of measuring sport-specific skills such as shooting, dribbling, and passing are beginning to appear (Vanlerberghe & Slock, 1987).

Issues that still require the attention of the scientist who is interested in adapted physical activity and the development of sports for the disabled include agreement on the principles of disability classification; peculiarities of exercise physiology and biochemistry in the disabled (including a suitable adaptation of test methods, the current fitness status, and the possibility of upgrading physical condition through appropriate training); biomechanical issues (abnormalities of movement patterns imposed by the disability, the design of equipment to maximize residual performance, the prevention of injuries, and considerations of ergonomics); psychosocial issues (including the impact of disability upon attitudes and personality, methods of encouraging enhanced activity, and the psychosocial benefits to be anticipated from greater physical activity); practical issues of program design (organization of coaching for various types and levels of disability and access to training facilities); and comparative aspects of adapted physical education in various cultures. Subsequent chapters will further explore each of these issues.

Key Ideas

1. A substantial proportion (5-10%) of most populations are affected by forms of physical or mental disability that limit both sport and occupational endeavors.

2. The majority of such individuals take less than an optimal amount of physical activity, with a consequent deterioration in the quality of their lives and an increase in their risk of hypokinetic diseases.

3. Normal wheelchair ambulation does not provide sufficient stimulus to restore or even to maintain physical condition.

4. Although devices such as laboratory ergometers and weight lifting can improve physical condition, many disabled subjects react more positively to suitably adapted forms of competitive sports.

5. The first major athletic initiative for a special population was the development of a sports organization for the deaf (CISS) in 1924. Subsequent to World War II, various other disability-specific organizations have emerged at national, regional, and international levels, including ISMGF, ISOD, CP-ISRA, IBSA, and the Special Olympics for the Mentally Retarded.

6. Many disabled individuals are now making dramatic demonstrations of their physical potential through adapted training prescriptions, and except in those individuals with a continuing disease process there has been a parallel improvement in prognosis over the past 2 decades.

Practical Applications

1. What are some of the diseases that complicate life in a wheelchair? Why have there been changes in their relative incidence over the past 2 decades?
2. Is it a good idea to expose the disabled to competition, knowing that they may face a further defeat that they could attribute to their disability?
3. Can you handicap a competition without stigmatizing the disabled?
4. What are some positive psychological aspects of sport for the disabled?
5. If you were the executive director of a sports organization catering to a specific disability, how would you minimize rivalry with other sports organizations for the disabled?

Chapter 3

Disability Classification

This chapter explores the logic of disability classification, proposes appropriate standards of qualification for examiners, and reviews current controversies between the various regulating bodies. The need for split classification is briefly discussed, and specific systems of classification are advanced for amputees, the blind, the cerebral palsied, les autres, and those with spinal lesions. Final sections consider the possibilities of integrated competition and open competition.

Justification of Handicaps

Disability classifications have been developed and refined for the various categories of athletic competition in an attempt to ensure that the "handicap" offered to individual participants is appropriate (see chapter 2), allowing those with "even the most severe disability to compete in a fair manner with other competitors with similar degrees of disability" (International Stoke Mandeville Games Federation, 1982).

Total fairness is perhaps an illusory goal, and quite plainly the process of arranging handicaps could be carried to excessive lengths. There has been vigorous discussion of the wisdom of granting "elite athlete" status to those who are severely disabled, particularly if they wish to undertake activities for which they have only a limited potential. Indeed, some people argue that competitions in any given type of sport should be restricted to those who can closely match the performance of an able-bodied individual. The debate has been particularly vigorous in connection with the Special Olympics, which long argued that self-esteem would be boosted if every competitor were a winner; the Canadian Association for the Mentally Retarded has suggested that all mentally retarded children should be allowed to attend national competitions, irrespective of their performance in local or regional contests. However, more recently even the Special Olympics has limited recognition to three medal winners and five ribbon recipients within a given category of event.

All disabled sports still incorporate either a handicap or a rigid categorization of contestants, but this does not necessarily detract from competition. The idea of allowing a substantial handicap, indeed, is not peculiar to contests for the disabled. Analogous adjustments are well recognized in many forms of athletic competition; for example, there is a careful age stratification of both Masters athletes and minor hockey league players and a weight categorization of wrestlers and boxers. On occasion, functional classifications are also adopted by the able-bodied; for example, competitions are arranged that distinguish novice, intermediate, and expert participants.

Limitations to Classification

Although existing classification procedures allow some equalization of prospects among disabled competitors, it is unrealistic to expect that examiners will have total success in matching what are highly individualized clinical problems. Inevitably, upper and lower limits exist in any given category of disability, and depending on their position within the permitted range some athletes will be at an advantage relative to other competitors.

Unfortunately, attempts to achieve greater fairness through a more precise categorization quickly become counterproductive. If the span from the upper to the lower limit of a given disability category is made too narrow, then a situation soon arises wherein the number of gold medals made available exceeds the likely number of competitors as calculated from the prevalence of the disability and the anticipated participation rate (Lindstrom, 1986). For example, current international regulations already allow 52 shot put classes for those with locomotor disabilities and a further six categories for blind shot-putters; if age and sex are also introduced as stratifying variables, the number of categories of competition rapidly becomes ridiculously large. Classification is thus designed to give all entrants a ''sporting chance'' of winning, but at the same time it is recognized that total fairness is not a practicable objective.

Qualifications of the Examiner

Unfortunately, as in sport for the able-bodied, classification decisions are increasingly disputed by the competitors, their coaches, and their rivals. Moreover, again making an unhappy parallel with able-bodied activities such as wrestling, entrants have in some instances attempted to mislead officials making the classifications, exaggerating the extent of their muscle weakness in order to gain a favorable categorization (Sherrill, Adams-Mushett, & Jones, 1986).

Thus classification must be undertaken by experienced examiners (the ISMGF maintains a register for this purpose) and the basis of decisions must be carefully documented against possible appeals. Nevertheless, the type of person who is best qualified to classify the extent of disability remains a matter of considerable discussion. The optimum choice of examiner (physician or certified classifier) depends in part on the type of classification that is to be made. Ideally, there should be combined input from a suitably experienced doctor or physical therapist and a doctoral-level specialist in adapted physical education and recreation.

Current Controversies of Classification

Given the wide range of disabling clinical conditions and the varying levels of disability encountered among those affected by any given disorder, the establishment of appropriate classification procedures has proved both difficult and controversial (Biering-Sorensen, 1983; Kessler, 1970; Kruimer, 1983; Lindstrom, 1986;

McCann, 1979a, 1979b, 1983, 1984; Sherrill, Adams-Mushett, & Jones, 1986; Strohkendl, 1985; Vorsteveld, 1985; Weiss & Curtiss, 1986).

There are currently four main systems for the classification of disability; these systems have been proposed respectively by ISMGF, ISOD, IBSA, and CP-ISRA. They address the needs of specific disability groups (ISMGF, spinal injuries; ISOD, amputees, the blind, and les autres; CP-ISRA, those with cerebral palsy). The Special Olympics uses the alternative tactic of requiring participants to arrive at a competition with previous times or distances validated by a coach or teacher; the meet director then assigns contestants to age and sex-specific heats, based also upon the reported abilities of other contestants.

Classification is relatively well developed for those with spinal injuries. Nevertheless, grading in most types of disability can be based on one or more of three possible approaches: (a) anatomico-medical (based on medical determinations of trunk balance and muscle strength and dependent upon the site of the lesion plus the completeness of transection in those with injuries of the spinal cord, (b) functional (based on the judgment of certified classifiers, supplemented where necessary by strength measurements and influenced by the quality and quantity of active muscle plus the ability to perform various sport-specific tasks), and (c) dynamic (based on the extent of habitual daily activity and characteristic patterns of voluntary energy expenditure).

Although the last tactic undoubtedly has value for epidemiological purposes (Kofsky, Davis, Jackson, Keene, & Shephard, 1983a; Kofsky, Davis, Shephard, Keene, & Jackson, 1980; Kofsky, Shephard, Davis, & Jackson, 1986), sports organizers have discussed mainly the merits of the first two approaches. There have been significant differences of opinion between the ISMGF and other agencies dealing with the wheelchair athlete (e.g., the Pan-American organization for Disabled Sports, the NWBA, and the NWAA; Weiss & Curtiss, 1986). In general, the ISMGF and the NWAA have leaned toward an anatomical type of classification, whereas other agencies such as ISOD, CP-ISRA, and German and several North American national groups (NWBA, NASCP, USAAA, and USABA) have favored a functional approach (Strohkendl, 1986).

Weiss and Curtiss (1986) argued that the functional approach penalizes athletes who have already optimized their performance through a combination of hard training, the development of coordination, and the learning of trick movements to maintain their balance. The ISMGF has, moreover, pleaded the uniqueness of those with spinal injuries and has excluded from their classification system other wheelchair groups such as amputees. On the other hand, a number of groups (particularly ISOD, ICC, and NWBA) have preferred an integrated approach to competitions (McCann, 1987); inclusion of a variety of disabilities in a given contest necessarily demands a functional classification rather than a rigid categorization by anatomical lesion level (see specifically the NASCP system for classifying both the cerebral palsied and les autres, Table 3.1).

Split Classifications

Irrespective of which classification system is adopted, disabled athletes have to date generally been awarded a single classification. However, in contrast with their able-bodied peers, many of those who are disabled enter a wide range of

Table 3.1   Classification System of NASCP for Competitors With Cerebral Palsy and Les Autres Conditions

Class	Functional ability
1	Motorized wheelchair. Severe involvement of all 4 limbs, limited trunk control, 25% range of motion, unable to grasp softball.
2	Wheelchair propelled by feet or very slowly by arms. Moderate to severe involvement of all 4 limbs, 40% range of motion, severe problems of motor control for accuracy. May have uneven function, 2U(pper) or 2L(ower) subclassifications.
3	Wheelchair propelled with short arm movements at fair speed. Moderate involvement in 3 or 4 limbs and trunk, 60% range of motion, can take a few steps with support.
4	Wheelchair propelled with forceful continuous arm movements. Excellent ability for wheelchair sports—only lower limbs involved, 70% range of motion and minimal control problems.
5	Walks with assistance from crutches, cane, or walker. Moderate to severe unilateral spasticity (hemiplegia) or both lower limbs (paraplegia), 80% range of motion.
6	Walks without support, but has obvious problems of balance and coordination. Moderate to severe involvement of 3 or 4 limbs, 70% range of motion in dominant arm.
7	Walks with slight limp. Mild to moderate spasticity (unilateral or all 4 limbs), 90 to 100% normal range of motion.
8	Runs and jumps without noticeable limp. Good balance, symmetric performance, normal range of motion, but obvious minimal problems of coordination.

competitions, including different types of sport (e.g., basketball and track events) and differing durations of activity (e.g., sprint and marathon races). From the viewpoint of fairness in competition, it might thus be appropriate to award different categorizations for different types of sport and even to distinguish different classes of contest within a given sport. Within the broad category of swimming events, for example, it might be useful to give disabled athletes differing classifications depending on the type of stroke (breaststroke, backstroke, or crawl) that they attempt (McCann, 1983; 1984).

In endurance sports, the impact of the lesion upon normal cardiorespiratory adaptations to exercise may be as important a limiting factor as any weakening of the active muscles. Wicks, Oldridge, Cameron, and Jones (1983) commented on differences in maximum heart rate and thus of peak oxygen intake between athletes with traumatic spinal cord injuries and those with poliomyelitis who would receive a similar disability categorization on the basis of residual muscle function. If spinally injured and poliomyelitic patients are to contest an endurance event, a classification based simply upon muscular strength will plainly be inappropriate and indeed will give the poliomyelitic a substantial advantage.

In other activities such as archery, fencing, bowls, and snooker, skill is more important than aerobic power or muscular strength. A precise classification of wheelchair competitors by level of spinal transection is then much less important. Account may need to be taken of spasm or athetoid movements, which can impose a substantial handicap. Nevertheless, if the number of entrants is small, some pooling of categories is possible and should be adopted for this group of sports. Finally, in sports such as basketball, procedures must be developed to match the average characteristics of entire teams that are heterogeneous in terms of their levels of disability.

Classification of Spinal Lesions

The classical ISMGF system adopts a combined anatomical and medical approach to classification. It stems from the clinical practice of evaluating the level of neural lesions by the testing of critical muscle groups (Long & Lawton, 1955; McDonald & Chusid, 1952). The main limitations of this method are practical difficulties in making adequate allowances for (a) the extent of lower-limb impairment, (b) any associated impairment of sensory function (Biering-Sorensen, 1980; Natvig, Biering-Sorensen, & Jorgensen, 1980), and (c) the cause of the lesion (e.g., congenital, infectious, or traumatic; Biering-Sorensen, 1980; Natvig, Biering-Sorensen, & Jorgensen, 1980). Competitors are generally classified in terms of the traumatized vertebral segment (e.g., sixth cervical, C6), and a descriptive adjective is sometimes added (e.g., complete, incomplete, or poliomyelitic). Refinements allow some differentiation of scoring between those with traumatic and poliomyelitic lesions (see Table 3.2). The current ISMGF system is thus quite well adapted to the classification of individuals with spinal injuries or poliomyelitis except in sports such as weight lifting, where the main criterion of performance is body mass.

ISMGF rules exclude not only those with minimal disability (e.g., chondromalacia patella or forefoot amputation) but also all non–spinal cord lesions (although above- and below-knee amputees have recently been admitted to wheelchair basketball). In principle, the ISMGF type of classification could apply to athletes with certain other types of disability, including not only the amputees but also those with brachial plexus lesions and the Guillain Barré syndrome (a diffuse infectious disease of the peripheral nerves that causes muscular weakness; Vorsteveld, 1985). However, McCann (1987) has argued it is not appropriate to the patchy and variable disability of cerebral palsy.

The ISMGF classification typically begins with observation of the quality of an individual's trunk and limb movements during warm-up or a practice game. Key trunk-control skills to watch include rotation (for the discus throw) and picking up a ball from the floor (in basketball). In essence, the objective of the examiner is to identify the anatomic level of a lesion, based upon the quality and quantity of muscle function that is conserved (Biering-Sorensen, 1980; Grosfield, 1980; Jackson & Frederickson, 1979; McCann, 1984, 1985). This information is supplemented as necessary by a consideration of the level of sensory loss, of the presence of any additional impairments such as amputations, spinal fusion, or muscle spasticity, and of the benefit gained from any orthotic devices that are worn.

Table 3.2   Anatomical/Functional Classification for Spinal Injuries, Based on International Stoke Mandeville Games Federation

Class	Cord level	Functional characteristics
IA	C4-6	Triceps 0-3 on MRC scale. Severe weakness of trunk and lower extremities, interfering with sitting balance and ability to walk.
IB	C4-7	Triceps 4-5. Wrist flexion and extension may be present. Generalized weakness of trunk and lower extremities, interfering significantly with sitting balance and ability to walk.
IC	C4-8	Triceps 4-5. Wrist flexion and extension may be present. Finger flexion and extension 4-5 permits grasping and release. No useful hand intrinsic muscles. Generalized weakness of trunk and lower extremities interfering significantly with sitting balance and ability to walk.
II	T1-5	No useful abdominal muscles (0-2). No functional lower intercostal muscles. No useful sitting balance.
III	T6-10	Good upper abdominal muscles. No useful lower abdominal or lower trunk extensor muscles. Poor sitting balance.
IV	T11-L3	Good abdominal and spinal extensor muscles. Some hip flexors and adductors. Weak or nonexistent quadriceps strength, limited gluteal control (0-2). Points 1-20, traumatic, 1-15 polio.
V	L4-S2	Good or fair quadriceps control. Points 21-40, traumatic, 16-35 polio.[a]
VI	L4-S2	Points 41-60, traumatic, 36-50 polio[a] (Class VI is a subdivision of V, applied only in swimming competitions).

[a]Each of the following muscle groups is awarded up to 5 points (5 = normal strength) per side: hip flexors, adductors, abductors and extensors, knee flexors and extensors, ankle plantar and dorsiflexors. Potential score, 40 points per side.

In activities such as archery, it is sufficient to distinguish the tetraplegic (quadriplegic) from the nontetraplegic, but in most sports the ISMGF has traditionally divided spinally injured athletes into eight categories—three levels of cervical lesion and five other categories. Although the boundaries of this classification system are now hallowed by history, they were originally adopted in a relatively arbitrary fashion, and the dividing lines between the various disability categories should probably be reconsidered, taking account of advances in knowledge of both wheelchair sports and electromyography of the disabled (McCann, 1979b; Steadward, 1979).

The classical ISMGF approach includes a functional element, as the strength of individual muscle groups is graded on a six-point scale (Daniels & Worthington, 1972). The marks that are assigned range from zero (a total lack of voluntary contraction) to 5 (a contraction of normal strength against full resistance throughout the full range of motion of a joint). A faint contraction without movement (Grade 1) and a contraction with very weak movement when gravity is eliminated (Grade 2) are not included when calculating the total amount of functioning tissue in a limb (see Table 3.2).

In practice, ISMGF Class IA is distinguished from Class IB mainly on the strength of the triceps, whereas Class IC is distinguished by the function of the hand muscles. Class IA subjects on average require twice the time of Classes IB and IC in order to complete a wheelchair dash movement (Steadward, 1979). However, this same unpublished report noted only minor differences of electromyographic function between Classes IB and IC (Steadward, 1979), and the need to distinguish these two categories from one another is thus debatable. Hand function is invaluable when grasping and releasing a discus, and in this sport Class IC has some advantage over Class IB. Trunk power contributes to rotation and a wind-up in throwing events; on the other hand, triceps function makes little contribution to this particular type of sport. When classifying athletes for either swimming or throwing events, it is probably important to consider the strength of the shoulder muscles.

The strength of the abdominal and spinal extensor muscles is important when distinguishing between ISMGF Classes II and III. The amount of balance (none, poor, fair, or good) is critical to the wheelchair competitor but is less vital for the swimmer. Classification of balance in a doctor's office is difficult, partly because a clinical examination bench differs greatly from a personalized wheelchair, partly because some athletes attempt to mask their true potential while being classified, and partly because those with long-standing lesions have had greater opportunity to learn tricks for conserving their balance than those who have recently been disabled. The final categorization must take account not only of residual function, but also of reaction time, any compensatory mechanisms that have been learned, innate coordination and training, spinal flexibility, spasticity, abnormal reflexes and reactions, and the motivation of the athlete.

In assessing Classes IV, V, and VI (swimming only), the muscles of the hip, knee, and ankle are evaluated and a point score is awarded. The critical score is higher for traumatic lesions than for poliomyelitis, because the latter patients conserve some sensation and do not face problems from residual spasticity. A trauma victim with more than 20 points or a poliomyelitis victim with more than 15 points is often capable of using the legs but will not necessarily do so in competition.

Partial Lesions

Since 1967, the athletic classification has made no attempt to distinguish partial from complete lesions, although it is generally agreed that the partial preservation of motor or sensory function distal to the nominal level of a lesion confers some competitive advantage. This issue is particularly important when victims of spinal cord trauma compete against amputees and patients affected by poliomyelitis.

In the "integrated" competitions of the NWAA, persons with spinal cord injuries and spina bifida are significantly underrepresented among the first-place winners relative to the overall membership of the association, whereas those with incomplete cord lesions, amputees, and poliomyelitis victims are overrepresented

(Weiss & Curtiss, 1986). However, it remains uncertain whether the problem of competitive inequality arises simply from the classification system itself or whether there are also difficulties in its enforcement.

The classification of patients with asymmetric lesions is a particularly difficult issue, as some sports use one side of the body more than the other. Competitors generally use the better preserved limb for events such as a shot put.

Problems of ISMGF Classification

Among potential sources of error in the ISMGF classification system (McCann, 1984), we may note recent injury (with incomplete adaptation or compensation), lack of appropriate rehabilitation or training, and deliberately half-hearted test efforts by the athlete in an attempt to obtain an unfair competitive advantage. Moreover, insufficient allowance is made for the benefits conferred by residual sensation in the paralyzed limbs; the extent of proprioception, in particular, can be quite an important issue in borderline classification (Weiss & Curtiss, 1986).

In some types of disorder, problems arise from residual spasticity. This may mimic voluntary muscular contraction, leading the examiner to overestimate muscle function. Because of its unpredictable extent, spasticity hampers precise athletic movements. Furthermore, it disturbs balance, particularly in field events, and it can cause a competitor to adopt unfavorable limb positions while swimming.

Improvements of performance could arise in individuals with high-level lesions if the trunk were to be stabilized in the wheelchair, either by the training and entrainment of accessory postural muscles (Daniels & Worthington, 1972) or by the use of supporting strapping. The latter is allowed in tetraplegic and novice archery competitions and in situations where a lack of restraints would expose the individual athlete or other contestants to a risk of injury.

Deformities such as fixed contractures and arthrodeses call for individual classification by an examiner well versed in both kinesiology and the sport to be contested. Although an arthrodesis of the spine might seem an advantage to an athlete with a high-level lesion (because it stabilizes the trunk), at the same time it reduces flexibility.

The use of a trunk or lower-limb orthosis is allowed in most types of competition, and hand orthoses are also permitted in archery (see Figure 2.2 in chapter 2). However, a competitor who wishes to use any type of orthosis must be observed and classified while wearing the supporting device.

Proposals for Team Sports

In sports such as wheelchair basketball, team members are likely to be heterogenous with respect to their type and level of disability. The problem of matching teams fairly has been dealt with by assigning arbitrary points to individual players based on their personal disability classifications (see Table 3.3) and by setting a ceiling of points for the entire team.

Unfortunately, the various sporting organizations have yet to agree upon details of the points to be awarded. For instance, McCann (1979a) suggested allowing 1 point for a player with ISMGF Classes I, II, and III, 2 points for Class IV, and 3 points for Class V. More recently, ISMGF has proposed an allowance of

Table 3.3 ISMGF Basketball Classification as Suggested by Strohkendl (1986)

		Functional test results		
Class	Level	Horizontal (sitting up)	Saggital (bending a/p)	Frontal plane (bending laterally)
I	T8 & up	—	—	—
II	T9 to L2	+	—	—
III	L3 to L5	+	+	—
IV	S1 to S2	+	+	+

Other classifications: ISMGF III (L2 to L5), IV (S1 to S2), NWBA II (T8 to L2), III (L3 and below, no class IV)

Note. Based on data from "The New Classification System for Wheelchair Basketball" by H. Strohkendl in *Sport and Disabled Athletes*, edited by C. Sherrill, 1986, Champaign, IL: Human Kinetics.

1 or 1.5 points for Class I, 2 or 2.5 points for Class II, 3 or 3.5 points for Class III, and 4 points for Class IV, the total number of points for a five-member team being limited to 14 (Strohkendl, 1985, 1986). United States rules adopted by the NWBA (McCann, 1979a; Strohkendl, 1986) use the traditional classification, awarding 1 point for ISMGF Classes I to III, 2 points for Class IV, and 3 points for Class V and allowing a maximum of 12 points for a team of five players.

In a new functional classification, Class I is reserved for athletes who have a lesion at T8 or above, with additional impairment in at least one arm (see Table 3.3); these athletes use a wheelchair with a high back, lose their balance when lifting both arms above their heads, and have difficulty in turning their heads backward. Class II is distinguished from Class III on the basis of hip joint control; individuals in the former cannot raise their trunks from their laps without using at least one arm, and they cannot wheel the chair at high speed while bouncing the ball. Class III is distinguished from Class IV because the former individuals lack control of abduction in at least one leg (Strohkendl, 1986); they also show limitations of trunk movements in the frontal plane.

Modified ISMGF Classification

There has recently been some rapprochement between the ISMGF anatomico-medical approach and the functional classifications favored by other organizations, this being reflected in the international basketball competitions held under ISMGF aegis. Strohkendl (1986) proposed a four-category system of categorization for the basketball competitor, based upon the control of trunk movement in the horizontal, saggital, and frontal planes (see Table 3.3).

Given the disabled person's potential to develop "trick" movements that can compensate for a poor intrinsic balance, the examiner directs particular attention to the quality of the movement. The examiner then obtains information from the coach and fellow team members, and this suffices for the classification of clear-cut cases. However, functional testing and medical examination may be required for contentious competitors (Strohkendl, 1985, 1986). Given the potential for recovery from some conditions, reexamination is recommended every 3 years (McCann, 1979a).

Alternative Methods for Classification of Spinal Injuries

In epidemiological studies, it may be difficult to obtain precise functional data, and an approximate topographic location of the lesion level may suffice. Several groups of investigators (Davis, Kofsky, Shephard, & Jackson, 1981; Fugl-Meyer & Grimby, 1971; Hjeltnes, 1984; Shephard, Davis, Kofsky, & Sutherland, 1983) distinguished four categories on a descriptive anatomical basis (C5-C8, tetraplegic; T1-T6, high-level paraplegic; T7-L1, mid-level paraplegic; L2-S2, low-level paraplegic).

A classification based upon patterns of habitual activity also has some attraction, as it may reflect the total consequences of a lesion, physiological and psychological. To date, a general association has been found between the reported daily activity and aerobic fitness (Kofsky et al., 1980, 1983a, 1986), although it remains unclear whether the normal energy cost of wheelchair ambulation is sufficient to provide an adequate training stimulus (Glaser, Laubach, Sawka, & Surprayasad, 1978; Gordon & Vanderwalde, 1956; Hjeltnes & Vokac, 1979; Nilsson et al., 1975; Voight & Bahn, 1969) (see chapter 5).

Comparison of two- (Davis, Tupling, & Shephard, 1986; Shephard et al., 1983), three- (Davis et al., 1981; Kofsky et al., 1983a), and four-level (Davis, Kofsky, Shephard, Keene, & Jackson, 1980; Jackson, Davis, Kofsky, Shephard, & Keene, 1981; Kofsky et al., 1980) categorization of habitual activity suggests that top level disabled athletes and recreational paraplegics differ significantly in peak oxygen intake and muscular strength, but that the latter show much smaller differences from inactive individuals with similar anatomical disabilities.

Correlation Between ISMGF Categorization and Physiological Data

Hulleman et al. (1975) observed a strong correlation between the classical ISMGF anatomico-functional category and the physical working capacity of the forearm muscles in a sample of 100 athletes attending the ISMGF Games of 1972. Other authors, also, described significant associations between functional category and aerobic fitness or arm strength (Cameron, Ward, & Wicks, 1978; Wicks, Lymburner, Dinsdale, & Jones, 1977; Wicks et al., 1983).

Some researchers, including myself, agree that Class I differs physiologically from Class II, but our laboratory has been unable to detect a significant effect of lesion level upon either peak arm ergometer oxygen intake or muscular strength over the range of ISMGF Classes I through V (Davis et al., 1980; Davis, Tupling, & Shephard, 1986; Jackson et al., 1981; Kofsky et al., 1980; Kofsky, Davis, Shephard, Keene, & Jackson, 1982; Kofsky, Shephard, Davis, & Jackson, 1986).

In contrast, the simplified descriptive/anatomical approach apparently distinguishes quite well between individuals in terms of both physiological (Davis et al., 1981) and psychological (Shephard et al., 1983) test scores.

Amputees

The current ISOD classification system for amputees (Biering-Sorensen, 1980; International Sports Organization for the Disabled, 1981; see Table 3.4) takes no account of etiology; the usual form of competition includes those with both congenital and acquired lesions. Originally, a complex 27-category classification of amputees was proposed, but it soon became apparent that this yielded too few competitors in most individual categories. Moreover, in certain sports the extent of an amputation has only a minor impact on performance, and an argument could be made for combination of some of the remaining nine categories (for example, 5 and 7 or 6 and 8 in track competitions).

Strohkendl (1986) proposed a simplified three-category classification of disability that allows heterogenous teams of amputees and the spinally paralyzed to participate in wheelchair basketball competitions. Bilateral amputations above the lesser trochanter are regarded as Class II lesions, bilateral amputations below the lesser trochanter are rated as Class III or IV (depending on residual trunk function), and unilateral amputees are rated as Class IV.

In winter sports (Benedick, 1985), alpine competitions are classed according to the number of skis and outriggers that are used—LW1 is 4-track (see chapter 2), LW2 is 3-track, LW3 is normal skiing with disability in both legs, LW4 is normal skiing with disability in one leg, LW5/7 is the use of normal skis with no poles, LW6/8 is the use of normal skis with one pole, and LW9 is a combination of arm and leg disability using equipment of the contestant's choice.

Table 3.4 ISOD and USAAA Classification Code for Amputees

Class	Type of lesion
A1	Double above knee
A2	Single above knee
A3	Double below knee
A4	Single below knee
A5	Double above elbow
A6	Single above elbow
A7	Double below elbow
A8	Single below elbow
A9	Combined lower and upper limb amputation

Blindness

Blind athletes are classified annually by a certified optometrist or ophthalmologist (Sherrill, Adams-Mushett, & Jones, 1986). The classification must be relatively precise (see Table 3.5), as an appreciable competitive advantage is conferred by the ability to distinguish shadows and light and darkness (Jackson & Frederickson, 1979). The scheme currently adopted by IBSA recognizes three categories of disability; Class I ranges from zero light perception to an inability to recognize objects or contours, Class II ranges from object recognition to a visual acuity of 2/60 as measured by Snellen test-type or a limitation of the visual field to an arc of 5°, and Class III covers visual acuities ranging from 2/60 to 6/60 or limitation of the field of vision to an arc of between 5 and 60°. Some have suggested that IBSA should modify rules to take account of the additional handicap imposed by the recent onset of blindness. In team sports such as goalball, competition is equalized by making all players wear blindfolds.

Cerebral Palsy

Cerebral palsy (CP) is characterized by nonspecific damage to areas of the brain controlling muscular tone and spinal reflexes. Some 61% of competitors with CP are affected primarily by spasticity, 17% by athetosis (alternating bouts of hyper- and hypotonus), and 10% by other disabilities (Sherrill, Adams-Mushett,

Table 3.5 Classifications of Blindness

Class	Functional ability
Medical	
Legal blindness	Vision 6/60 (20/200); able to see at 6 meters (20 feet) what the normal eye can see at 60 meters (200 feet)
Travel vision	Vision 1.5-3/60; (5-10/200)
Motion perception	Vision 0.9-1.5/60; (3-5/200)
Light perception	Vision <0.9/60; (<3/200); able to see strong light but unable to detect hand movement at 0.9 meters (3 feet)
Total blindness	Unable to recognize strong light shone directly into eye
International Blind Sports Association	
I	Total blindness to inability to recognize objects or contours
II	Object recognition to visual acuity 2/60 (6.7/200), or limitation of visual field to arc <5 degrees
III	Visual acuity 2/60 to 6/60 (6.7 to 20/200) or limitation of visual field to arc of 5-60 degrees

& Jones, 1986), although many CP athletes have both spasm and athetoid movements. Depending on the etiology of the disorder, there may be associated problems such as abnormal reflexes, hyperkinesia, impulsiveness, epileptic seizures, attentional deficiencies, learning disabilities, perceptual-motor disorders (which make it difficult for a competitor to stay in the appropriate lane or to hit targets), deafness (particularly if the disorder is due to incompatibility of Rh blood grouping), and visual difficulties such as far sightedness, inwardly crossed eyes (esotropia), or blindness in half of the visual field (homonymous hemianopia).

Some 88% of the population who are affected by CP have a combination of three or more disabilities (Sherrill, Adams-Mushett, & Jones, 1986). It has thus been argued by ISMGF that such patients cannot compete fairly with the spinally paralyzed. Nevertheless, those with CP who wish to participate in wheelchair competitions generally have less in the way of associated handicaps than those who do not have such ambitions. For instance, 30 to 70% of the general CP population have some degree of mental retardation, but only 10 to 15% of CP athletes have a low intelligence quotient. The 1983 manual of the now-defunct NASCP and more recently the 1987 manual of the U.S. Cerebral Palsy Athletic Association (USCPAA) recognized this distinction, specifying that the CP sports are intended for those who are not eligible for the Special Olympics (Sherrill, Adam-Mushett, & Jones, 1986).

The CP-ISRA system of classification (MacGregor, 1980; Cerebral Palsy International Sports and Recreation Association, 1983) has been developed specifically for the patient with cerebral palsy (see Table 3.6). Classification is inevitably much more difficult than for a patient with spinal injury or an amputee, as the lesion is located in the brain rather than in accessible muscles. Individual competitors are categorized after interviews with the athlete and coach, followed by field observation of such factors as posture, locomotion, throwing, grasping, and mobility in water (Kruimer, 1985). Where possible, the examiners determine those

Table 3.6   Classification System of Cerebral Palsy International Sports and Recreation Association (CP-ISRA)

Class	Method of ambulation
1	Quadriplegic—motorized wheelchair
2	Quadriplegic—manual wheelchair
3	Weak quadriplegic or triplegic—wheelchair propelled with one or two arms slowly
4	Diplegic—wheelchair used for normal daily activities and sports
5	Diplegic or moderate to severe hemiplegic—ambulant, with or without cane(s) or crutch(es)
6	Quadriplegic athetoid—ambulant
7	Moderate to minimal hemiplegic or moderate to minimal quadriplegic—ambulant
8	Minimal handicap—ambulant

features of CP most likely to affect performance and make appropriate allowances for any associated disorders (Sherrill, Pope, & Arnhold, 1986) (see Table 3.1 for details). Eight tests examine function of the arms and torso, and a further four tests evaluate leg function and stability. Account is taken of response time, speed, coordination, accuracy of movement, and range of motion rather than strength, the simplest form of classification noting the ease of locomotion. There are eight basic categories for this type of disability (see Table 3.6). Individuals falling into the first four of these categories require a wheelchair for both sports and normal daily activities. Some 80 to 85% of competitors are awarded a constant category across different types of sport (Kruimer, 1983).

Les Autres

The ISOD classification for les autres (International Sports Organization for the Disabled, 1981; Natvig et al., 1980) is functional and shows some similarity to that proposed for CP (International Sports Organization for the Disabled, 1981). Table 3.7 shows the schema that have been developed for field events; differing specifications have been adopted for swimming and table tennis.

Many difficulties arise both in matching the wide range of admissible conditions and in deciding which competitors are eligible for a les autres classification (International Sports Organization for the Disabled, 1981). Potential candidates include patients with various types of ankylosis; arthrodesis or arthrosis of major joints; ankylosing spondylitis; Guillain-Barré syndrome; brachial plexus lesions with arm

Table 3.7 ISOD Les Autres Classification System for Field Events

Class	Characteristics
L1	Wheelchair bound. Reduced muscle strength, mobility and/or spasticity in throwing arm. Poor sitting balance.
L2	Wheelchair bound. Normal function in throwing arm with poor to moderate sitting balance, or reduced function in throwing arm but good sitting balance.
L3	Wheelchair bound. Normal arm function and good sitting balance.
L4	Ambulant with or without crutches or braces, or reduced function in throwing arm and problems of balance. Note: an athlete is allowed to use orthosis or crutches if desired. The throw can be made from a standstill or a moving position in classes L4 and L5.
L5	Ambulant with normal function in throwing arm, but reduced function in lower limbs or balance problem.
L6	Ambulant with normal function in throwing arm, but minimal trunk or lower limb disability sufficient to give a locomotor disadvantage relative to able-bodied athletes in throwing events.

paresis or complete paralysis; arthrogryposis (a congenital contracture syndrome affecting a number of large joints); dwarfism (physical growth departing from the age-related norm by more than three standard deviations); congenital hip dislocation; congenital disorders of bone and connective tissue such as osteogenesis imperfecta (brittle bones that fracture frequently) and the Ehlers Danlos syndrome (hyperextensibility of the joints, with an increased tendency to dislocation of the affected joints); developmental disorders of the limbs (dysmelia, or absence of arms or legs; phocomelia, or absence of the middle segment of a limb, anisomelia, or at least 7 cm of asymmetry between the limbs, 10 cm difference in swimming); locomotor problems (caused by tuberculosis, hemophilia, neoplasms, burns, fractures, or injuries of the musculoskeletal or nervous systems); multiple sclerosis; muscular dystrophies; polyneuritis; syringomyelia; polyarthritis; and Friedrich's ataxia (see the glossary for brief descriptions of these conditions).

Les autres classification does not make specific provision for those with severe mental disability, nor does it offer clearly defined handicaps for those individuals having cardiac, respiratory, abdominal, cutaneous, auditory, or visual problems without locomotor disability (Biering-Sorensen, 1983). Whereas CP-ISRA is content with three broad categories of event (track, field, and swimming), ISOD offers detailed functional descriptions for each of the 16 sports it currently recognizes. ISOD also tends to be more elitist than CP-ISRA, maintaining that a proportion of the disabled lack the capacity to participate in certain types of competition. For instance, it maintains that those needing artificial flotation devices should not be allowed to take part in swimming contests (Lindstrom, 1986).

Integrated Classifications

Integrated classification schemes represent attempts to allow athletes with one type of disability to compete on an equal basis against those with another type of disability. The scale of handicaps is relatively arbitrary for many sports, although adjustments can be devised quite readily for activities such as archery and shooting.

ISOD has strongly supported an integrated approach to disabled sports, arguing that the resultant increase in the scale of competition is helpful in attracting both media and audience attention. The 1984 games in New York City offered shooting events, table tennis, and weight-lifting competitions on an integrated basis (Lindstrom, 1986). However, an analysis by Williamson (cited by Sherrill, Adams-Mushett, & Jones, 1986) suggests that amputees tend to dominate most categories of integrated competitions (implying that present classification systems give them an unfair advantage).

Open Competition

The ISMGF and the NWAA have open competitions in which persons of any classification can enter. However, the incorporation of events for wheelchair competitors into open track meets for the able-bodied is a relatively recent development (M.W. Clark, 1980), and it has created some controversy among both able-bodied participants and officials.

Able-bodied runners have complained that the wheelchair contingent is seeking to exploit what was previously "their" competition in order to gain publicity. Runners have raised issues of safety, but the main basis of concern is undoubtedly that modern developments in wheelchair design now allow disabled individuals to complete events such as marathon races at faster speeds than the able-bodied (Brandmeyer & McBee, 1986; Goode, 1978; Lebow, 1983; Marshall, 1982). Those able-bodied runners who have been embarrassed by such successes have argued that wheelchair athletes should be competing against cyclists! In other forms of competition, the disabled person is likely to perform more poorly than the able-bodied individual, and the direct comparison of achievements inherent in an integrated competition may have a negative psychological impact upon some disabled competitors (A.N. Witt, 1973).

Winter Sports

Classification schemes for winter sports participants are still in their infancy. Categories are assigned mainly on the extent of modifications to skis and poles that are required by the individual competitor (Benedick, 1985).

Key Ideas

1. The objective of classification schemes for disabled athletes is to match competing individuals in terms of functional impairment.

2. Many methods of classification have been proposed, including anatomico-medical, functional (the ability to perform key tasks), and dynamic (based on habitual activity patterns). European groups tend to favor the anatomico-medical approach, whereas North Americans are more strongly influenced by residual function.

3. Classification systems depend not only upon the experience of the examiner but also the honesty of the athlete. It is, regrettably, possible to simulate disability while being classified.

4. Suitably weighted adaptations of current classification schemes allow entire teams to be matched for games such as wheelchair basketball.

5. Physical performance of the spinally injured differs strikingly between ISMGF Class I (tetraplegia) and Classes II to V (paraplegia). But intercategory differences in peak arm ergometer oxygen intake and muscle strength are small between ISMGF Classes II through V.

6. The classification of amputees can be adapted to allow fair participation in contests for the spinal cord injured.

7. Assessment of blindness depends very much on the athlete's cooperation, but competition between the visually impaired can be made equitable by the wearing of blindfolds.

8. In cerebral palsy, the handicap of paralysis is worsened by unpredictable spasticity or athetoid movements. Often, there is also the handicap of mental retardation, although such individuals compete in the Special Olympics rather than the CP-ISRA events.

9. A classification scheme is available for les autres, although it remains very difficult to match what are a diverse range of clinical conditions.

10. Integrated classifications allow athletes with various types of disability to compete against one another. Such a pattern of organization is helpful in reducing the number of contests and assuring a reasonable number of entrants in each category of competition.

Practical Applications

1. How well do handicaps operate in sports for the able-bodied? Can one achieve total fairness in competitions between the disabled?

2. If you were to certify examiners for wheelchair sports classification, what qualifications would you seek?

3. What are the relative merits of anatomical versus functional classifications of disability?

4. What differences in disability pattern are conferred by a congenital origin as opposed to a traumatic or infectious etiology?

5. Should wheelchair sports be confined to the spinally injured? What arguments have been used to exclude those with other types of disability from events for the wheelchair disabled?

6. Why have there been objections to wheelchair participation in marathon events for the able-bodied? Are the reasons that have been advanced valid?

Chapter 4

Fitness Assessment

Appropriate techniques for the quantitative assessment of fitness are important in gauging not only individual progress but also the success of entire training programs (Wessel, 1983). This chapter considers possible methods of testing the disabled. As in an able-bodied population (see chapter 1), a full examination of fitness for physical activity and sport would include at least an assessment of clinical status, leisure habits (Compton, Witt, & Ellis, 1983), anaerobic power and capacity, aerobic power, electrocardiographic response to exercise, muscle strength and endurance, body composition, and flexibility. Normative data for these various measurements are summarized briefly in Appendix B.

Unfortunately, much of the information to date simply concerns methods for the assessment of physical performance and aerobic power. We shall consider separately the specific problems that arise when testing the wheelchair confined and those with other types of disability. Those wishing technical details of individual procedures are referred to the short monograph by Werder and Kalakian (1985).

The Wheelchair Disabled

Even a measurement as simple as body mass requires special consideration if the person to be measured is confined to a wheelchair. Kofsky et al. (1986) described a portable device built from two standard bathroom scales; it allows the individual to be weighed while sitting in a wheelchair, and the weight of the wheelchair is then subtracted from the total recorded mass. Given that there is often considerable wasting of the limbs below the level of a spinal cord lesion, it is difficult to decide whether the subject is overweight or not relative to an actuarial table of "ideal" weights (see Table B.1 in Appendix B).

Skinfold readings provide a better guide to obesity. Measurements are taken as for a nondisabled person, but because of changes in limb dimensions and bone density, some question whether the formulas for the prediction of percentage body density and body fat that have been developed on able-bodied people (Durnin & Womersley, 1974; Shephard, 1978a) can be applied to the paraplegic or indeed to those with other categories of disability such as amputees and the cerebral palsied (see Appendix B). It is often preferable to interpret data in terms of the directly measured skinfold thicknesses.

Anaerobic Power and Capacity

In principle, there seems no reason why a test of the type described by Bar-Or and Inbar (1978) could not be carried out by lower-limb disabled subjects using an arm ergometer with a suitable adaptation of flywheel loading to assure an optimal force/velocity relationship. However, to my knowledge the anaerobic performance of the arms has not yet been evaluated except in average healthy adults (Ben Ari, Inbar, & Bar-Or, 1978), elite able-bodied athletes (Patton & Duggan, 1985), and a small sample of 6 spinally injured subjects (Coutts & Stogryn, 1987).

Lakomy, Campbell, and Williams (1987) recently drew attention to the lactate threshold (the percentage of the maximum oxygen intake developed at a blood lactate concentration of 4 mmol/L) as a further useful test of ability to operate a wheelchair over a 5-km distance; in their data for 10 paraplegic and 2 tetraplegic spinally injured athletes, the coefficient of correlation with 5-km times was 0.87, compared with only 0.61 for maximum oxygen intake.

Muscle Strength

Although clinical observations of muscle strength are used extensively when classifying the disabled for competition (see chapter 3), rather fewer measurements of muscle strength have been made using standard physiological techniques. Wakim, Elkins, Worden, and Polley (1949), Nilsson et al. (1975), and Gairdner (1983) all described the ability to lift free weights. Zwiren and Bar-Or (1975), Beal, Glaser, Petrofsky, Smith, and Fox (1981), Wicks et al. (1983), Kofsky, Davis, and Shephard (1983b), and Kofsky et al. (1986) described the use of the handgrip dynamometer. Gersten, Brown, Speck, and Grueter (1963), Zwiren and Bar-Or (1975), Davis et al. (1980), Wicks et al. (1983), Wiles and Karni (1983), and Kofsky et al. (1983a, 1983b, 1986) applied cable tensiometry to elbow and shoulder movements. More recently Grimby (1980), Davis et al. (1980), Gandee et al. (1981), Jackson et al. (1981), Wicks et al. (1983b), and Kofsky et al. (1983b, 1986) discussed application of the Cybex isokinetic dynamometer to determinations of isokinetic strength and endurance for the shoulder, elbow, and wrist muscles.

Static handgrip force has been considered a good predictor ($r = .80$) of more general measures of muscle function in able-bodied subjects (H.H. Clarke, 1966), although much of the observed correlation between hand and general body strength reflects a mutual dependence of the measured variables upon body mass. In the spinally injured population, researchers observed a correlation of .79 between dominant handgrip force and total upper body isokinetic strength (Davis, Jackson, & Shephard, 1984a; Jackson et al., 1981), although they also observed interindividual differences of predictive ability, depending upon the quantity of functional muscle mass and motivational factors. Moreover, the combined scores for dominant handgrip force (A), static shoulder extension force (B), and static elbow extension force (C) were moderately well correlated ($r = .82$) with total isokinetic strength for the upper limb (D) according to the following equation (Kofsky et al., 1983a): D (Nm) $= 1.71\ A$ (N) $+ 0.134\ B$ (N) $+ 0.397\ C$ (N) $+ 79.3$.

The average discrepancy between laboratory and field tests was 12.9%, and after allowing for "attenuation" of the correlation by errors in the isokinetic data, the researchers found the error of the field test to be about 9%. It thus seems possible to use isometric estimates of muscle function in field situations in which isokinetic equipment is not available.

Aerobic Power

As in the able-bodied individual, aerobic power is the main determinant of a disabled person's ability to undertake endurance events such as distance road races. Issues to examine in the context of assessment include (a) differences of test response induced by the use of upper- as opposed to lower-limb exercise, (b) the significance of absolute data versus figures expressed relative to body mass, (c) the relative merits of wheelchair and arm ergometer tests, and (d) details of specific test protocols.

Features of Upper Limb Exercise

Sawka (1986) recently compared the immediate impact of upper- and lower-limb exercise upon the cardiorespiratory function of healthy, able-bodied subjects. Although substantial differences of acute response become apparent if data for the two types of activity are compared at a given absolute oxygen consumption, many of these differences disappear if values are examined at the same fraction of the respective limb-specific peak oxygen intakes. Peak heart rates are generally lower for arm than for leg exercise (see Table 4.1). The ratio of arm to leg peak oxygen intake has ranged from 0.36 to 0.89 in various reports, with an average value of 0.73. However, in subjects who have undertaken specific training of the upper body muscles, the ratio can rise as high as 0.90; possibly, an increase of local muscular strength allows exercise to continue to a higher level of cardiorespiratory performance before activity is halted by an inadequate blood flow to the working muscles and resultant local fatigue (see chapter 1).

Although blood lactate levels seem comparable at a given relative intensity of arm or leg exercise (Pimental, Sawka, Billings, & Trad, 1984; Sawka, Miles, Petrofsky, Wilde, & Glaser, 1982b), the anaerobic threshold is somewhat lower for arm than for leg work (Davis, Vodak, Wilmore, Vodak, & Kurtz, 1976; Reybrouck, Heigenhauser, & Faulkner, 1975). Peak intramuscular concentrations of lactic acid at exhaustion are probably similar for arm and leg exercise, but because the active muscle mass is smaller, lower peak blood lactate concentrations may be anticipated for arm than for leg work.

During submaximal activity, the cardiac output may be either a little higher (Miles et al., 1984; Reybrouck et al., 1975) or a little lower (Åstrand et al., 1965; Bevegard et al., 1966) for arm than for leg work, but the arm value is plainly much the greater if it is expressed per unit mass of active muscle (Clausen, Klausen, Rasmussen, & Trap-Jensen, 1973). In consequence, both systolic and diastolic pressures are greater (Åstrand, Ekblöm, Messin, Saltin, & Stenberg, 1965; Bevegard, Freyschuss, & Strandell, 1966; Miles et al., 1984) and peak

Table 4.1   Comparison of Maximum Heart Rates for Arm and for Leg Exercise

Maximum heart rate (beats/min)		
Arms	Legs	Author
177	190	Åstrand & Saltin (1961)
173	195	Bar-Or & Zwiren (1975)
176	198	Bergh et al. (1976)
183	186	Bouchard et al. (1979)
184	193	Davis et al. (1976)
167	190	DeBoer et al. (1982)
174	185	Fardy et al. (1977)
172	184	Franklin et al. (1983)
174	195	Magel et al. (1978)
169	179	Sawka et al. (1982a)
169	179	Shephard et al. (1988)
178	179	Simmons & Shephard (1971b)
178	188	Stenberg et al. (1967)
169	177	Vander et al. (1984)
174.5	187.0	Unweighted average

Note. Based in part on data from "Exercise Testing, Training and Arm Ergometry" by B.A. Franklin, 1985, *Sports Medicine, 2,* pp. 100-119.

cardiac output is smaller for arm than for leg work. Other factors that contribute to the higher peripheral resistance during arm exercise include a greater relative secretion of catecholamines (Davies et al., 1974), isometric exercise associated with the need for torso stabilization (Clausen et al., 1973; Sawka et al., 1982a) and a greater tendency to hemoconcentration (Pimental et al., 1984).

The higher heart rates during submaximal arm work suggest a greater sympathetic drive (Davies et al., 1974). However, perhaps because of differences in cardiac filling, contractility indices are much as for leg work (Miles et al., 1984).

Pulmonary ventilation at any given power output is greater for arm than for leg work. Possible contributory factors include a low peak oxygen intake (and thus a high relative work rate during submaximal effort), a high blood lactate, a greater proportion of isometric activity, and a greater neurogenic drive from muscles of the upper limbs (Sawka, 1986). Perhaps because the surface area/mass ratio favors the dissipation of locally produced heat from the arms, both rectal temperature and sweating rate at a given relative intensity of effort are less for arm than for leg exercise (Sawka, Pimental, & Pandolf, 1984).

Gamerale (1972) suggested that the perception of exertion was greater for arm than for leg work. This is theoretically conceivable, partly because the body normally receives a greater sensory input from the upper limbs, and partly because most skilled tasks with a proprioceptive component are based on the use of the arms rather than the legs (Pandolf, Billings, Drolet, Pimental, & Sawka, 1984). Ratings of effort during arm work certainly have a large peripheral muscular component (Shephard, Vandewalle, Bouhlel, & Monod, 1988), but at any given fraction of the corresponding peak oxygen intake there does not seem any great difference in global ratings of exertion between arm and leg work.

Arm and leg exercises seem equally effective methods of eliciting symptoms and signs of myocardial ischemia, such as anginal pain and a deep horizontal or down-sloping depression of the ST segment of the electrocardiogram. However, angina apparently develops at a higher rate-pressure product when using the arms (Clausen & Trap-Jensen, 1976; Lazarus, Cullinane, & Thompson, 1981; see Table 4.2). By way of explanation, it is probable that the smaller venous return associated with arm work leads to a diminution of ventricular end-diastolic dimensions and (through the law of LaPlace) to a decrease of ventricular wall tension. This both facilitates myocardial perfusion and reduces the workload of the heart, postponing the onset of angina for a given atherosclerotic narrowing of the coronary vessels.

Absolute Data Versus Relative Values

The peak oxygen intake of the arm muscles, as measured in the laboratory, is augmented by postural activity in the trunk. The key variable is thus the usable power output of the arms rather than the maximum quantity of oxygen consumed by arms plus trunk (Bar-Or & Zwiren, 1975; Shephard et al., 1988). Because wheelchair activity is weight supported, some have argued that the aerobic performance of a wheelchair competitor should be presented in absolute units (watts)

Table 4.2   A Comparison of Ischemic Responses to Arm Ergometry Versus Cycle Ergometry, Based on Rate–Pressure Product for the Two Modes of Exercise

Rate–pressure product		
For angina	For ST depression	Authors
Greater with arm	—	Clausen & Trap-Jensen (1976)
—	Same for arm & leg	DeBusk et al. (1978)
Greater with arm	—	Lazarus et al. (1981)
Same for arm & leg	Same for arm & leg	Schwade et al. (1977)
Same for arm & leg	—	Wahren & Bygdeman (1971)

Note. Based in part on data from "Physiology of Upper Body Exercise" by M.N. Sawka, 1986, *Exercise and Sport Science Reviews,* **14**, pp. 175-211.

rather than in relative units (W/kg). When choosing between absolute and relative power output, much depends upon the type of situation examined. In a level wheelchair race, energy is expended against friction from the ground surface and wheel bearings (both of which forces are proportional to the total mass of the subject plus wheelchair), against air resistance, and against any head wind. However, if a hill is to be climbed, a major part of the work performed is attributable to the raising of the chair and body mass against the force of gravity. Thus, for the high-speed racer the absolute power output is the most relevant statistic, but for the average wheelchair subject who is climbing a hill to the corner store the relative power output may be of greater importance.

Nevertheless, practical difficulties remain in calculating the relative power of the disabled individual (Greenway, Houser, Lindan, & Weir, 1970). Particularly in those who are confined to a wheelchair, the lean mass of the body is reduced by a loss of muscle protein from the lower limbs (Cooper, Rynearson, MacCarty, & Power, 1950), a loss of bone mineral from both the upper and the lower limbs (Lussier, Knight, Bell, Lohman, & Morris, 1983), and disturbances of intra- and extracellular fluid volumes secondary to changes in serum protein concentrations (Arieff, Pysik, Tigay, & Bernsohn, 1960; Shizume et al., 1966). At the same time, an inactive lifestyle may lead to a substantial accumulation of body fat. Moreover, both the loss of muscle protein and the increase in body fat content vary from one individual to another, being related to the duration of disability. The end result of these various processes is that a differing relative aerobic power may be calculated for subjects who have upper limbs of comparable absolute power but differing lesion levels or differing periods of wheelchair confinement (Greenway et al., 1970; Greenway, Littell, Houser, Lindan, & Weir, 1965).

Wheelchair Ergometer Versus Arm Ergometer Tests

Data on aerobic power has been collected using various forms of wheelchair ergometer and arm ergometer (Davis et al., 1981; Franklin, 1985). For reasons we do not fully understand, the peak oxygen intake is similar for the two types of test (Glaser, Sawka, Laubach, & Surprayasad, 1979; Wicks et al., 1977), but the peak heart rate is 7% higher, the peak blood lactate concentration is 2 mmol/L higher, and the peak power output is 30 to 200% higher when using the arm ergometer (Glaser, Sawka, Brune, & Wilde, 1980a; Sawka, 1986; Wicks et al., 1983).

During submaximal exercise, cardiac output, stroke volume, blood pressure, respiratory minute volumes, and plasma lactate concentrations are also significantly lower for arm ergometry than for wheelchair operation (Glaser et al., 1979; Wicks et al., 1977-78). Factors favoring performance on the arm ergometer include inherent neural pathways that are adapted to asynchronous limb movements (Glaser et al., 1980; Marincek & Valencic, 1978), a lesser need for isometric activity in trunk stabilization (Marincek & Valencic, 1978; Steadward, 1980), better gearing ratios (Engel & Hildebrandt, 1974; Glaser, Young, & Surprayasad, 1977), transmission of torque by a handle rather than pressure on the wheel rim (Engel & Hildebrandt, 1974; Wicks et al., 1983), and an improved application of potential arm force to the process of locomotion (including the movements of both extension and flexion; Glaser, Foley, Laubach, Sawka, & Surprayasad, 1978a). The end result is a greater mechanical efficiency for the arm ergometer than for the wheelchair, a factor that must be noted when maximal power outputs are compared for the two types of device.

Free-Wheeling Wheelchair. The simplest and most realistic approach to wheelchair testing is to collect data while the subject is propelling a normal wheelchair over flat ground (Brattgard, Grimby, & Hook, 1970; D. Crews, Purkett, Wells, & McKeeman, 1982). Alternatively, the wheelchair can be mounted on a broad-belted, inclined treadmill fitted with safety supports (Engel & Hildebrandt, 1973; Gass & Camp, 1979; Gass, Camp, Davis, Eager, & Grout, 1981; Horvat, Golding, Beutel-Horvat, & McConnell, 1984; Voight & Bahn, 1969), or it can be run over low-friction rollers (Brouha & Korbath, 1967; Gandee, Winningham, Deitchman, & Narraway, 1980; Lundberg, 1980). The obvious advantage of such methods is that the findings have immediate relevance to the daily life of the wheelchair disabled and to many forms of wheelchair competition (Glaser & Collins, 1981; Horvat et al., 1984).

Wheelchair Ergometers. Several laboratories have now developed wheelchair ergometers. The subject drives such machines by pushing the hand against large-rimmed flywheels (see Figure 4.1) or in one case (Higgs, 1987) by turning small cranks where the push rim would normally be located. In some designs, the normal conditions of wheelchair operation are mimicked rather closely (Dreisinger & Londeree, 1982; Thacker, O'Reagan, Aylor, & Brubacker, 1980; Whiting, Dreisinger, & Hayden, 1984), whereas in others the flywheels of the chair are coupled to a standard type of cycle ergometer (Glaser et al., 1978a, 1978b; Sawka, Glaser, Wilde, & Von Luhrte, 1980; Wicks et al., 1983).

The net mechanical efficiency of operation (see chapter 1) is quite low for most types of wheelchair ergometer (Dreisinger & Londeree, 1982; Fisher & Gullickson, 1978; Knowlton, Fitzgerald, & Sedlock, 1981). Depending somewhat upon the design of the chair and the experience of the user (Glaser, Giner, & Laubach, 1977; Glaser et al., 1978), typical figures for young and able-bodied but experienced volunteers rise from 6.5 to 10.5% over the power output range of 5 to 25 watts.

Rather similar net efficiencies have been reported for disabled adults when they propel a standard wheelchair over hard indoor surfaces (7.7% net efficiency at a speed of 4 km/hr) (Hildebrandt, Voight, Bahn, Berendes, & Krager, 1970); even lower figures (3.3-4.5% net efficiency) have been observed when able-bodied subjects who are not accustomed to propelling a wheelchair have attempted a similar task (Glaser, Young, & Surprayasad, 1977; Glaser et al., 1979).

Arm Ergometry. The main advantage claimed for arm ergometry is that it provides a readily standardized and nonspecific measure of cardiorespiratory performance that can be performed by a paraplegic or an amputee (Bergh, Kanstrup, & Ekblöm, 1976; Hjeltnes, 1977; Mangum, Ribisl, & Miller, 1983; Strauss, Haynes, Ingram, & McFadden, 1977). The mechanical efficiency is higher (~ 18.5%) and more consistent than for a wheelchair ergometer (Brattgard et al., 1970). In longitudinal training experiments, the majority of subjects enter a study

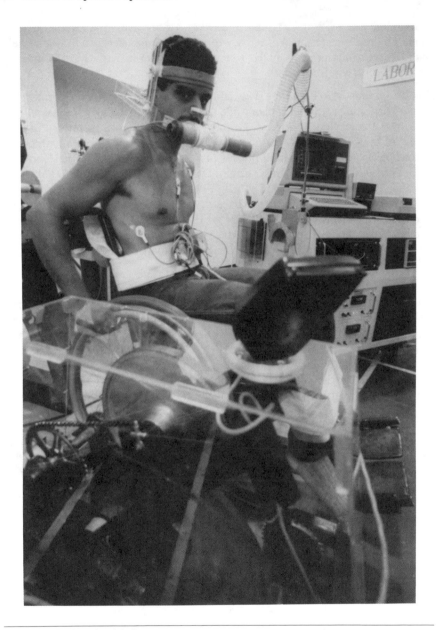

Figure 4.1. A wheelchair ergometer.

with no previous experience of this particular device. Researchers must thus make allowance for habituation (a lessening of anxiety) and test learning as the experiment proceeds. Moreover, if power output rather than oxygen consumption is measured, researchers must allow for a reduction in the efficiency of operation by those subjects with high level cord lesions (Kofsky, Davis, & Shephard, 1983b) or significant spasticity (see Table 4.3).

Many arm ergometers are simple adaptations of devices originally designed for leg operation. Some have a mechanical loading, and others are electrically braked. The former are typically "rate-dependent" devices like the Monark ergometer, with which the power output depends on both flywheel speed and loading. In contrast, a number of the electrically braked ergometers claim to be "rate-independent" machines; they adjust the external power output (although not necessarily the subject's rate of energy expenditure) to a predetermined value, irrespective of cranking rate. Most arm ergometers are operated by using the limbs alternately (see Figure 4.2), as in leg ergometry, although there are some designs (Bobbert, 1960; Cummins & Gladden, 1983; Secher, Ruberg-Larsen, Binkhorst, & Bonde-Petersen, 1974; Shaw et al. 1974) that require both arms to be thrust forward simultaneously. Marincek and Valincec (1978) found little difference of physiological cost between synchronous and asynchronous patterns of cranking, although they commented that most subjects preferred the latter due to the associated reduction of trunk movements in the sagittal plane.

The crank shaft of a forearm ergometer is usually positioned at shoulder level (Hellerstein & Franklin, 1984). I. Åstrand et al. (1968) found that the physiological strain imposed by a rhythmic task such as hammering was increased if the arms were lifted above the head. J.A. Davis et al. (1976) suggested that in

Table 4.3 The Relationship Between Forearm Power Output (Watts) and Oxygen Intake of Male Subjects, Classified by ISMGF Category

ISMGF classification	Slope (ml/min/W)[b]	Intercept (ml/min)	Intercept (Mets)[c]	Correlation coefficient	Mechanical efficiency
1	3.7	696	(2.9)	.12	[a]
2	13.5	544	(2.3)	.68	13.0
3	17.5	447	(1.9)	.89	14.7
4	20.0	299	(1.3)	.93	14.7
5	19.6	356	(1.5)	.89	15.0
6	16.7	468	(2.1)	.83	16.3

Note. Based in part on data from "Field-Testing—Assessment of Physical Fitness of Disabled Adults" by P.R. Kofsky, G.M. Davis, R.W. Jackson, G.C.R. Keene, and R.J. Shephard, 1983, *European Journal of Applied Physiology, 51*, pp. 109-120 and "Muscle Strength and Aerobic Power of the Lower-Limb Disabled" by P.R. Kofsky, G. Davis, and R.J. Shephard, 1983, *Annali del I.S.E.F., 2*, pp. 201-208.

[a]Value not calculated because of low correlation coefficient. [b]Calculated as delta efficiency (i.e., L/slope times thermal equivalent of oxygen). [c]Mets = ratio of observed oxygen consumption to assumed basal oxygen intake of 3.5 ml/kg • min STPD.

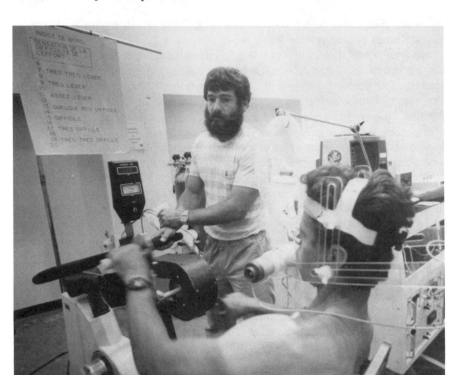

Figure 4.2. An arm-crank ergometer.

ergometry, the anaerobic threshold was reached sooner but the peak oxygen intake was unchanged if the arms were positioned above heart level. Pendergast, Cerretelli, and Rennie (1979) further found a decrease of peak oxygen intake when the subject's arms were raised, but this may merely have reflected the difficulty of exercising from the supine position that had been adopted in the experiments. A further variable is the extent of the torso restraint and thus involvement of the shoulder muscles in overhead work (Cerretelli, Pendergast, Paganelli, & Rennie, 1979; Cummins & Gladden, 1983; Davies & Sargeant, 1974). Some have argued that if activity is carefully restricted to the arms by an appropriate system of harnesses, then responses are affected surprisingly little by variations of arm position relative to the heart (Cummins & Gladden, 1983).

Specific Protocols.   The arm ergometer testing procedure has varied quite widely from one laboratory to another (Franklin, 1985; Sawka, 1986; see Tables 4.4 and 4.5). There have been advocates of both continuous and discontinuous protocols, the latter having recovery intervals ranging from 1 (deBusk et al., 1978; Washburn & Seals, 1983) to 20 minutes (Miles et al., 1984) between individual increments of loading. The continuous protocol offers a substantial saving of time for both patient and physician, whereas advantages that have been claimed for an intermittent test (Franklin, 1985) include an opportunity to counter local fatigue, a period when the subject is relatively stationary (facilitating blood pressure and ECG recording), and a lesser likelihood of carrying a test to a dangerous level of myocardial ischemia. In practice, rather similar physiological results are yielded by continuous and discontinuous techniques (Sawka, Foley, Pimental, Toner, & Pandolf, 1983a; Washburn & Seals, 1983).

Cranking rates have varied quite widely from 30/min (Glaser, Sawka, Brune, & Wilde, 1980a; Sawka et al., 1983b) and 40/min (Magel et al., 1975; Shaw et al., 1974) to 90/min (Powers, Beadle, & Mangum, 1984). Based partly on the manufacturer's recommendation (Odeen, 1972) and partly on subjective preference (Davis et al., 1980; Keene, Davis, Jackson, & Shephard, 1979), our laboratory has adopted a rate of 80/min, although figures of 50 to 60/min are perhaps more commonly adopted in other laboratories. One possible issue when choosing an optimal rate of cranking is the ease with which the frequency of limb movement entrains the breathing frequency (Cowell et al., 1986). Sawka, Foley, Pimental, Toner, and Pandolf (1982a, 1983a) noted that the higher crank rates yielded larger peak oxygen intakes. Possible factors causing this effect include not only a decrease of mechanical efficiency at higher crank speeds (Powers et al., 1984) but also a reduction of peak crank force, the latter change facilitating perfusion of active muscles in the limbs (Kay & Shephard, 1969; Petrofsky, Phillips, Sawka, Hanpeter, & Stafford, 1981; Sawka, Foley, Pimental, & Pandolf, 1983b). Because the active muscle mass is small during arm exercise, the work rates that are chosen must also be quite low; typical increments of loading for a progressive test are 17 to 25 watts per stage. The duration of individual stages has varied widely from 1 (Powers et al., 1984) to 6 minutes (Wahren & Bydgeman, 1971). J. Williams, Cottrell, Powers, and McKnight (1983) proposed a schedule of loading that is related to body mass; using their plan, power output is increased by one MET (ratio to resting metabolic rate) per minute for all subjects, irrespective of their body size.

Despite use of an appropriate test protocol, the arm effort of many subjects becomes limited by local muscle fatigue before a plateau oxygen consumption has been realized; Kofsky, Davis, Jackson, Keene, and Shephard (1983a) commented that only 15 of 49 paraplegics reached a classical oxygen plateau where oxygen intake increased by less than 2 ml/kg for a further 5% increase of power output.

DiRocco (1986) proposed using tethered swimming to test the cardiopulmonary fitness of nonambulatory individuals. In principle, the various types of swimming tests used in the able-bodied seem practicable, with the answer probably reflecting overall cardiovascular function rather than the power output that can be developed when sitting upright in a wheelchair.

Field Tests.   In principle, the usual design of arm ergometer is sufficiently small that it can be transported to the homes of severely disabled patients for purposes of field testing, but in practice problems can arise in stabilizing the ergometer relative to the subject's normal seat or wheelchair. According to Mangum et al. (1983), the maximal power output as measured on such a device can be combined with a figure for body mass to yield an estimate of peak oxygen intake having a standard error of 2.3 ml/kg • min and only a small tendency to systematic overprediction of the true peak oxygen transport. Coutts, Rhodes, and McKenzie (1983)

Table 4.4 Test Protocols for Continuous Effort Arm Ergometry

Crank rate (rpm)	Initial power output (watts)	Increment (watts)	Time at each load (min)	Crank height	Authors
50	73-122	24	2	Shoulder	Bar-Or & Zwiren (1975)
—	—	—	2	Shoulder[a]	Cerretelli et al. (1979)
80	0	8.5	1	Shoulder	G.M. Davis et al. (1981)
50	0	12	1	60-70° angle	J.A. Davis (1976)
60	0	25	2	Shoulder	DeBoer et al. (1982)
50	20	20	3	Shoulder	Huang et al. (1983)
60	15-40	15-40	3	Shoulder	Kavanagh et al. (1973)
—	5-33	11-33	6	—	Knuttson et al. (1973)
80	40% of age-predicted max	20% of age-predicted max	5	Shoulder	Kofsky et al. (1983a)
60	25	16	3	Shoulder	Lazarus et al. (1981)
70	Based on heart rate	17	3	Sternum	Pimental et al. (1984)

60-70	—	16	2	—	Pollock et al. (1974)
90	15	15	1	Shoulder	Powers et al. (1984)
30-70	75	25	3	Shoulder	Sawka et al. (1983b)
50	0	24	3	—	Schwade et al. (1983)
60-80	Based on heart rate	16	2	—[b]	Secher et al. (1974)
40	33	16	3	Shoulder	Shaw et al. (1974)
50-60	24	24	3	—	Vander et al. (1984)
60	—	40	3	—	Vrijens et al. (1975)
—	—	16-24	6	—	Wahren & Bygdeman (1971)
60	25-40	5-40	2	Shoulder	Washburn & Seals (1983)
50-60	0	16	—	—	Wicks et al. (1983)
50	Based on heart rate	24	2	Shoulder	Zwiren & Bar-Or (1975)

Note. Based in part on data from "Exercise Testing, Training and Arm Ergometry" by B.A. Franklin, 1985, *Sports Medicine*, **2**, pp. 100-119 and "Physiology of Upper Body Exercise" by M.N. Sawka, 1986, *Exercise and Sport Science Reviews*, **14**, pp. 175-211.

[a]With torso restraint; [b]Using synchronous arm movements.

Table 4.5 Test Protocols for Intermittent Effort Arm Ergometry

Crank rate (rpm)	Initial power output (W)	Increment (W)	Time at each load (min)	Recovery period (min)	Crank height	Authors
60	74-118	6	3	10	3 levels[ab]	Cummins & Gladden (1983)
80	Corr. to 115 beats/min	Corr. to 132, 153 beats/min	6-7	2		Davis et al. (1981)
—	24	24	3	1	Shoulder	DeBusk et al., (1978)
60	24	24	4	2	Tabletop	Fardy et al. (1977)
30	Corr. to 75% max heart rate	10	4	7	Shoulder	Glaser et al. (1980a)
40	39	20	4	10	—	Magel et al. (1978)
45	25	20	7	20	Mid-sternum	Miles et al. (1984)
60	0	15-30	5	4	Gleno-humeral joint	Reybrouck et al. (1975)
45	Corr. to 75% max heart rate	20	7	20	Mid-sternum	Sawka et al. (1982a)

50	Corr. to 70% max heart rate				
	25	3	15	Shoulder	Sawka et al. (1983b)
60	–	–	–	Shoulder	Seals & Mullin (1982)
50	16	3	1	Shoulder	Schwade et al. (1977)
60	–	5	5	Shoulder	Simmons & Shephard (1971b)
60	87	5	10	–	Stamford et al. (1978)
60	Based on heart rate 10-20%	3	5	Shoulder	Vokac et al. (1975)
60	25-40 5-40	2	1	Shoulder	Washburn & Seals (1983)
60	Based on body mass	2	0.25	–	J. Williams et al. (1983)

Note. Based in part on data from "Exercise Testing, Training and Arm Ergometry," by B.A. Franklin, 1985, *Sports Medicine*, **2**, pp. 100-119 and "Physiology of Upper Body Exercise," by M.N. Sawka, 1986, *Exercise and Sport Science Reviews*, **14**, pp. 175-211.

[a]With torso restraint; [b]Using synchronous arm movements.

also noted that peak oxygen intake could be predicted quite well ($r^2 = .86$) from the maximal power output (Ẇmax) during incremental ergometry to exhaustion (V̇O$_2$peak $= 0.108 + 0.267$ Ẇmax).

Other authors have found a relatively close correlation between power output and oxygen consumption during submaximal exercise ($r = .85-.88$; see Table 4.3; and also chapter 7), although in some instances the intercept on the ordinate (oxygen consumption at zero load) has been larger and the slope of the relationship (Δ efficiency) shallower (Franklin, Vander, Wrisley, & Rubenfire, 1983; Kofsky, Davis, Jackson, Keene, & Shephard, 1983; Kofsky, Davis, & Shephard, 1983b) than that found by Coutts et al. (1983).

Procedures for the prediction of maximum oxygen intake (Shephard, 1977, 1982b) from submaximal data were originally developed for leg exercise. During arm work, problems might be anticipated from a differing relationship of power output and oxygen consumption or from a lower peak heart rate (Davis & Shephard, 1988; Simmons & Shephard, 1971b). However, in practice, the prediction procedures seem to work surprisingly well—at least for amputees and paraplegics with lesions below the level of sympathetic outflow. Kavanagh and Shephard (1973) applied the standard Åstrand nomogram to data for eight amputees and found a close correspondence between the average directly measured peak oxygen intake (17 $\pm$ 4 ml/kg • min) and the corresponding nomogram prediction (18 $\pm$ 6 ml/kg • min). Kofsky, Davis, Jackson, Keene, and Shephard (1983a) also evaluated the Åstrand type of prediction in a larger sample of paraplegics; the researchers were able to use submaximal heart rate and the corresponding power output to predict oxygen intake with a standard deviation of 14.5% in women and 12.5% in men, a precision judged sufficient for an approximate field categorization of fitness. Glaser, Foley, Laubach, Sawka, and Surprayasad (1978a) are a third group of investigators who predicted fitness from the submaximal heart rate and power output of subjects performing arm ergometry.

Rhodes, McKenzie, Coutts, and Rogers (1981) suggested that the field testing of aerobic power could be based on a wheelchair analogue of the Cooper (1968a, b) 12-minute running test, the observer measuring the maximum distance travelled around a 400-m track in 12 minutes. Prediction equations (see Table 4.6) that accounted for a half to three-quarters of the variance in the data ($r^2 = .48$ to .77) were based on the distance covered by the subject, blood pressure, and physical characteristics (age, height, and body mass).

More recently, Gairdner (1983) proposed a 6-minute wheelchair endurance test. Although these techniques have some promise for field surveys, significant difficulties must be overcome when making any precise interpretation of the data. Problems include variance attributable to differences in wheelchair design and mass, experience of the subject in the technique of fast wheeling, knowledge of an appropriate pace to assure maintenance of maximal performance over a 12-minute period without premature exhaustion, and the impact of changes in ground and environmental conditions upon the speed of movement. Moreover, any field measure of the amount of physical work performed that is based upon the distance covered over a specified time necessarily assumes a constant mechanical efficiency from one individual to another.

Table 4.6 Relationship Between Wheelchair Distance Covered in 12 Minutes and Peak Oxygen Intake

Distance (km)	Peak oxygen intake (ml/kg • min)
<1.0	<12
1.0-1.4	13-17
1.4-1.7	18-28
1.7-2.0	29-35
>2.0	>36

Based in part on data from "A Field Test for the Prediction of Aerobic Capacity in Male Paraplegics and Quadraplegics" by E.C. Rhodes, D.C. McKenzie, K.D. Coutts, and A.R. Rogers, 1981, *Canadian Journal of Applied Sport Sciences,* **6**, pp. 182-186.

Coefficients of correlation: all subjects, $r = 0.80$ (excluding tetraplegics where $r = 0.54$). Multiple regression equations:

All subjects $= 0.98(D) + 0.011(BP_s) - 0.009(BP_D) + 0.007(M) - 1.051$ ($r = 0.85$)

Paraplegics $= 0.30(D) + 0.007(BP_s) = 0.022 (BP_D) + 0.011(A) + 0.013(H) + 0.360$
     ($r = 0.69$)

Where D is distance in km, BP_s and BP_D are the corresponding blood pressures, M is the body mass in kg, A is the age in years and H is the height in cm. Note that the multiple regression equations do not improve substantially on the simple distance prediction. The average 12-minute distance is 1.62 km (or 1.87 km, excluding the tetraplegics).

However, it seems likely that in practice the technique of wheelchair propulsion will be poor and the efficiency of movement will be less than average in subjects with high-level lesions or significant spasticity. It also seems likely that efficiency will be influenced by the speed of movement. Winnick and Short (1984) described adaptations of the usual high school performance tests such as arm hang, pull-ups, shuttle run, softball throw, and distance run suitable for field testing of the wheelchair confined; their paper reported results obtained on 141 spinally injured students aged 10 to 17 years.

Other Disabilities

A number of other disabilities can complicate the satisfactory completion of a standard, able-bodied exercise test protocol. Problems include difficulties in motivating the subjects, together with changes of mechanical efficiency caused by the disorder.

Blind subjects can be trained to run around a track, holding either a guide rail or the hand of a sighted guide (C. Buell, 1982, 1984), but if a specific performance such as a 600-yd run (Titlow & Ishee, 1980) is to be used as a field measure of aerobic power, considerable time must be allowed to ensure that the subject has gained sufficient confidence to run at maximum speed. Moreover, the guiding hand tends to alter running posture and thus the efficiency of movement (see chapter 7). Even greater problems are encountered in explaining the use of a device such as an ergometer (Lee, Ward, & Shephard, 1985) or a treadmill (Jankowski & Evans, 1981) to the sightless individual. Anxiety may cause considerable tachycardia and hyperventilation during an initial laboratory visit. This can be countered by prolonged learning and habituation to the test environment (Shephard, 1969a), but if account is not taken of these two processes, a misleading impression of the extent of the training may be gained from the decrease of exercise heart rate observed over a longitudinal experiment.

Whether measuring field performance or muscle force or encouraging a final minute of treadmill running, the development of all-out effort depends greatly upon the urging of the investigator. Unfortunately, this type of feedback is difficult to arrange for deaf subjects (Hattin et al., 1986), although some attempt can be made with written instructions and prearranged hand signals (Pender & Patterson, 1982; Winnick & Short, 1986). Because of associated vestibular problems, rapid movement may also lead to disorientation and loss of balance in deaf children (Winnick & Short, 1986).

Subjects with severe mental retardation may have difficulty in understanding not only the required test procedures but also the need for maximal effort. However, Bar-Or et al. (1971) reported that 15% of mentally retarded subjects failed to complete a maximum treadmill test, due mainly to refusals. Researchers need to take extra time and patience to familiarize the subject with the laboratory and its equipment while creating a feeling of participation in the laboratory's endeavors; more attention must also be paid to test safety, including the use of harnesses or well-trained treadmill "spotters" (Fernhall & Tymeson, 1988). If oxygen consumption is not measured, such problems as a limited ability to learn test cadence, poor adherence to the required rhythm, variations of mechanical efficiency over the test, and lack of motivation to perform maximally (Seidl, Reid, & Montgomery, 1987) may arise.

Neither Sengstock (1966) nor Londeree and Johnson (1974) observed any problems of motivation in a 600 yd walk-run. However, Nordgren (1971) found difficulty in carrying out even a submaximal cycle ergometer test on some 25% of his subjects; not only was the required rhythm not followed, but often a second work stage was incomplete, leading to difficulties in extrapolating the data. Similarly, Bundschuh and Cureton (1982) noted poor motivation in cycle ergometry, Reid, Montgomery, and Seidl (1985) reported that 18% of their subjects were unable to conform to the required stepping rhythm of the Canadian Home Fitness Test, and Tomporowski and Jameson (1985) observed problems of rhythm in both cycle ergometer and rowing ergometer tests. Because of these difficulties, scores may vary greatly from one test to another (Montgomery, Reid, & Seidl, in press). The best solution with a mentally retarded population may be to impose an exercise cadence by use of a treadmill (Seidl et al., 1987).

Finally, in field situations where estimations of power output replace direct measurements of oxygen consumption, due account must be taken of alterations in mechanical efficiency due to such factors as muscle imbalance, vestibular disturbances, spasticity, athetoid movements, arthrodeses, and other sources of unusual movement patterns. The wide variety of performance tests that have been proposed for disabled subjects (de Potter, 1987; Findlay, 1981; Roswall, Roswall, & Dunleavy, 1986; Short & Winnick, 1986; J.U. Stein, 1975; Tilley, Mosher, & Sinclair, 1987; Werder & Kalakian, 1985; Winnick & Short, 1985) indicates something of the practical problems that researchers encounter when using this approach to make field measurements on special populations (Fait, 1983). Details of individual test procedures are found in the references cited.

Although physical performance tests are superficially attractive to both the schoolteacher and the clinician who lacks laboratory facilities, in practice their results can be quite misleading. In addition to problems of terrain, environmental conditions, and test details, which plague the use of such procedures in able-bodied subjects, performance may be hampered by (a) lack of opportunity to practice the required skills, (b) poor motivation or comprehension of the test, and (c) a short stature relative to an able-bodied person of the same age (a major problem, as scores depend heavily on body dimensions; Cumming, 1971). Although performance tests may have some place as a simple means of goal setting, school placement, or providing feedback of training responses to the individual, we need more precise laboratory data for serious research.

Key Ideas

1. As with the able-bodied, fitness assessment of the disabled should examine anaerobic capacity and power, aerobic strength, electrocardiographic response to exercise, muscle strength and endurance, body composition, and flexibility.

2. Amputation, muscle wasting, or failures of limb development restrict lean mass and thus complicate the prediction of ideal body mass.

3. Anaerobic capacity and power in the lower-limb disabled can be tested by 30 seconds of all-out exertion on an arm ergometer.

4. Muscle strength must be assessed over a substantial range of joint movements, as the active disabled person shows a local development of the muscles used in ambulation. Isometric test scores seem fairly closely correlated with isokinetic data, offering the possibility of field testing of those individuals who find difficulty in visiting the laboratory.

5. The aerobic power of the lower-limb disabled can be tested by either an arm ergometer or a wheelchair ergometer; the operating characteristics of the former are more readily standardized, but performance on the latter type of machine has more relevance to sport and the activities of daily living. When interpreting results, researchers must take due account of physiological differences between arm and leg exercise.

6. During wheelchair exercise, the effort expended against ground friction and the ascent of any slope is proportional to body mass, but the load imposed by air resistance and a head wind is relatively independent of body mass. The relative importance of these factors influences the method of presenting fitness data—absolute units or values expressed relative to body mass.

7. Protocols for the testing of aerobic power vary widely from one laboratory to another, and such factors as the rate of limb movement, stage duration, and load increments need to be standardized.

8. Disabilities other than spinal cord injury can complicate commonly accepted exercise test protocols, due to difficulties of comprehension, motivation, and changes of mechanical efficiency caused by the disorder itself.

Practical Applications

1. What are the main physiological differences between arm and leg exercise? Does arm position modify performance on an arm ergometer?

2. What are the relative merits of an arm ergometer versus a wheelchair ergometer for assessing the aerobic fitness of the spinal cord injured? In what circumstances would you recommend one or the other approach?

3. Is there such a thing as an ideal weight for an amputee or a paraplegic? Should fitness be expressed in absolute units or relative to body mass?

4. How important are field procedures when seeking representative data on the physical condition of the disabled? What practical problems limit interpretation of the wheelchair distance covered in a specific time?

5. What practical problems might be anticipated when testing the fitness of those with disabilities other than paraplegia?

Chapter 5

Current Fitness Status

In this chapter, we shall examine available information on the current fitness status of the disabled, including physical characteristics, resting physiological data, muscular strength, cardiorespiratory responses to submaximum exercise, maximum performance, and daily habitual activity. The first section presents findings for the wheelchair disabled and the second part presents data for individuals with various other categories of disability.

Fitness of the Wheelchair Disabled

Some authors (Cowell et al., 1986, Greenway et al., 1970; Hjeltnes, 1977) have described quite extensive changes in body composition with spinal injury, including decreases in lean body mass, increases in the percentage of body fat, and increases in the proportion of extracellular fluid (see Table 5.1). For example, Winnick and Short (1984) reported skinfolds averaging 15.7 mm in young boys, 12.7 mm in young girls, 15.5 mm in older boys, and 20.5 mm in older girls with spinal neuromuscular problems. Others have found considerable interindividual variability but little average difference from a normal mesomorph (Bulbulian, Johnson, Bruber, & Darabos, 1987). Hjeltnes (1977) observed that the average body mass of eight paraplegics was only 80% of the value that would be predicted for able-bodied subjects of the same height. In the later stages of spinal injury, when the atrophied muscles are replaced to a variable extent by connective tissue, lipids, and water, an increase of overall body mass is sometimes observed (Claus-Walker & Halstead, 1981). A low HDL cholesterol also increases the risk of a heart attack by 90% relative to controls (LaPorte et al., 1983).

However, there is often some self-selection of test volunteers. Thus, the physical characteristics of those who volunteer for laboratory experiments may remain surprisingly similar to figures for the general population. Kofsky et al. (1986) reported data for 163 male and 97 female lower-limb disabled adults; although all were well enough to volunteer for exercise testing, an attempt was made to recruit broadly from various housing, sporting, and recreational facilities and associations for the disabled. Lesion levels ranged over ISMGF Classes II through V. In the males, the average height was 170.0 ± 13.5 cm, the body mass was 68.4 ± 13.8 kg, and the average thickness of four skinfolds was 11.5 ± 5.7 mm;

Table 5.1   Body Composition of Paraplegic and Quadriplegic Individuals

Variable	Paraplegic	Quadriplegic
Age (yr)	28	31
Height (cm)	180	175
Body mass (kg)	66.2	67.3
Lean body mass (kg)	52.4	45.4
Body fat (%)	20.8	17.7
Body water (L)	37.7	32.6

Note. Based on data from "Long Term Changes in Gross Body Composition of Paraplegic and Quadriplegic Patients" by R.M. Greenway, H.B. Houser, O. Lindan, and D.R. Weir, 1970, *Paraplegia,* **7**, pp. 310-318.

in the females the corresponding figures were 158.2 ± 12.6 cm, 57.8 ± 12.0 kg, and 14.5 ± 5.8 mm. These figures coincided fairly closely with Toronto norms for able-bodied subjects of similar age (Shephard, 1977).

On average, the Toronto sample of spinal cord disabled was apparently slightly shorter, lighter, and less obese than some previously reported paraplegic groups (Gass & Camp, 1979; Greenway et al., 1970; Zwiren & Bar-Or, 1975). One reason for this discrepancy is undoubtedly subject selection; many of the earlier authors tested fairly small samples, focusing on in-patients and people who were completely free of recreational pursuits. A second factor contributing to the particular characteristics of the Toronto sample was the inclusion of a proportion of subjects whose growth had been limited by congenital or childhood conditions such as spina bifida or infantile poliomyelitis (DiNatale, Pierrynowski, Tupling, & Forsyth, 1984).

Coutts (1986) found that among more active patients, both body mass (71.6 kg vs. 75.1 kg) and average skinfold thickness (7.6 mm vs. 11.3 mm) differed substantially between marathon participants and basketball players. Habitual physical activity patterns of the disabled plainly affect body composition, particularly the relative amounts of fat and muscle. Zwiren and Bar-Or (1975) also noted that wheelchair athletes were significantly thinner than their inactive counterparts. Likewise, Davis et al. (1986) found a 5.5-kg greater body mass but a 1.6-mm thinner average skinfold in provincial or national wheelchair athletes relative to a less active group of subjects with similar age and disability level.

Such data have two practical implications. First, if a wasting of the lower limbs occurs subsequent to spinal injury (as seems likely), then the normalcy of overall lean mass in the wheelchair athletes suggests that this loss of lean tissue has been matched by a hypertrophy of muscles in the upper half of the body. Such muscular development is particularly obvious in those individuals who have trained themselves to a national or a provincial level of competition. Second, the average wheelchair disabled person who volunteers for laboratory exercise testing is no fatter than a sedentary but otherwise able-bodied North American of similar age.

Nevertheless, even a small quantity of surplus fat adds to the load that must be propelled, and it is thus probable that some locomotor advantage would be gained if the average paraplegic aimed for the thinner skinfolds found in top level endurance competitors.

Resting Responses

Heigenhauser, Ruff, Miller, and Faulkner (1976) noted that both the resting oxygen consumption (2.8 ml/kg • min) and the resting cardiac output (46 ml/kg • min) of a group of paraplegic subjects was less than that of able-bodied controls. This presumably reflects the wasting of lean tissue in the paralyzed lower limbs, and if so, the extent of the deficit would reflect the balance between hypertrophy of the arm and shoulder muscles and atrophy in the legs. Davis, Shephard, and Leenen (1987) applied M-mode echocardiography to a group of paraplegic patients, finding similar ventricular dimensions and indices of contractility to those observed in able-bodied subjects (see Tables 5.2 and 5.3). The important practical lesson to be learned from these several studies seems that cardiac function can be restored by an appropriate conditioning regimen. Indeed, in contrast to the discouraging findings of Logan, Rubal, Raven, English, and Walters (1981), Francis and Nelson (1981) noted that the 1980 wheelchair marathon record holder showed significant ventricular hypertrophy.

The cardiac function of the individual with spinal injury is influenced by lesion level. In the able-bodied person, diastolic filling and thus the output of the heart depends heavily upon venous tone and thus the return of blood to the heart. Tilt-table tests (Corbett, Debarge, Frankel, & Mathias, 1975; Corbett, Frankel, & Harris, 1971; Guttmann, Munro, Robison, & Walsh, 1963; Wolf & Magora, 1976) show that in subjects with spinal cord lesions at a high enough level to cause a disturbance of sympathetic venomotor tone (at and above T5 for the upper limb, T10 for the lower limb), cardiac performance is initially handicapped by a relaxation of peripheral veins (with pooling of blood in the dependent parts of the body; Hjeltnes, 1977). Interruption of adrenal innervation (T5-T9) also causes a loss of catecholamine secretion (which normally increases ventricular contractility, augmenting stroke volume for a given diastolic filling of the ventricle; Mathias, Christensen, Corbett, Frankel, & Spalding, 1976a; Mathias, Frankel, Christensen, & Spalding, 1976b; Munro & Robinson, 1960).

As recovery from injury occurs (a spontaneous process covering several weeks in humans), the body becomes more responsive to available catecholamines (Frewin, Levitt, Myers, Co, & Downey, 1973; Mathias et al., 1976a, b), probably through an increase in the density of beta-adrenergic receptors, and an increased output of the hormone renin from the kidneys also helps to restore blood pressure (Johnson & Park, 1973). At this stage the system becomes hypersensitive, and stimuli such as exposure to cold can cause a massive reflex hypertension via the spinal cord (Mathias, Hillier, Frankel, & Spalding, 1975), with a secondary compensatory increase in output of the blood pressure–decreasing hormone prostaglandin E. In the cerebral palsied and in the spinally injured with lower-level lesions, sympathetic function remains intact, but there is still some tendency to venous pooling because of poor physical condition and lack of skeletal muscle tone.

Table 5.2   M-mode Echocardiographic Variables at Rest: Initial Values and Results After 8 and 16 Weeks of Endurance Training

Subject group	Disabled adults			Normal values	
	0 weeks	8 weeks	16 weeks	(i)	(ii)
L. Ventricular end-diastolic diameter (mm)					
C	48 ± 3	49 ± 3	47 ± 3	48 ± 4	37-56
E	46 ± 2	46 ± 2	46 ± 2		
L. Ventricular end-systolic diameter (mm)					
C	32 ± 2	33 ± 2	30 ± 2	33 ± 5	22-40
E	29 ± 1	29 ± 2	29 ± 2		
L. Ventricular mass (g)					
C	238 ± 38	240 ± 39	234 ± 39	189 ± 18	
E	242 ± 24	250 ± 24	249 ± 25		
L. Ventricular diastolic volume (ml)					
C	112 ± 19	120 ± 20	109 ± 20	107 ± 27	
E	100 ± 11	102 ± 11	107 ± 12		
L. Ventricular systolic volume (ml)					
C	34 ± 8	39 ± 8	29 ± 5	55 ± 16	
E	25 ± 4	26 ± 4	26 ± 4		
Stroke volume (ml)					
C	78 ± 12	81 ± 13	80 ± 15	52	60-69
E	76 ± 8	76 ± 7	80 ± 9		

Note. C = Control, E = experimental subjects. Based on data from "Cardiac Effects of Short-Term Arm Crank Training in Paraplegics: Echocardiographic Evidence" by G.M. Davis, R.J. Shephard, and F.H.H. Leenen, 1987, *European Journal of Applied Physiology,* **56,** pp. 90-96 for wheelchair-disabled subjects and "normal" adults of (i) Zeppilli et al. (1980) and (ii) Abbasi (1981).

In individuals with a partial or complete paralysis of the phrenic nerve (lesions affecting C3-C5 and above) or with severe disruption of the intercostal nerves, an impairment of normal respiratory mechanics creates additional problems (Fugl-Meyer & Grimby, 1971; Ohry, Molho, & Rozin, 1975; Silver, 1963; see Table 5.4). This not only has an adverse effect on dynamic lung volumes and alveolar gas exchange, but also disturbs the normal "thoracic pump," further hampering the normal processes of venous return.

Responses to Submaximal Exercise

Much of the available physiological data on the exercising paraplegic refer to maximal performance. However, wheelchair operation and most of the activities of daily living demand fairly heavy submaximal rather than maximal exercise (Glaser, Simsen-Harold, Petrofsky, Kahn, & Surprayasad, 1983; Sawka et al., 1981).

Table 5.3   M-mode Echocardiographic Indices of Left Ventricular Performance at Rest and During Isometric Exertion

Variable	Disabled subjects		
	0 weeks	8 weeks	16 weeks
Resting values			
Fractional shortening (%, normal values 29-39)			
C	35 ± 1	32 ± 2	36 ± 1
E	38 ± 1	38 ± 2	37 ± 2
Ejection Fraction (%, normal values 55-70)			
C	73 ± 1	69 ± 2	73 ± 1
E	74 ± 1	76 ± 2	75 ± 1
Velocity of circumferential fiber shortening (circ • s^{-1}, normal values 0.89-1.60)			
C	1.10 ± 0.04	1.01 ± 0.05	1.13 ± 0.08
E	1.28 ± 0.09	1.36 ± 0.15	1.29 ± 0.04
Isometric exercise (3 min at 30% of maximum force of handgrip)			
Functional shortening (%)			
C	31 ± 2	32 ± 2	36 ± 2
E	35 ± 2	36 ± 2	35 ± 2
Ejection fraction (%)			
C	68 ± 2	69 ± 2	73 ± 1
E	72 ± 2	73 ± 2	72 ± 3
Velocity of circumferential fiber shortening (circ • s^{-1})			
C	1.13 ± 0.17	1.08 ± 0.06	1.17 ± 0.16
E	1.30 ± 0.10	1.31 ± 0.15	1.22 ± 0.11

Note. C = Control, E = experimental subjects. Based on data from "Cardiac Effects of Short-Term Arm Crank Training in Paraplegics: Echocardiographic Evidence" by G.M. Davis, R.J. Shephard, and F.H.H. Leenen, 1987, *European Journal of Applied Physiology,* **56**, pp. 90-96 for wheelchair-disabled subjects and "normal" adults of (i) Zeppilli et al. (1980) and (ii) Abbasi (1981).

Performance of submaximal tasks is influenced by such factors as the mechanical efficiency of arm work (Glaser, Laubach, Sawka, & Surprayasad, 1978b) and knowledge of wheelchair technique (Steadward, 1980; Tupling, Davis, & Shephard, 1983; Tupling et al., 1986) together with circulatory and cellular responses to any conditioning that has already been undertaken. Concepts of mechanical efficiency are discussed further in chapter 7.

Power Output/Heart Rate Relationship

Emes (1978) compared the wheelchair responses of paraplegic basketball players with those of able-bodied basketball enthusiasts. No greater efficiency of submaximal effort was seen among the habitual wheelchair users. Respective power

Table 5.4 Influence of Lesion Level on Pulmonary Function

Variable		Lesion level and percent function			
		Cervical	T1-T6	T7-T12	Lumbar
FVC	(a)	31.7	43.4	47.8	69.9
	(b)	40.8	54.8	66.7	92.2
$FEV^{1.0}$	(a)	37.4	56.7	44.7	58.3
	(b)	51.2	72.7	73.7	82.8

Note. All data are expressed as percentage of normal values for able-bodied adults of similar age, height, and sex. Based on data from "Alterations of Pulmonary Function in Spinal Cord Injured Patients" by A. Ohry, M. Molho, and R. Rozin, 1975, *Paraplegia, 13,* pp. 101-108. (a) = before and (b) = after 6 months of physiotherapy.

outputs at a heart rate of 170 beats/minute were 91.4 watts (1.45 W/kg) and 103.7 watts (1.34 W/kg), suggesting that the physical condition of the two groups was similar.

Likewise, Marincek and Valencic (1978) found very similar heart rates (93, 112, and 137 beats/min) and oxygen intakes (0.80, 1.11, and 1.37 L/min) with surprisingly high net mechanical efficiencies (16.1-20.7%) when nonathletic individuals with spinal injuries were compared with sedentary but otherwise able-bodied subjects at forearm power outputs of 25, 50, and 75 watts. A second experiment from the same laboratory compared wheelchair basketball players with healthy university students (Marincek, 1980); again, responses to submaximal arm cranking were similar in the two groups.

On the other hand, Tahamont, Knowlton, Sawka, and Miles (1986) observed a higher mechanical efficiency in wheelchair-confined women than in their able-bodied peers. They suggested this was because the able-bodied women made strong isometric contractions of their leg muscles in an attempt to stabilize themselves in the wheelchair, whereas the spinally injured group could only use the weaker arm muscles for this purpose.

Heart Rate

Whiting, Dreisinger, and Abbott (1983a) commented that whereas amputees and paraplegic subjects showed a normal cardiac acceleration as power output was increased, tetraplegic and hemiparetic subjects demonstrated a loss of "chronotropic reserve" (i.e., the latter two groups had only a limited tendency for heart rate to increase at higher work rates). The residual mechanisms available for an increase of heart rate in those with high level lesions (e.g., an increase of venous return from the working muscles or the secretion of catecholamines) are themselves impaired and in any event have a relatively long time constant (Knutsson, Lewenhaupt-Olsson, & Thorsen, 1973; Nilsson et al., 1975).

During light activity, compensation for the lack of heart rate increase remains possible through an increase of stroke volume, but if submaximal exercise is sustained, the stroke volume diminishes. At this stage, the tetraplegic patient becomes vulnerable to circulatory strain, with a danger of disturbances of cardiac rhythm (particularly premature ventricular contractions) and other electrocardiographic warnings of myocardial oxygen lack, including T-wave inversion, ST depression, and in some cases cardiac arrest (Blocker et al., 1983; Frison, Sanchez Massa, Garmacho, & Gimeno, 1979; Van Alste et al., 1985a, b). Subjects should not pursue exercise in the face of increasing chest pain, an increasing frequency of "extra beats," or a falling blood pressure. Adverse ECG signs include a horizontal or downsloping depression of the ST segment of 2 mm or more and polyfocal premature ventricular complexes of varying waveform occurring before the end of the T wave.

Cardiac Output and Stroke Volume

G.M. Davis et al. (1987) noted that all of their spinally injured subjects (ISMFG Classes II-VI) were capable of increasing their cardiac outputs as the power output was increased, the mechanism being an essentially normal increase of heart rate and little change of stroke volume (see Figure 5.1). However, at any given heart rate the stroke volume was 38 to 44% greater for athletes than for inactive subjects; moreover, the athletes developed a larger oxygen consumption (40-49%) and a greater power output (56-96%; Davis & Shephard, 1988) than the inactive individuals relative to the heart rate. Indeed, the athletic subjects still developed a 16 to 22% larger stroke volume than their inactive peers if a covariance analysis was used to adjust for their larger oxygen intakes at any given fraction of peak power output.

Likewise, the active group enjoyed a 13 to 23% advantage of their estimated maximum cardiac output (estimated by extrapolation to peak heart rate, 14.4 L/min, vs. 10.2 L/min for inactive subjects). The apparent benefit of training shown by cross-sectional comparisons within the spinally injured group may be compared with the 8% gain of maximum cardiac output that was seen when able-bodied subjects undertook 4 weeks of forearm ergometer training (Simmons & Shephard, 1971a).

Possible explanations of any larger training response in the wheelchair disabled include a cross-sectional design with some selection of athletes, several years of training in the serious competitors, and the potential of the spinally injured to correct an initially "hypokinetic" circulation through (a) increases of venous tone and thus a reduction of pooling in the lower half of the body, (b) an increased use of lower body movements, serving as a "muscle pump" that increases venous return from the lower half of the body, (c) a reduction of cardiac afterload, due to an increase in cross section of active muscles in the upper limbs, and (d) a correction of vasodilation in the inactive lower limbs (Burkett et al., 1988). Longitudinal experiments argue most strongly in favor of the third of these explanations.

Heigenhauser et al. (1976) and Hjeltnes (1977, 1980) observed hypokinetic cardiac responses to forearm cranking among their samples of paraplegics, although somewhat larger (and thus more "normal") cardiac outputs have been

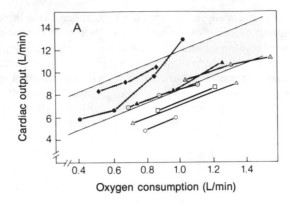

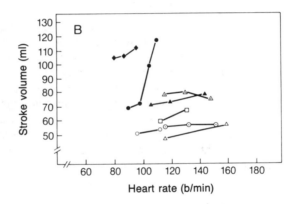

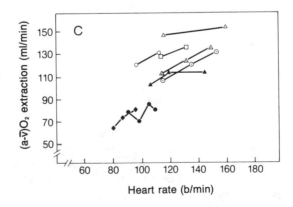

Figure 5.1. The relationship between (A) oxygen intake and cardiac output, (B) heart rate and stroke volume, and (C) heart rate and arteriovenous oxygen difference during steady-state exertion for disabled subjects from several studies. Based on unpublished data of G.M. Davis (1985).

described by others using wheelchair ergometry (Glaser et al., 1978b; Sawka et al., 1980; Wicks et al., 1977; Wilde et al., 1981); possibly, fewer inactive subjects were tested in the wheelchair ergometer experiments. Heigenhauser et al. (1976) commented that the cardiac output response to graded forearm cranking was on average 68% smaller in traumatic paraplegics than in their able-bodied counterparts. Likewise, Hjeltnes (1977) observed that in general both the stroke volume and the cardiac output response to submaximal work were lower in spinally injured than in healthy subjects; the author attributed the hypokinetic response to a pooling of blood in the lower limbs. In support of the pooling hypothesis, Hjeltnes (1980) demonstrated that exercise performance was improved if venous return was facilitated by the use of an abdominal corset and elastic leg bandages. Van Loan, McCluer, Loftin, and Boileau (1987) found both a small stroke volume (peak 52ml) and a low maximum heart rate (109 beats/min) in quadriplegic subjects; they attributed their findings to a combination of impaired cardiac sympathetic stimulation and a small active muscle mass.

As the oxygen cost of submaximal exercise is unchanged in the face of a hypokinetic cardiac output, the disabled patients studied by Hjeltnes (1980) must necessarily have developed larger arteriovenous oxygen concentration differences than their able-bodied peers at any given power output. Bruin and Binkhorst (1984) also found a smaller stroke volume in disabled subjects, although in their sample there was a compensatory tachycardia, so that the cardiac output at a given rate of forearm cranking was the same as in an able-bodied group of swimmers.

In contrast to these reports, Sawka et al. (1980) found that the stroke volume, cardiac output, and arteriovenous oxygen difference of a paraplegic group were in the normal able-bodied range for a comparable intensity of forearm ergometry. However, the heart rate, cardiac output, and systolic blood pressure response were greater during wheelchair propulsion than when developing a comparable power output on the forearm ergometer. Because of the apparent economy of cardiac effort, the researchers suggested that a forearm crank might be a more appropriate method of driving a wheelchair than hand thrusting on the usual push rim; this issue is discussed further in chapter 6. Wilde et al. (1981) found similar cardiovascular responses in the wheelchair disabled and in able-bodied individuals while performing light work; in their experiments, the stroke volumes of spinally injured paraplegics were as large as 107 to 114 ml at an oxygen intake of 10.5 L/min.

Most studies of the disabled have tested male subjects. Tahamont and Knowlton (1981) confirmed that relative to able-bodied peers, disabled women also developed a hypokinetic response, showing a smaller stroke volume and cardiac output at a given oxygen intake or power output. However, probably because of local muscular development in the upper limbs, the disabled group developed a lower blood lactate than the able-bodied during steady-state work.

One important variable that may explain some of the discordant results (particularly a normal vs. a hypokinetic circulation) is the duration of exercise. The stroke volume of the spinally injured person seems time dependent, perhaps because of a difficulty in sustaining central blood volume during prolonged exercise. Thus Fitzgerald, Sedlock, Knowlton, and Schneider (1982) found that although the initial cardiovascular response of spinally injured subjects to wheelchair ergometry was as in the able-bodied, after 20 minutes of exercise at 50 to 55% of maximum oxygen intake, stroke volume and cardiac output both decreased relative to controls, with a matching increase of arteriovenous oxygen difference.

Arteriovenous Oxygen Difference

The overall arteriovenous oxygen difference at any given intensity of exercise reflects (a) total cardiac output, (b) the distribution of total blood flow between active and inactive tissues, and (c) the activity of aerobic enzymes within the working tissues. Wakim et al. (1949) compared the peripheral vascular responses of able-bodied and paraplegic subjects to a 10-minute isotonic exercise that consisted of rhythmic flexion and extension of the shoulder and elbow muscles against an external resistance. In this situation, the paraplegic group seemed able to sustain a somewhat greater local perfusion of the active tissues than did the able-bodied group. Respective increases of hand and forearm flow for able-bodied and paraplegic individuals were 128 and 152%. In contrast, increases of blood flow to the legs and feet were 33 and 11% for the two subject groups. The differences of blood flow distribution observed in the spinally injured group probably reflect a hypertrophy of the arm and shoulder muscles (with easier perfusion of the working tissues) and an atrophy of muscles in the lower half of the body consequent upon life in a wheelchair.

Some authors (Bruin & Binkhorst, 1984; Sawka et al., 1980; Wilde et al., 1981) support the idea that the upper limbs of the spinally injured subjects are well perfused, finding arteriovenous oxygen differences of 67 to 90 ml/L during rhythmic submaximal exercise. Tahamont et al. (1986) commented further that in wheelchair-confined women, the blood lactate at 80% of peak oxygen intake was substantially lower than in able-bodied women, suggesting that the paraplegic group had a better local blood flow to the upper limbs.

In contrast, Hjeltnes (1977) found high arteriovenous oxygen extractions (140-200 ml/L) and above anticipated lactate levels (3.5-4.5 mmol/L) when paraplegic subjects performed submaximal exercise at an oxygen cost of 0.8-1.0 L/min. A second study from the Norwegian laboratory (Hjeltnes, 1980) confirmed high arteriovenous oxygen extractions and blood lactate levels in relation to the vigor of exercise. The findings of Hjeltnes (1977) do not necessarily contradict data from other laboratories, as it could be argued that training of his sample would have given the upper limb muscles a potential to extract more oxygen from the arterial blood, while permitting an improved perfusion of the working tissues during intense isometric efforts.

Fitzgerald et al. (1982) related a part of any increase of arteriovenous oxygen extraction among the disabled to a substantial hemoconcentration during prolonged exercise. After 90 minutes of submaximal effort, plasma volumes decreased 6.8 and 4.5% for spinally injured and able-bodied women, respectively. Gass et al. (1981) also noted a 6% decrease of plasma volume in active male wheelchair users over 60 minutes of exercise at 52% of their peak oxygen intake. Presumably, when the arterial blood pressure is increased by exercise, the tendency to fluid loss is greater in paralyzed than in able-bodied limbs.

Muscular Strength

A substantial development of strength in certain of the upper limb muscles might be anticipated in the lower-limb disabled, as force must be applied repeatedly either to wheelchair push rims (Tupling et al., 1983) or to crutches. However, much depends on motivation, and the severely disabled may be so inactive that muscle strength is actually lost from the arms and trunk (Nilsson et al., 1975).

Muscle development is important to sustained aerobic performance, as muscle perfusion depends on the fraction of peak isometric force exerted (Kay & Shephard, 1969), the peak power output during arm exercise is limited largely by local muscular sensations (Kofsky et al., 1983a; Shephard et al., 1988), and peak oxygen intake is fairly closely correlated with local muscular strength. Peak arm forces are even more important to brief all-out effort, for instance when a wheelchair must mount a curb or a ramp. However, the muscle function of the disabled has received surprisingly little attention to date.

One notable exception is the careful laboratory evaluation of isometric strength that the Danish Infantile Paralysis Association has carried out on victims of polio- myelitis (Asmussen, 1968; Asmussen & Molbech, 1954; Asmussen & Poulsen, 1966; Asmussen, Poulsen, & Bøgh, 1964). A prime concern of this group of investigators was to define the minimum levels of strength needed for daily tasks such as operating a normal or a modified automobile.

Isometric and Isokinetic Strength

Research from our laboratory has shown surprisingly little correlation between the level of cord injury and muscle performance over the ISMGF Disability Classes II through V (Kofsky et al., 1983a). Nevertheless, paraplegics as a group show an upper body isometric strength that is above the average for sedentary, able-bodied individuals. Moreover, this can be correlated with their level of habitual activity (Cameron, Ward, & Wicks, 1978; Grimby, 1980). Likewise, isokinetic measures of peak moment are highly correlated with the extent of an individual's participation in sport and fitness programs (G.M. Davis, Kofsky, Shephard, & Jackson, 1981; G.M. Davis, Shephard, & Ward, 1984b; G.M. Davis et al., 1986; see Figure 5.2).

Handgrip Force

A number of reports discuss the handgrip force of the wheelchair disabled. Winnick and Short (1984) noted a poor grip strength in 141 paraplegic children and adoles-cents. Nakamura (1973) compared the handgrip force of 280 lower-limb disabled subjects with able-bodied peers who were working at similar industrial tasks (see Table 5.5). The average grip force of those disabled by trauma, which was 382 newtons (the Standard International unit of force)[1], was greater than that of either

---

[1]Those unfamiliar with the Standard International Units of measurement should consult *Units, Symbols and Abbreviations: A Guide for Biological and Medical Editors and Authors* by G. Ellis (Ed.), 1971. London: Royal Society of Medicine.

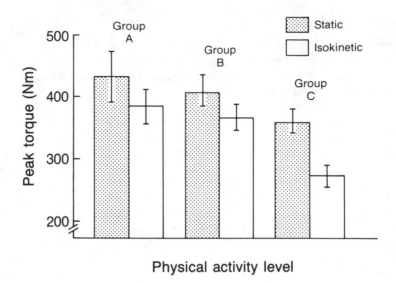

Figure 5.2. Relationship of static and isokinetic strength to habitual activity. Data for 42 lower-limb disabled men. Group A = national caliber athletes (n = 9); Group B = recreational sportsmen (n = 15); and Group C = inactive (n = 18). Based on data from Davis, Jackson, & Shephard (1984).

Table 5.5   Isometric Muscle Force and Industrial Absenteeism

Type of disability	Right handgrip force (N)	Right arm flexion force (N)	Absenteeism (1971, %)
Spinal injury	382	283	4.2
Cerebral palsy	231	68	7.3
Poliomyelitis	314	191	2.0
Progressive muscular dystrophy	151	4	5.2
Spinal tuberculosis	343	162	8.6
Control	354	237	—

Note. Disabled athletes had 4.0% absenteeism and wages of $132/month. Other disabled had 5.7% absenteeism and wages of $108/month. Based on data from "Working Ability of the Paraplegics" by Y. Nakamura, 1973, *Paraplegia*, **11**, pp. 182-193.

able-bodied (354 N) or poliomyelitic subjects (314 N). However, scores were substantially smaller for those with cerebral palsy (321 N) or progressive muscular dystrophy (151 N).

Zwiren and Bar-Or (1975) reported scores that were averaged over dominant and nondominant hands. The grip force was 569 newtons for able-bodied athletes,

504 newtons for elite disabled, 535 newtons for inactive disabled, and 475 newtons for sedentary normals, suggesting only a minor effect of either normal or competitive wheelchair operation upon grasping force. Likewise, Gass and Camp (1979) found only a slightly above-average score of 588 N for elite wheelchair athletes. Beal et al. (1981) noted that synchronous wheelchair ergometry demanded a lesser grip force than forearm cranking, and they argued that ordinary daily wheelchair propulsion made insufficient physical demands to increase grip strength above "normal" values. Biomechanical studies (Tupling, Davis, Pierrynowski, & Shephard, 1986) confirmed that some wheelchair athletes propel their chairs using a "strike" rather than a "grasp" of the driving rim (see chapter 7), and at least in those individuals using a strike, no increase of grip strength would be anticipated from normal ambulation.

Lesion level in itself apparently has little influence on handgrip force, at least over the middle range of disabilities (ISMGF Classes II-V). In support of the observations of Kofsky et al. (1983a), Wicks et al. (1983) found little difference of handgrip (517-548 N for men, 344-359 N for women) over ISMGF Classes II to V. However, as Kofsky et al. (1983) also noted, values were 62 to 74% smaller for tetraplegics than for paraplegics.

Kofsky, Davis, Shephard, Keene, and Jackson (1982) found little relationship between grip strength and peak oxygen intake. Nevertheless, a substantial association can be shown between habitual physical activity and grip strength (Davis et al., 1980; Jackson et al., 1981; Kofsky et al., 1983a, 1983b, 1986). Indeed, Coutts (1986) observed a 20% difference of grip strength between distance performers such as wheelchair marathoners and sprint athletes such as basketball players. Moreover, the grip force of the dominant hand seems a good predictor of combined upper body strength (Davis et al., 1980, 1981; Kofsky et al., 1983a).

Cable Tensiometry.   Despite the limited influence of daily wheelchair activity upon maximum handgrip force, wheelchair ambulation seems to affect arm strength. Stoboy and Wilson-Rich (1971) reported that the elbow strength of older disabled adults (42-63 years) was actually greater than that of younger able-bodied individuals (23-45 years). One expression of the associated muscle hypertrophy is an altered relationship between the integrated EMG signal and muscle force. Thus, Stoboy and Wilson-Rich (1971) observed that when developing an elbow flexion force of 200 newtons, wheelchair users who covered a daily distance of 7.2 km demonstrated a 40% lower electrical activity in their biceps muscles, and a lower heart rate (82 vs. 105 beats/min), but a similar oxygen cost to that observed in able-bodied subjects.

Likewise, Nakamura (1973) observed that relative to the able-bodied, the spinal cord injured had an advantage of elbow flexion strength (maximum force 283 vs. 237 N) and endurance (tolerance of sustained isometric contraction 225 vs. 132 s). On the other hand, workers who had been disabled by poliomyelitis or spinal tuberculosis developed lesser elbow flexion forces than the able-bodied (191 vs. 162 N), with a lesser endurance (127 vs. 109 s), whereas very poor performances were demonstrated by those subjects affected by cerebral palsy or muscular dystrophy (scores 68 and 4 N; 94 and 0 s, respectively). Nakamura (1973) commented that poor upper body strength was adversely related to industrial performance (see Table 5.5); wheelchair athletes had less absenteeism (5%

compared with 5-8%) and fewer work-related symptoms than their inactive peers. Although this suggests a practical benefit from training, the possibility nevertheless remains that a better clinical status allowed both regular productive attendance at work and participation in competitive sports.

Kofsky et al. (1982, 1983a) reported that the sum of several isometric force measurements (elbow flexion, elbow extension, and shoulder extension) was quite closely correlated with isokinetic total upper body strength ($r = .82$; see chapter 4); they thus suggested that the isometric measurements could be used to assess dynamic strength under field conditions. However, the correlation between isometric data and peak oxygen intake ($r = .65$) was lower, implying that arm strength was not a major factor limiting aerobic performance. The total static strength of inactive subjects (275 N) was significantly lower than that of either participants in recreational sports (368 N) or elite disabled athletes (385 N). On the other hand, total muscle strength was unaffected by lesion level over ISMGF Disability Classes II through V. As in the able-bodied population, men were 40% stronger than women.

Cameron et al. (1978) also found minimal differences of strength with disability grade among participants in the Toronto olympiad of 1976. In contrast, strength varied considerably with type of contest. For instance, competitors in weight-lifting and throwing events had a 50% advantage over the average participant with respect to both elbow flexion and extension strength; this characteristic was associated with a greater muscle mass in the arms. Wheelchair track competitors demonstrated a high triceps force despite their relatively low overall body mass, but participants in skill events such as wheelchair archery and table tennis showed low values for all measurements of isometric strength.

Isokinetic Data.   Isokinetic data in general confirm some increase of arm muscle strength among the active wheelchair population. Grimby (1980) reported that paraplegic basketball players and amputee swimmers developed a 49% greater isokinetic elbow flexion force and a 63% greater elbow extension force than their able-bodied peers. The 5 subjects who were biopsied showed a selective hypertrophy of slow twitch fibers, perhaps because of their interest in swimming. (We may note that the very rapid movements of wheelchair basketball might be expected to cause a selective hypertrophy of fast twitch fibers; Tesch & Karlsson, 1983, certainly described such a selective development of Type II fibers in their sample of wheelchair basketball players.) In keeping with the finding of slow twitch fiber hypertrophy, Grimby's (1980) group of subjects showed a greater training-induced gain of torque at slow than at rapid speeds of isokinetic elbow rotation. During arm abduction, the peak torque was 20 to 30% greater in paraplegics than in moderately trained able-bodied men.

G.M. Davis et al. (1981) argued that if sports participation were responsible for differences of isokinetic strength, it should be possible to classify patterns of habitual activity using a discriminant function based upon the strength data. They demonstrated that the habitual activity of 90% of disabled men and women could be classified correctly on the basis of seven measures of isokinetic strength and endurance. Moreover, the maximum impulse the subject could apply to the wheelchair was related to the peak moment recorded by the isokinetic dynamometer (Tupling et al., 1983; Tupling et al., 1986; see chapter 7).

G.M. Davis et al. (1986) went on to compare isokinetic strength and endurance between wheelchair athletes and less active paraplegics (see Figure 5.3). Two points of technique should first be noted. Because the subjects had some problems of balance, measurements were made with the subjects lying supine on a padded table. Yet most of the data for the able-bodied has been obtained with the subjects in an upright or a semirecumbent position (Kanehisa & Miyashita, 1983a, b). Second, no gravity corrections were applied to the isokinetic force reading, as the technique of doing this for the upper limbs has yet to be finalized. Winter, Wells, and Orr (1981) suggested that gravitational and inertial factors could cause errors of 26 to 510% in the recording of early force peaks for the movements of knee flexion and extension. G.M. Davis et al. (1986) commented that it was necessary to adjust their data for a small difference of stature between active and inactive individuals. The inactive group tended to be smaller, possibly reflecting both the selection of tall subjects for basketball and the inclusion in the inactive sample of a higher proportion of individuals with atraumatic, growth-impairing lesions such as spina bifida (DiNatale, Pierrynowski, Tupling, and Forsyth, 1984).

When a four-category classification of sports participation was made, no difference of isokinetic strength was seen between highly athletic and recreational sports participants nor between totally inactive subjects and those with limited mobility (G.M. Davis et al., 1980; Jackson et al., 1981; Kofsky et al., 1983a). However, researchers found a clear difference of strength between the first two and the last two categories. Individuals in the two more active categories demonstrated advantages of peak moment (14-29%), peak power (peak moment × angular velocity, 17-41%), average power (15-39%), and total work performed (10-57%) at all angular velocities from 60 to 300 degrees/s, the advantage being relatively greater at the higher angular velocities. This last observation suggests fast twitch hypertrophy, and it may be linked to the selective hypertrophy of fast twitch fibers in the medial deltoid muscles of Olympic-caliber wheelchair basketball players, which was described by Tesch and Karlsson (1983).

Perhaps because of mechanical limitations inherent in the Cybex dynamometer (Sapega, Nicholas, Sokolow, & Sarantini, 1982; Winter et al., 1981), discrimination between active and inactive individuals was clearest when using data for average power rather than peak power, peak moment, or total work. Typical equations for the prediction of average power were:

Shoulder flexion (W) = 0.33 (V) + 5.82 (A) + 0.13 (AV) + 0.001 (H^2) − 1.00 (r^2 = 0.77)

Elbow extension (W) = 0.29 (V) + 2.00 (A) + 0.09 (AV) + 0.001 (H^2) − 15.52 (r^2 = 0.82)

where V is the angular velocity (degrees/s), A is the activity group (1 = athletic, 0 = inactive), and H is the standing height (cm).

Differences between active and inactive subjects were larger for shoulder abduction (37-50%) than for shoulder flexion, elbow flexion, elbow extension, or

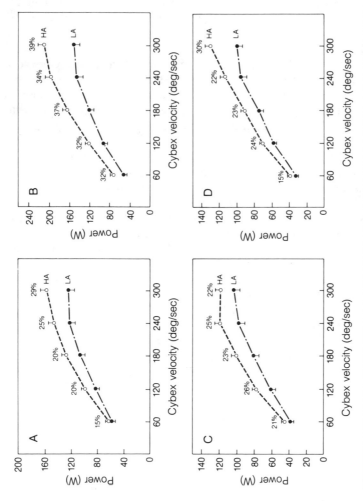

Figure 5.3. The relationship between angular velocity of isokinetic device (Cybex II) and (A) shoulder flexion average power, (B) shoulder extension average power, (C) elbow flexion average power, and (D) elbow extension average power, for highly active (HA) and less active (LA) disabled males. Values are adjusted means ± *SE* from analysis of covariance. Percentages indicate significant differences between groups ($p < .05$). Based on data of G.M. Davis et al., 1986.

shoulder adduction (22-29%; G.M. Davis et al., 1986), but activity-related differences also tended to be somewhat greater for shoulder extension (advantage 22-34%) than for shoulder flexion (24-29%). These findings suggest that a specific development of shoulder abductors and extensors was induced by training for wheelchair competition. Grimby (1980) also commented on the importance of the anterior and medial heads of the deltoid to wheelchair competition, noting that the shoulder abduction torque as measured by an isokinetic dynamometer was 20 to 100% higher in male paraplegics than in moderately trained normal subjects.

One puzzling finding from the study of G.M. Davis et al. (1986) was that with the exception of the abductor/adductor comparison, differences of strength between the athletes and the less active group were similar for movements generally regarded as wheelchair specific (shoulder flexion and elbow extension) and for nonspecific movements. This may be because movement patterns in long-distance track events are not the same as in normal wheelchair ambulation (Coutts, 1986). Moreover, a substantial proportion of the athletes selected were swimmers or basketball players rather than track competitors; in swimming and in team sports, general muscular development may offer some competitive advantage. Coutts (1986) compared a small sample of three wheelchair marathoners and three wheelchair basketball players, finding that the former had an advantage of 40% for elbow flexion but only 20% for shoulder extension strength. The researchers commented that the type of training undertaken by the marathon group was relatively specific; they were using chairs with a narrow push rim (see chapter 7) and included uphill wheeling as an important part of their training program.

Few differences of isokinetic strength can be traced to a differing etiology of limb paralysis or (over the middle-range of lesion levels) to a differing severity of disability. Wicks et al. (1983) noted that tetraplegics with upper-limb atrophy developed low scores for both elbow flexion and extension, but little variation in scores existed (flexion 60-65 Nm in males, 32 Nm in females; extension 42-57 Nm in males, 27 Nm in females) over ISMGF Classes II through V. Likewise, Kofsky, Davis, Jackson et al. (1983a), Kofsky, Davis, and Shephard (1983b), and Davis et al. (1986) found that lesion level has little impact on isokinetic strength over the ISMGF disability Classes II through V.

Muscular Endurance

In distance sports, the tolerance of repeated contractions (muscular endurance) may be more important than the force that can be developed during a single vigorous effort. Winnick and Short (1984) noted poor scores for flexed arm hang and pull-ups in 141 paraplegic children and adolescents. Davis et al. (1986) examined the influence of habitual activity on the isokinetic endurance of wheelchair-confined subjects. When endurance was expressed as the final force relative to the strength of the initial contraction, the researchers saw no relationship between the drop-off score during 50 maximal contractions and habitual activity patterns. Both highly active and less active individuals showed a 45 to 56% decrease over their initial score with repeated use of the various muscle groups (see Table 5.6).

Table 5.6   Endurance "Drop-Off" Scores for Wheelchair-Disabled Males With Highly Active and Less Active Lifestyle Patterns

Muscle activity (W)	Percentage drop-off*	
	Highly active group (n = 15)	Less active group (n = 15)
Shoulder extension		
Peak power	57.4 ± 4.2	64.5 ± 4.3
Average power	50.7 ± 3.9	56.1 ± 4.1
Shoulder flexion		
Peak power	56.2 ± 3.1	56.9 ± 3.2
Average power	48.4 ± 3.4	45.4 ± 3.5
Elbow extension		
Peak power	60.5 ± 4.6	60.8 ± 4.8
Average power	56.3 ± 4.9	59.4 ± 5.0
Elbow flexion		
Peak power	51.1 ± 3.5	51.0 ± 3.6
Average power	47.7 ± 3.6	49.8 ± 3.7

*Values are mean percentage decrease in power ± SE over 50 repeated contractions at 3.14 rad • s^{-1}. Based on data of G.M. Davis (1985), see note to Table 5.8, and G.M. Davis, S. Tupling, & R.J. Shephard (1986). Dynamic strength and physical activity in wheelchair users, pp. 139-145. In: Sherrill, C. (Ed.), Sport and disabled athletes. Champaign, IL: Human Kinetics.

Muscle Fiber Characteristics.   Grimby (1980) found a positive relationship between shoulder abduction torque and deltoid fiber diameter in the wheelchair population. Many wheelchair-disabled subjects develop extremely large diameter fibers in their arm muscles (Tesch & Karlsson, 1983). In Tesch and Karlsson's (1983) sample, the medial head of the triceps showed significant hypertrophy of both Type I and Type II fibers; the paraplegics also displayed a higher proportion of slow twitch (Type I) fibers (69%) than able-bodied controls (41%). In support of the researchers' view that hypertrophy is localized to aerobic (Type I) fibers, deltoid muscle biopsies actually showed lower levels of the glycolytic marker phosphofructokinase than those found in able-bodied controls. Although the shortage of glycolytic enzymes probably reflects largely a "dilution" of anaerobic activity by the overall hypertrophy, it does also mean that after training there would be a lesser tendency to anaerobic breakdown of glycogen per unit of muscle mass.

Taylor et al. (1979) and Taylor (1981) observed that the triceps muscle of wheelchair athletes demonstrated significant hypertrophy of both Type I and Type II fibers relative to able-bodied Olympic athletes (see Table 5.7). However, as subsequently supported by the data of Grimby (1980) and Corcoran et al. (1980), enzyme profiles showed that per unit mass of muscle, concentrations of marker enzymes for both the oxidative (SDH) and glycolytic (PFK) pathways were low or at best average values.

The observations of Tesch and Karlsson (1983) concerning the fiber composition in the medial head of the deltoid muscle of wheelchair basketball players have been noted previously. The proportion of fast twitch (Type II) fibers (47%) found in these researchers' experiments was similar to that of physically active young soldiers, but it was higher than that observed in Olympic kayak paddlers (30%). The size of both Type I and Type II fibers (average 7100 μm^2) was larger than in either of the active able-bodied groups (4900-5500 μm^2). In contrast to the work of Grimby (1980) and Taylor et al. (1979), the researchers found a tendency to selective hypertrophy of Type II fibers, as in able-bodied subjects who undergo heavy resistance training (Edstrom & Ekblöm, 1972; Gollnick, Armstrong, Saubert, Piehl, & Saltin, 1972) or who undertake activities requiring both strength and speed (Thorstensson, Larsson, Tesch, & Karlsson, 1977). The observed pattern of hypertrophy presumably represents a response to the stimuli of daily walking on crutches, weight training, or participation in sports that require rapid, forceful movements (e.g., wheelchair basketball and throwing events).

Skrinar, Evans, Ornstein, and Brown (1982) found relatively low initial glycogen levels in muscle biopsies taken from wheelchair athletes. Samples from the anterior head of the deltoid showed an average concentration of only 92.5 mmol/kg versus the anticipated figure of 120 to 140 mmol/kg in able-bodied adults. The authors attributed this finding to a reliance upon anaerobic effort during normal wheelchair ambulation; the disabled thus had little opportunity to replenish glycogen stores. Because the aerobic power of the disabled was generally small, the rate of utilization of carbohydrate during prolonged exercise was slower than in the able-bodied. Nevertheless, high plasma-free fatty acid and glycerol levels confirmed that during prolonged bouts of physical activity, the switch to fat as a metabolic fuel occurred earlier than would be anticipated in able-bodied individuals.

Table 5.7   Muscle Fiber Characteristics of the Wheelchair Confined Before and After Training

Muscle fiber	Nonathletes		Athletes
	Before training	After training	
Slow twitch			
Percent	48.0	56.6	49.2
Fiber area (μm^2)	6,361	8,180	10,883
Fast twitch			
Percent	52.0	43.4	50.8
Fiber area (μm^2)	9,803	10,150	16,148

Note. Based on data from "Physical Activity for the Disabled" by A.W. Taylor, 1981, *Report of the Research Priority Development Conference*, pp. 15-21. Ottawa: Fitness & Amateur Sport.

Maximal Performance and Cardiorespiratory Fitness

Wheelchair-confined individuals differ widely in their cardiorespiratory fitness. Whereas some individuals are seriously incapacitated, with a very limited aerobic power, others can match or even surpass the attainments of sedentary able-bodied adults (see Tables 5.8 and 5.9).

In able-bodied subjects, the peak oxygen intake during arm work is generally about 70% of that for leg work (Franklin, 1985; Simmons & Shephard, 1971a) (see Table 5.10). The peak heart rate is also somewhat lower than in the able-bodied (Hjeltnes & Vokac, 1979; Sawka et al., 1981), in part because of the use of arm exercise (80-99% of normal leg maxima). Zwiren, Huberman, and Bar-Or (1973) and Zwiren and Bar-Or (1975) compared maximum responses to arm cranking in 20 spinally injured and 21 able-bodied young men. The peak oxygen intake of the wheelchair athletes was 8% less than that of able-bodied athletes drawn from national sports teams that were analogous to those of the wheelchair competitors. However, the wheelchair athletes achieved scores 44% greater than those for an inactive wheelchair group. There were no intergroup differences of maximum heart rate, but the active wheelchair group also held an advantage over their inactive peers in terms of average maximal respiratory minute volume and peak oxygen pulse and had a lower heart rate when performing any given submaximal task.

Our data for elite wheelchair competitors (Kofsky et al., 1983a) showed a higher peak oxygen intake than in some previous investigations of wheelchair athletes (Gass & Camp, 1979; Hullemann et al., 1975). Likewise, the less active group had a better performance than earlier samples of completely untrained, spinally injured subjects (Hjeltnes, 1977; Pollock et al., 1974). Possibly we were more successful in motivating our subjects to all-out effort, or perhaps the International Year of the Disabled triggered a secular trend to improvement of physical condition in all categories of wheelchair-confined subjects. Certainly, the margins of peak oxygen intake, peak power output, and aerobic endurance between the elite and the average wheelchair user observed by Kofsky et al. (1983a) (44%, 57%, and 34%, respectively) were much as in the original study of Bar-Or and Zwiren (1975).

The peak blood lactate concentration of the spinally injured subject (7.8-11.7 mmol/L; Burkett et al., 1988; Glaser et al., 1980a; Marincek & Valencic, 1978) is generally quite high relative to able-bodied data for maximal arm work. In addition to good motivation on the part of some wheelchair athletes, this may reflect an increase of arm muscle volume, secondary to the substantial isometric effort that is required when stabilizing the trunk and gripping the rim of the wheelchair or the handle of an arm ergometer (Davis et al., 1984b; Nelson et al., 1974; Sawka et al., 1980; Wicks et al., 1977). Beal et al. (1981) commented that the static handgrip force is significantly related to both the intensity of forearm ergometer cranking and the speed of wheelchair propulsion.

As in able-bodied individuals, the advantage of the disabled athlete over an inactive person with spinal injury depends largely upon the type of competitor that has been recruited. Measuring peak oxygen intake by means of a wheelchair ergometer, Cameron et al. (1978) found the highest values among those competing in track (37.4 ml/kg • min) and swimming events (34.6 ml/kg • min) with much lower scores for those involved in contests of strength and skill (25.6 and 24.4 ml/kg • min, respectively). Likewise, Coutts (1986) indicated an average aerobic power of 43.9 ml/kg • min for three wheelchair marathoners but a score of only 31.6 ml/kg • min for three wheelchair basketball players. Gandee et al. (1980) noted a forearm crank figure as high as 64 ml/kg • min for a unilateral amputee who was a world-class marathon racer, R.S. Francis and Nelson (1981) quoted a value of 51.8 ml/kg • min for the 1980 record holder (115 min to complete the marathon), and Gass and Camp (1979) reported peak oxygen intakes of 42 to 49 ml/kg • min in top Australian track participants. The one atypical data set is from Lundberg (1980); he observed an average peak oxygen intake of 47 ml/kg • min in Swedish wheelchair basketball players, but this surprisingly high figure may not be representative of their sport, as team members had adopted the unusual tactic of using a wheelchair ergometer as a means of aerobic conditioning.

Studies from the University of Toronto confirm that the gradient of peak oxygen intake extends over the full range of habitual activity from the top wheelchair athlete to the very inactive patient (see Figure 5.4). Jackson et al. (1981) demonstrated that both peak power output and peak oxygen intake were higher in disabled subjects who were classed as athletic (undertaking sports or fitness training at least 4 times per week) or active (exercising 2 to 3 times per week) than in inactive or severely limited individuals. Kofsky et al. (1983a) suggested that paraplegic subjects of athletic or active habits (the latter undertaking regular exercise at least once per week) had rather similar levels of peak oxygen intake (2.52 and 2.42 L/min, respectively). However, in a second study using a much larger sample, Kofsky et al. (1986) found it more appropriate to categorize subjects into elite athletes and recreationally active or inactive categories (see chapter 6); peak oxygen intakes for these two activity categories ranged from 32 to 46 and 22 to 33 ml/kg • min, respectively. G.M. Davis and Shephard (1988) further found significant differences of maximum power output (57%), endurance time to exhaustion (34%), peak oxygen intake (44%), and peak respiratory minute volume (53%) between disabled subjects who were classed as active or inactive.

The only direct measurements of aerobic performance in women seem to be the wheelchair ergometer data of Tahamont et al. (1986). Six young but inactive wheelchair-dependent women had a peak oxygen intake averaging no more than 14.9 ml/kg • min, perhaps because they were able to realize a maximum heart rate of only 150 beats • min.

Davis and Shephard (1988) attempted to estimate the peak cardiac output of their sample from the observed maximal heart rate and the stroke volume as measured during submaximal exercise, assuming there would be no more than a minor decrease of stroke volume from submaximum to peak power output. In support of this type of calculation, Åstrand and Rodahl (1977) observed only a 4% decrease of stroke volume on moving from submaximal to maximal leg ergometer exercise (both tests being carried out from a sitting position). Our values, as calculated by such an extrapolation, substantiate the conclusions drawn from more direct observations of cardiac output during submaximal work. In particular, the estimated maximal cardiac output differs substantially between active and inactive individuals.

Table 5.8   Cross-Sectional Studies of Physically Disabled Subjects: Maximal Cardiorespiratory Responses During Forearm Cranking

Study (year)	Group	Disability	(n)	HRmax (b/min)	POmax (W)	$\dot{V}O_2$max (L/min)	$\dot{V}O_2$max (ml/kg · min)	$\dot{V}_E$max (L/min)
Kavanagh & Shephard (1973)								
42-59 yr	NA	Amp				1.29		
64-69 yr	NA	Amp				0.82		
71-79 yr	NA	Amp				0.78		
Hullemann et al.[a] (1975)								
	A	II	(4)	151	74	0.96		
	A	III	(13)	154	104	1.27		
	A	IV	(10)	157	95	1.41		
	A	V	(6)	147	113	1.28		
	A	VI	(4)	158	127	1.54		
Zwiren & Bar-Or (1975)								
	A	T_7-L_2	(13)	183		2.07	35.0	78.5
	NA	T_7-L_2	(9)	174		1.38	19.6	56.5
Hjeltnes (1977)	NA	T_2-T_{12}	(9)	179	100-120	1.47		
Wicks et al. (1977, 1983)								
	A	Ia	(8)	143	33.7	0.93	13.7	50.9
	A	II	(11)	174	98.0	1.62	23.0	70.6
	A	III	(10)	179	112.7	1.97	28.0	96.0
	A	IV	(17)	177	115.8	2.01	31.0	92.4
	A	V	(10)	184	120.9	2.26	37.7	97.4
Marincek & Valincec (1978)	NA	T_3-T_{12}	(3)	180	100	1.78		
Wicks et al. (1978)	NA	C_7-L_1	(2)	183		1.63		98.5
Gandee et al. (1980)	World class	Amp	(1)	176		3.21	64.0	150.9
Glaser et al. (1980a)	NA	Mixed	(6)	169[a]	79.4[a]	1.33[a]		58.8[a]
Grimby (1980)	A	Para	(4)	167		1.50	20.8	
	A	Amp	(3)	188		2.03	28.5	

Study	Activity	Lesion	n					
Hjeltnes (1980)	NA	C_5-C_8	(8)		42[a]		14.5	
	NA	T_7-L_1	(14)		123[a]		28.2	
Jackson et al.[a] (1981)	A	Mixed	(6)	191	98.0		38.8	
	Active	Mixed	(20)	172	93.3		36.5	
	NA	Mixed	(18)	171	72.3		26.5	
	Poor	Mixed	(5)	161	48.7		23.4	
	Mixed	I	(8)	127	40.1		15.9	
	Mixed	II	(7)	189	89.3		30.6	
	Mixed	III	(9)	185	81.1		32.9	
	Mixed	IV	(11)	183	85.3		33.3	
	Mixed	V	(7)	175	92.7		36.2	
	Mixed	VI	(7)	180	102.0		40.4	
Taylor (1981)	A	III-IV	(5)	160	106.7	2.14	26.3	
	NA	Mixed	(5)	170	83.3	1.58	27.4	
Nag et al. (1982)	NA	Polio	(9)	186		0.78	16.5	52.0
Kofsky et al. (1983a)	A	Mixed	(8)		100.1	2.52		
	Active > 1/wk	Mixed	(16)		95.2	2.42		
	NA	Mixed	(18)		71.1	1.63		
Gass & Camp (1984)	Active	II-V	(10)	181		1.96	30.1	66.4
Goswami et al. (1984)	NA	Polio	(7)	180		1.15	29.2	
Ward & Fraser[a] (1984)	Untrained	C_5-T_1	(31)	123	21.5	11.1	17.5	
	Trained	C_5-T_1	(11)	129	42.0			
Burke et al. (1985)	A	T_8-T_{10}	(4)	182	129.1	2.20	29.5	67.9

Note. Values are for male subjects unless otherwise noted. C_7-S_2 represents site of spinal cord lesion. Ia-VI represents ISMGF classification. A = athletic. NA = inactive. Based largely upon reports accumulated by G.M. Davis (1985). *Cardiovascular fitness and muscle strength in lower limb disabled males.* Unpublished doctoral dissertation, University of Toronto.

[a]Subjects were 24 males and 18 females.

Table 5.9 Cross-Sectional Studies of Physically Disabled Subjects: Maximal Cardiorespiratory Responses During Wheelchair Ergometry

Study (year)	Group	Disability	(n)	HRmax (b/min)	POmax (W)	$\dot{V}O_2$max (L/min)	$\dot{V}O_2$max (ml/kg · min)	$\dot{V}_E$max (L/min)
Cameron et al. (1978)	WC. track	Mixed	(13)				37.4	
	Swimming	Mixed	(11)				34.6	
	Skill	Mixed	(10)				24.4	
	Strength	Mixed	(8)				25.6	
Wicks et al. (1978)	NA	C_7-L_1	(2)	184		1.76		110.5
Gass & Camp (1979)	A	C_7-S_2	(16)	179		2.04	33.6	60.7
Glaser et al. (1980a)	NA	Mixed	(6)	156	61.7	1.24		48.5
Sawka et al.[a] (1980)								
20-30 yr	NA	Mixed	(6)	160-200	70-100	1.92	27	
50-60 yr	NA	Mixed	(6)	110-130	15-22	0.73	10	
80-90 yr	NA	Mixed	(6)	90-110	5-18	0.55	7	

Study								
Francis & Nelson (1981)	A	Amp	(1)			3.13	51.8	
Gass et al. (1981)	A	T_4-L_1	(7)	174		1.97	29.5	61.9
Rhodes et al. (1981)	Mixed	para	(20)	143		2.10	30.0	40.5
Crews et al. (1982)	A	III-IV	(4)	173		2.17	31.0	91.7
Wicks et al. (1977, 1983)	A	Ia	(8)	146	8.2	1.00	14.7	39.1
	A	II	(11)	172	33.8	1.55	22.0	75.9
	A	III	(10)	178	41.2	1.95	27.8	93.6
	A	IV	(17)	177	42.2	2.02	31.2	84.6
	A	V	(10)	178	40.2	2.16	36.1	103.3
Gass & Camp (1984)	Active	II-V	(10)	179		2.04	33.6	60.7

Note. Based on data from *Cardiovascular fitness and muscle strength in lower-limb disabled males* by G.M. Davis, doctoral dissertation, University of Toronto. Values are for male subjects unless otherwise noted. C_7-S_2 represents site of spinal cord lesion. Ia-VI represents ISMGF classification. A = athletic. NA = inactive.

[a]Subjects were 24 males and 18 females.

Table 5.10   Percentage of the Leg Maximum Oxygen Intake Attained During Arm Exercise

Percent	Author
Normal men	
70	Åstrand & Saltin (1961)
66	Stenberg et al. (1967)
72	Simmons & Shephard (1971b)
78	Vokac, Bell, Bautz-Holter, & Rodahl (1975)
81	Vrijens et al. (1975)
73	Bergh et al. (1976)
64	J.A. Davis et al. (1976)
70	Fardy, Webb, & Hellerstein (1977)
80	Franklin et al. (1983)
Normal women	
79	Vander, Franklin, Wrisley, & Rubenfire (1984)
Male paddlers	
89	Vrijens, Hoestra, Bouckuert, & Uytvanck (1975)
95	Cermak, Kuta, & Pařízková (1975)
77	Dransart (1977)
87	Tesch, Piehl, Wilson, & Karlsson (1984)
89	Vaccaro, Clark, Morris, & Gray (1984)
Female paddlers	
100	Cermak et al. (1975)

Influence of Age, Type, and Severity of Lesion

It seems likely that the age of the subject and the type, duration, and severity of the lesion will influence cardiorespiratory fitness. However, in practice it is difficult to disentangle such factors from the influence of differences in habitual activity and limitations of performance imposed by some primary disease process.

Age. Sawka et al. (1981) attempted to infer the rate of aging of cardiorespiratory fitness in the wheelchair confined, using a small sample of cross-sectional data (18 subjects). Despite some design flaws (e.g., the etiology of disability was not comparable for the three age groups), Sawka et al. estimated coefficients for the aging of oxygen transport and power output that (at least in percentage terms) were similar to those seen in the able-bodied population; the absolute decreases in peak oxygen intake and peak power output amounted to 2.6 ml/kg • min and 42 watts, respectively, per decade of life. However, the apparent decrease of peak heart rate (33 beats/min per decade) was greater than in able-bodied individuals.

Lesion Level. Peak oxygen intake readings for individuals with traumatic tetraplegia are generally much lower than for those with traumatic paraplegia;

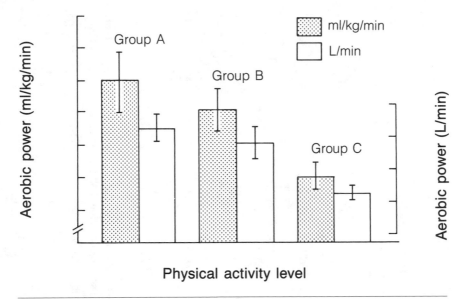

Figure 5.4. Peak oxygen intake of male wheelchair users. Group A = national caliber athletes (n = 9); Group B = recreational sportsmen (n = 15); and Group C = inactive (n = 18). Based on data of G.M. Davis and Shephard, 1988.

for instance, Ward and Fraser (1984) found a peak oxygen transport as low as 17 to 20 ml/kg • min among a tetraplegic sample, whereas Van Loan et al. (1987) reported an average of only 12 ml/kg • min in eight paraplegics. Hullemann et al. (1975) noted significant differences of peak oxygen transport and peak power output with lesion level. In their sample, the peak oxygen intake increased from 0.96 L/min in ISMGF Class II subjects to 1.54 L/min in Class VI subjects. Peak power output also increased, from an average of 74 watts in ISMGF Class II to 118 watts in ISMGF Classes V to VI. Likewise, Wicks et al. (1977; 1983) and Cameron et al. (1978) observed a relationship between lesion level and the peak oxygen intake observed during either forearm cranking or wheelchair ergometry. Some effects of lesion level have also been reported in field test scores; thus Rhodes et al. (1981) found a 12-minute wheelchair distance of 1.62 km in paraplegics but only 1.14 km in tetraplegics.

Much presumably depends upon the range of disabilities studied and the maximization of potential within a given category. Our laboratory found a significant difference of predicted maximum oxygen intakes only for those patients with Class I disabilities (see Table 5.11); subjects falling into Classes II through VI had similar peak oxygen intakes (31-40 ml/kg • min), peak heart rates (175-189 beats/min) and peak power outputs (80-102 W). Any difference from the earlier studies may reflect the fact that we tested a very diverse population that displayed a wide range of fitness levels within a given disability category. The sample comprised, necessarily, volunteers who were willing to visit our laboratories for nonclinical reasons, and there may also have been a selective recruitment of the fit or the highly motivated among those with high-level lesions.

Table 5.11 Mean Values (± *SE*) of Other Cardiorespiratory Variables at Peak Oxygen Intake

Variable	ISMGF classification						
	I	II	III	IV	V	VI	All
Peak heart rate (b/min)	127.6	188.8	182.9	185.7	171.8	178.2	172.5
	11.9	±2.0	±1.4	±3.6	±2.3	±1.7	±2.4
% theoretical heart rate*	66	97	95	96	91	92	89
	±5.9	±1.2	±1.4	±3.6	±2.3	±1.7	±2.4
Respiratory gas exchange ratio (RER)	.95	.99	1.01	.98	.95	.96	.98
	±.02	±.04	±.04	±.04	±.04	±.04	±.01
Final minus penultimate oxygen consumption (ml/kg · min)	2.5	4.4	2.3	4.3	2.9	3.4	3.3
	±.07	±1.5	±0.6	±1.3	±0.5	±0.4	±0.9
Peak oxygen intake							
Observed	**	.14	.14	.13	-.27	-.17	-.07
Predicted (L/min)		±.24	±.21	±.26	±.16	±.20	±.10

Note. Based on data from *Cardiovascular fitness and muscle strength in lower-limb disabled males* by G.M. Davis, doctoral dissertation, University of Toronto. Values are for male subjects unless otherwise noted. C_7-S_2 represents site of spinal cord lesion. I-VI represents ISMGF classification.

*Based on age-related maxima of Jones and Campbell (1982). **Prediction not possible because of bradycardia.

Etiology.   The nature of the primary pathology sometimes has an effect upon aerobic power. However, G.M. Davis et al. (1981) saw no difference of function between individuals with traumatic, prenatal atraumatic (spina bifida), and infantile atraumatic (poliomyelitis) spinal lesions. Hjeltnes (1980) found that in cases in which tetraplegia was of traumatic origin, patients could develop only a third of the maximal power and a half of the peak oxygen uptake found in traumatic paraplegic subjects of similar age and body mass. In this study, peak blood lactate levels for both subject groups (6.5 and 10.7 mmol/L) were quite high relative to able-bodied figures for arm work (Shephard et al., 1988). On the other hand, nontraumatic tetraplegics sometimes develop peak oxygen intake values as large as their paraplegic peers (Wicks et al., 1977-78; 1983). In the studies of Wicks and associates, the peak oxygen intake, peak heart rate, and peak power output were 1.23 L/min, 163 beats/min, and 35.5 watts for patients with poliomyelitic tetraplegia, but only 0.74 L/min, 119 beats/min, and 31.0 watts for those with traumatic tetraplegia.

Grimby (1980) observed that unilateral thigh amputees were able to develop a 37% greater peak oxygen transport than spinal cord–injured subjects of similar age. Little information is available on the performance of hemiplegic patients. One report (Brinkmann & Hoskins, 1979) used the Åstrand nomogram to predict the maximum oxygen intake of hemiplegics before and after 12 weeks of cycle ergometer training. Respective results were 1.07 and 2.46 L/min in five women and 2.85 and 3.08 L/min in two men.

Energy Demands in Normal Ambulation

Estimates of the energy cost of self-paced wheelchair propulsion vary substantially with the nature of the floor (G.A. Wolfe, 1978). Figures for propulsion over smooth and level surfaces range widely from 9 to 55% of maximum oxygen transporting power, the precise percentage depending on both the age and the initial fitness level of the subject (Glaser et al., 1983; Hildebrandt et al., 1970; Traugh, Corcoran, & Reyes, 1975; G.A. Wolfe, Waters, & Hislop, 1977). Plainly, for some people normal ambulation is quite light work. Hjeltnes and Vokac (1979) suggested that the typical paraplegic (lesion level T2 to T12) taxed only 15 to 20% of the heart rate reserve during normal daily life in a wheelchair; in essence, these findings mirror the situation of sedentary, able-bodied office workers, who rarely develop a heart rate greater than 100 beats/min. Over an average of 13.5 waking hours, six paraplegics exceeded 50% of their heart rate reserve for an average of only 36.9 minutes per day; these episodes were attributable to ambulation on crutches and participation in high-intensity sports such as wheelchair basketball, swimming, and distance wheelchair racing.

It seems unlikely that the usual intensity of daily wheelchair activity is sufficient to influence the training status of either a disabled athlete (Wicks et al., 1983) or a healthy young person with spinal injury (Burke, Auchinachie, Hayden, & Loftin, 1985; Hildebrandt et al., 1970; Sawka et al., 1981). On the other hand, normal ambulation may have an impact upon the physical fitness of an elderly, deconditioned wheelchair user (Sawka et al., 1981). The likelihood of a training effect naturally increases with the speed of movement.

Although the energy cost of wheelchair ambulation is less than that of walking at low speeds of operation, at speeds of over 4 km/hr, movement in a wheelchair becomes more costly than walking (Glaser, Sawka, Wilde, Woodrow, & Surprayasad, 1981; see chapter 7). One study of a crank-operated tricycle found subjects used 68% of their peak oxygen intake at a speed of 8.5 km/hr (Nag, Panikar, Malvankar, Pradhan, & Chatterjee, 1982). Usually, the speed that can be developed and thus the oxygen consumption developed depends upon the amount of residual musculature. Gordon and Vanderwalde (1956), for example, found that those individuals who had retained good control over their trunks and a fair amount of control of their legs were able to reach quite high wheelchair speeds and oxygen consumptions, but those who were more severely disabled had a very low maximum speed.

Sport.   Wheelchair basketball makes substantial aerobic demands upon the average paraplegic. Burke et al. (1985) found an energy expenditure averaging 36 kJ/min over 30 minutes of typical wheelchair basketball participation.[2] In their sample, this averaged 77% of peak oxygen intake.

Crews et al. (1982) attempted to simulate the racing pace of four wheelchair marathoners on a 400-m track. The rate of energy expenditure observed under these conditions (43 kJ/min) was at the surprisingly high level of 94% of peak oxygen intake; probably, the subjects were stimulated to some increase over racing pace by the fact that measurements were being made, and it seems unlikely that they could sustain so high an energy usage over a 2-hour event. Able-bodied marathoners typically hold their oxygen consumption to about 75% of maximum oxygen intake in an attempt to avoid anaerobic activity.

Fitness of Amputees

Obviously, physical condition differs greatly between the traumatic amputee (who may well have been highly active prior to injury) and an ischemic amputee with continuing diabetes or peripheral vascular disease (who may have been inactive initially or who may have become so as the result of the primary disease; Najenson & Levy, 1971).

Following trauma, the twin aims of a rehabilitation program are (a) to restore and if possible to improve both cardiorespiratory and muscular fitness and (b) to assure perfect adaptation to any prosthesis that is fitted. However, in older amputees with continuing cardiovascular disease the potential for restoration of function may be quite limited, and in such people the encouragement of alternative forms of ambulation such as the use of a wheelchair may be a more effective and a more successful therapeutic objective (see chapter 7).

Associated Lesions

The ability to make a full return to the activities of independent daily living is adversely affected if the individual suffers from other clinical problems such as

---

[2]The kilojoule (kJ) is the SI unit of energy. One kilocalorie = 4.186 kJ. Energy expenditure is usually derived indirectly from measurements of oxygen consumption (see chapter 1).

concomitant myocardial ischemia or cerebrovascular disease (Cruts, Van Alste, de Vries, & Huisman, 1985; E.A. Hamilton & Nichols, 1972; Kavanagh & Shephard, 1973; Najenson & Levy, 1971; Peizer, 1961; Van Alste et al., 1985a, 1985b).

Kavanagh and Shephard (1973) noted that peripheral vascular disease was the most common reason for amputation among a group of patients who attended the Toronto Rehabilitation Centre. The average age of this group was quite high, and only 48 out of 166 lower-limb amputees (29%) had received surgery for conditions other than vascular disease (auto accidents, malignancy, or infections). The young, traumatic amputees usually had no complications. On the other hand, of the 62 older vascular amputees who were willing to be tested in the exercise laboratory (average age of 66 years), 28 had additional medical conditions worsening their prognoses (diabetes, 10 cases; vascular emboli, 3 cases; osteomyelitis, 1 case; essential hypertension, 1 case; gangrene, 1 case; popliteal aneurysm, 1 case; cerebral vascular disease, 4 cases; blindness, 1 case; deafness, 1 case; gross obesity, 1 case; and chronic alcoholism, 4 cases).

Moreover, 30 of the 62 had a history of some previous heart trouble, including myocardial infarction (22 cases); cardiac failure (3 cases); angina (3 cases), and a need for regular digoxin treatment (18 cases). Twenty-eight of the 62 vascular amputees also showed electrocardiographic abnormalities, including evidence of previous myocardial infarction, T-wave abnormalities, arrhythmias, and various degrees of heart block. Twenty-three of the group had a diastolic blood pressure of more than 100 mm Hg, 13 of these being from the subgroup of 30 with cardiac problems.

Body Build

It is difficult to determine excess body mass after a limb has been amputated. Kavanagh and Shephard (1973) commented that some of their male patients were substantially underweight relative to actuarial norms, even after data had been arbitrarily corrected by 4% for below-knee and 10% for above-knee amputations. The average discrepancy was -1.7 ± 8.2 kg for the men but +1.6 ± 1.4 kg for the women. The low body mass most probably is a sign of lean tissue atrophy secondary to disease or amputation.

Aerobic Power

Some problems of safety and practicality exist with amputees when making the tests of aerobic power that would be applied to the able-bodied. Ghosh (1980) predicted maximum oxygen intake using a double step (18 to 23 cm per riser) with hand rail support. Subjects climbed for 5 minutes at 20 ascents per minute. A maximum oxygen intake of 36 ml/kg • min was estimated in young Indian workers who had required either below- or above-knee amputations following industrial trauma.

Van Alste et al. (1985a) used what they described as a rowing ergometer to make direct measurements of aerobic power in amputees. In some respects, a rowing device would provide a more satisfactory test of cardiovascular function than the usual arm crank, as the subject could then apply back and shoulder muscles to the task. The Van Alste ergometer consisted of two short cranks mounted at close to shoulder height and rotated by alternate thrusting and pulling movements. Van Alste et al. (1985a) found an average maximum power output of 63 watts, with a maximum heart rate of only 124 beats/min in a series of 39 elderly patients (aged 43-92 years, average 67 years). They commented that the maximum heart rate was only 80% of the age-predicted value, and this result was not changed when patients receiving beta-blocking drugs were omitted from their average. Possibly, some subjects had insufficient time to familiarize themselves with the testing device or were not motivated to all-out effort, and for 14 of the group the test was halted because of ST depression. Among those continuing to voluntary exhaustion, complaints included general fatigue (59%), arm fatigue (18%), and difficulty in sustaining the required cadence (23%).

Kavanagh and Shephard (1973) demonstrated that in their sample of amputees, the Åstrand cycle ergometer nomogram could be applied successfully to arm ergometer data. Their results suggested that the aerobic power of the elderly amputee was quite low. Male values averaged 1.29 L/min at an average age of 50 years, 0.82 L/min at an average age of 67 years, and 0.78 L/min at an average age of 75 years. In women, an average of 0.81 L/min was seen at an average age of 66 years. Moreover, many of the group were unable to reach even these low predicted peak values because of myocardial ischemia. The majority of amputees halted the ergometer test at a power output of 45 watts or less.

The question was thus posed as to whether attempts at upright ambulation using a prosthesis might be not only impractical but even dangerous. It was concluded that many elderly amputees might need to content themselves with mastering the tactics of life using crutches or even a wheelchair.

Electrocardiographic Abnormalities

In addition to the electrocardiographic abnormalities previously noted, 6 of the 62 patients studied by Kavanagh and Shephard (1973) showed premature ventricular contractions (PVCs) at rest. Van Alste, la Haye, Huisman, de Vries, and Boom (1985) also commented on the frequency of PVCs in the resting electrocardiograms of elderly amputees.

In the series of elderly subjects tested by Kavanagh and Shephard (1973), many individuals developed quite a severe horizontal or downward sloping ST segmental depression during exercise, even at the lowest power output (24 W). Eighteen of 27 individuals who completed the arm ergometer test demonstrated clinically significant evidence of myocardial ischemia (a horizontal or downsloping ST depression of more than 0.10 mV during maximal effort). Van Alste et al. (1985a, 1985b) likewise found that 14 of their 39 patients had significant exercise-induced ST depression. Such changes presumably reflect on the one hand a large increase of cardiac work rate as weak arm muscles attempt to sustain effort by contracting at a large percentage of maximum voluntary force and on the other hand impairment of the coronary circulation due to atherosclerotic vascular disease.

Fitness and Blindness

Most studies of the blind have noted a poor physical work capacity. Researchers have also described delays in the appearance of various motor skills (Adelson & Fraiberg, 1974) along with poor balance (Gipsman, 1981; Leonard, 1969; Ribadi, Rider, & Toole, 1987), gait, and locomotion (A.N. Buell, 1979; Emes, 1984), and problems of central information processing (Shingledecker, 1978). In some instances, balance is poorer in the partially sighted (who incorporate incomplete visual cues) than in the totally blind (who must rely more on development of muscular or proprioceptive feedback for balance; Gipsman, 1981). Scores on the Kraus-Weber physical performance test battery have been poor (Seelye, 1983), whereas physical working capacity and maximal oxygen intake have been reported as below normal values for subjects of comparable age (Cartmel & Banister, 1968; Cumming et al., 1971; Hopkins, Gaeta, Thomas, & Hill, 1987; Jankowski & Evans, 1981; Sündberg, 1982; see Table 5.12).

Researchers attribute these various handicaps not to any genetic limitation of performance but rather to overprotection and discouraging attitudes on the part of parents or teachers (Winnick, 1985; Nixon, 1988). It is thus important to stress that 80% of those classed as "legally blind" have residual vision that can be exploited by appropriate training (Liska, 1974). A further factor among those who have been blind from birth is a difficulty in conceptualizing the movement patterns required for specific types of physical activity (Dodds & Carter, 1983).

Table 5.12 Maximum Oxygen Intake of Blind Children

Age range	Maximum oxygen intake (ml/kg • min)		Authors
	Boys	Girls	
8-12	44.6	37.4	Cumming et al. (1971)
13-17	44.6	33.6	Cumming et al. (1971)
4-18	29.0	29.0	Jankowski & Evans (1981)
8-14	45.3	36.8	Sündberg (1982)
11-18	49.8	37.0	Lee et al. (1985)
11-18	53.2*	36.0*	Lee et al. (1985)
7-17			Hopkins et al. (1987)
(vision 5-20%)	41.6	41.6	
(<5%)	42.0		
(blind)	35.0		

*Selecting out experiments with "good" maximum effort.

Body Build

Lee et al. (1985) examined body build in a sample of sightless adolescents who attended a residential school for the visually handicapped that had a strong interest in maintaining the physical condition of its pupils. Relative to normal Canadian children of similar age, the blind students were approximately 5 cm shorter, and they also had a lighter body mass.

The estimated body fat of the boys (16.1%) was less than the average for a representative sample of normally sighted age-matched students, as reported by the Canada Fitness Survey (1983), whereas the figure for the girls (25.9%) corresponded closely with the Canada Fitness Survey norms. The lean mass per centimeter of stature was a little below the population average in both sexes. In contrast to these findings, Hopkins et al. (1987) found that totally blind children who attended normal elementary schools in the Auckland area of New Zealand had almost twice the skinfold fat of those children who were normally sighted.

Aerobic Power

The aerobic power of the blind students examined by Lee et al. (1985) was well up to Canadian norms. The average score was 49.8 ml/kg • min in the boys and 37.0 ml/kg • min in the girls. Taking results only from those subjects who made a good maximum effort, figures rose to 53.4 ml/kg • min in the boys, but scores were unchanged in the girls.

We may conclude that to the extent that earlier figures for blind students showed obesity and a poor level of aerobic fitness, the students concerned were probably receiving an inadequate school program of physical education. This hypothesis is borne out both by the training and detraining experiments of DiNatale, Lee, Ward, and Shephard (1985), as discussed in chapter 6, and by the correlation between habitual activity and maximum oxygen intake observed by Hopkins et al. (1987) in visually impaired students.

Fitness and Deafness

Several reports suggest that deaf children are inferior to normals with respect to static equilibrium, dynamic equilibrium, motor coordination, speed, and power (Boyd, 1967; Cratty, Cratty, & Cornell, 1986; Lindsey & O'Neal, 1976; Myklebust, 1964; Padden, 1959; Pender & Patterson, 1982; Pennella, 1979), in part because of social withdrawal (Fait & Dunn, 1984; Sherrill, 1981). Some studies found that considerable compensation for sensory deficiencies is possible through the use of visual cues (Lindsey & O'Neal, 1976; Pennella, 1979), but others disagreed (Carlson, 1972).

In terms of scores on simple performance tests and ability to undertake daily activities, poor balance and coordination lead to an ineffective use of muscle strength and cardiorespiratory power. Brunt and Broadhead (1982) found that deaf students had significant deficits on such simple psychomotor tasks as standing on the preferred leg, walking forward heel-to-toe on a balance beam, jumping up and clapping the hands, and response speed (see Table 5.13). Others found a

Table 5.13   Psychomotor Responses of Normal and Deaf Children

Variable	Age (yrs)	Boys Normal	Boys Deaf[a]	Girls Normal	Girls Deaf[a]
Standing on one leg on balance beam (s)	7	8.1	3.5	8.4	3.1
	10	9.2	5.8	9.3	6.8
	14	9.6	6.4	9.3	8.0
Forward walk on balance beam (steps)	7	4.4	1.0	4.5	0.9
	10	5.1	1.0	5.4	2.8
	14	5.1	3.1	5.8	3.0
Jump up and clap hands (claps)	7	1.8	1.8	1.8	1.7
	10	2.8	1.9	2.3	2.7
	14	3.4	2.7	3.3	2.5
Response speed	7	6.0	2.9	5.4	4.0
	10	10.1	8.5	9.7	8.3
	14	11.7	8.4	11.3	8.0

Note. Based on data from "Motor Proficiency Traits of Deaf Children" by D. Brunt and G.D. Broadhead, 1982, *Research Quarterly, 53*, pp. 236-238.
[a]Hearing loss >60 decibels.

substantial shortening of the normal postrotatory nystagmus (Potter & Silverman, 1984). One problem of the deaf seems a delayed response to a disturbance of balance (Brunt, Layne, Cook, & Rowe, 1984). In contrast, the performance of deaf subjects is superior to that of normal children on items that involve visual-motor control.

Boyd (1967) commented that the deterioration of balance was shown equally by those with congenital deafness and by those whose hearing defect had an infective etiology. However, Myklebust (1964), Lindsey and O'Neal (1976), Brunt et al. (1984), and Butterfield (1987) attributed any associated deterioration of balance to an effect of the primary lesion upon vestibular mechanisms. For instance, poor balance was often a sequel to an infectious meningitis (see Table 5.14) and poor balance was more common in idiopathic than in genetically determined deafness (Butterfield & Ersing, 1986). The lack of balance inevitably had a negative impact upon most tests of skilled motor performance (Butterfield, 1986, 1987), although the hearing loss itself, measured in decibels, was not correlated with performance test scores. A further factor that adversely influences performance in some tests requiring a motor response is that the attention of a totally deaf student may be directed to the examiner or track official rather than to a more specific cue for a response (such as a light or a starter's pistol).

The one exception in this litany of poor coordination is visual motor control; on items such as drawing a straight line or copying a circle, the deaf students are sometimes superior to their peers who have normal hearing. Brunt and Broadhead

Table 5.14   Influence of Etiology on Balance of Deaf Children

	Arbitrary score	
Etiology of deafness	Static balance	Dynamic balance
Genetic	7.0	3.5
Rubella	5.3	3.1
Meningitis	4.2	1.9
Idiopathic	4.0	2.0
Other	6.1	2.3

Note. Based on data from "The Influence of Age, Sex, Hearing Loss, Etiology, and Balance Ability on the Fundamental Motor Skills of Deaf Children" by S.A. Butterfield, 1987, in M. Berridge and G. Ward (Eds.), *International Perspectives in Adapted Physical Activity* (pp. 43-51). Champaign, IL: Human Kinetics.

(1982) attributed this advantage to a special education that emphasizes the recognition of visual cues. If their view is correct, then the performance of other types of skill might also be enhanced by encouraging a greater reliance on visual cues.

Body Build

Hattin et al. (1986) collected data on deaf children having an average age of 13.5 years. Relative to a sample of blind children also studied in our laboratory (discussed previously), the deaf boys were actually a little fatter (average figures were 18.4% body fat in the deaf boys and 26.0% body fat in the deaf girls). In the report of Cumming et al. (1971), the corresponding figures for deaf students were 18.0 and 23.4% body fat. Winnick and Short (1986) examined a large sample of deaf and hearing-impaired students aged 10 to 17 years; girls (but not boys) showed a progressive increase of skinfold readings from the hearing to the hearing impaired and the deaf. Hattin et al. (1986) commented that in both sexes, the lean mass of the deaf was lower than that of blind students.

Muscle Strength and Flexibility

Winnick and Short (1986) noted that with one minor exception, they observed no differences of grip strength between hearing, hearing-impaired, and deaf students. However, possibly because of vestibular involvement or a greater difficulty in motivating the subjects, muscular endurance (as tested by speed sit-ups) was poorer in the deaf than in those with normal hearing. Pender and Patterson (1982) reported an insignificant trend in the same sense. In the girls (but not in the boys), flexibility (as assessed by a sit-and-reach test) was also impaired in the deaf.

Aerobic Power

Problems of communication plainly restrict the participation of deaf students in some types of sport, and on this account a low level of aerobic fitness might be anticipated. However, Sündberg (1983) found normal lung volumes (forced expiratory volume and forced vital capacity), and one report (Cumming, Goulding, & Baggley, 1971) observed a much higher level of aerobic fitness in deaf children than in those who were blind or mentally retarded; from this set of data the authors hypothesized that a lack of sensory stimulation had encouraged the deaf children to engage in a more than usual amount of leisure-time physical activity, with a resultant maximization of their aerobic potential.

Although some evidence exists that deaf children induce deliberate cerebral stimulation by rocking movements, a critical examination of the results of Cumming et al. (1971) shows that the intercategory differences that they reported were attributable to a low maximum oxygen intake in their groups of blind and mentally retarded students rather than to a high average figure for the aerobic power of the deaf. Pennella (1979) concluded that deaf students attending residential schools with a good physical education program had relatively normal fitness levels, although day students were often at a disadvantage relative to those with normal hearing.

Hattin et al. (1986) conducted maximum effort tests on a cycle ergometer (see Table 5.15). In their sample of deaf boys they found a 9.5% disadvantage of peak power output and a 17.3% disadvantage of maximum oxygen intake relative to blind students, despite identical maximum heart rates. On the other hand, in their sample of girls, both maximum power output (+6.6%) and maximum oxygen intake (+9.5%) were a little higher in deaf than in blind individuals. Actual performance data for the Toronto sample of deaf students (peak oxygen transport and peak power output 43.6 ml/kg • min, 3.45 W/kg in the boys; 37.0 ml/kg • min, 2.93 W/kg in the girls) and for the PWC_{170} (2.43 W/kg in the boys, 2.02 W/kg in the girls) corresponded very closely with the supposedly high figures reported earlier by Cumming et al. (1971).

Winnick and Short (1986) found no significant effect of deafness on either a 50-yd dash or a 12-minute run. However, the distance covered by the Toronto students during a 12-minute all-out run was shorter in the deaf than in the blind (a 13% disadvantage in the boys and a 14% disadvantage in the girls; Hattin et al., 1986).

Recent data thus do not support the idea that deaf children have an unusually high level of either physical activity or aerobic fitness as a compensation for their deafness. Indeed, lack of socialization tends to give poor fitness levels with an accumulation of body fat, and difficulties of motivation may also restrict performance relative to capacity.

Fitness and Cerebral Palsy

The physical performance of a subject with cerebral palsy may be limited by muscle spasm, athetoid movements, rigidity, lack of coordination (ataxia), tremor,

Table 5.15 Fitness of Deaf Children

| Variable | Hattin et al. (1986)[a] | | Cumming et al. (1971)[a] | | | |
	Boys 13.4	Girls 13.5	Boys 8-12	Boys 13-17	Girls 8-12	Girls 13-17
Height (cm)	156	153	144	164	149	161
Body mass (kg)	45.3	45.3	37.3	57.2	46.3	52.3
Body fat (%)	18.4	26.0	16.0	18.0	25.5	23.4
PWC_{170} (W/kg)	2.43	2.02	2.38	2.50	1.90	1.95
Maximum oxygen intake (ml/kg · min)	43.6[b]	37.0[b]	43.8	45.2	37.0	37.6

[a]Age measured in years. [b]Extrapolating values for students with low maximal heart rate.

or a general lack of muscle tone. In 50% of patients, the predominant feature of the disease is spasm; the main physiological findings are then limitation of muscle strength and endurance. However, in about a quarter of patients the major clinical feature is athetosis; fine motor skills are then greatly handicapped, but strength and walking ability are less affected (Huberman, 1976). Unfortunately, much of the available empiric data has failed to specify clearly the type, severity, and extent of disability, using an objective scale such as that developed by CP-ISRA.

Submaximal Work Performance

During standard forms of submaximal exercise, the mechanical efficiency of the patient with cerebral palsy can be very low (e.g., around 12% for those with predominantly spastic lesions and 16% for those with predominantly athetoid lesions) compared with an average of 22% for normal controls performing a comparable cycle ergometer task (Lundberg, 1975, 1976). The high ratio of oxygen consumption to work performed in patients with cerebral palsy reflects the energy "wasted" in developing both spasm and athetoid movements, effort expended in overcoming the spasticity of antagonist muscles, and sometimes abnormal reflexes that lead to an exaggeration of movements that the subject would otherwise find easy to perform (Berg & Bjure, 1970).

As a consequence of these several handicaps, the heart rate is high during submaximal exercise, and a misleading impression of the limitation of aerobic power may be obtained if maximum oxygen intake is predicted from the power output and heart rate during a submaximal test (Lundberg, 1973). The situation is further complicated by the variable nature of muscle spasms. There is a need for empiric research that examines the influence of major competition on muscle tone and spasm in each of the various CP-ISRA categories. Some influence of cerebral arousal might be anticipated, and at least one report suggested an enormous increase of spasm immediately prior to a major athletic competition, limiting performance further relative to estimates made in the base laboratory (Huberman, cited by Rotzinger & Stoboy, 1974). Others who have worked in contests for the cerebral palsied have not been impressed subjectively by any worsening of spasm at the meet.

Habitual Activity

Perhaps in part as a reaction to the high energy cost of ambulation (Molbech, 1966), adolescents with cerebral palsy often become progressively less willing to undertake normal ambulation as they become older. Physical condition thus deteriorates, and in some instances the heart rate corresponding to a given cycle ergometer power output may rise by as much as 10 beats/min per year (Lundberg, 1973). Reported daily energy expenditures vary widely from 4.0 to 14.7 MJ, figures being much higher for lean and dyskinetic individuals than for those who are spastic and obese (Berg & Olsson, 1970).

Aerobic Power

Measurements of peak power output and maximum oxygen intake in patients with cerebral palsy have generally shown figures 10 to 30% below normal standards for those of the same age and sex (Bar-Or, Inbar, & Spira, 1976; Lundberg, 1978). However, the interpretation of such data is complicated by failure to detail the type and extent of the palsy and by associated abnormalities of body build and composition. Children with cerebral palsy not only are short for their age but also have an increased body water and a reduced body cell mass (Berg & Isaksson, 1970). If due allowance is made for these various differences, the aerobic power of a well-trained person with cerebral palsy is essentially normal.

Fitness in Muscular Dystrophies and Multiple Sclerosis

Formal research on fitness levels in muscular dystrophies and multiple sclerosis is quite limited. Nevertheless, it is recognized that muscular dystrophies progressively rob the growing child and adolescent of muscle strength, endurance, and aerobic power. Likewise, multiple sclerosis gives rise to progressive weakness and a poor tolerance of strenuous workouts.

Muscular Strength and Anaerobic Performance

The muscular strength of an able-bodied boy shows a major spurt at puberty. However, in patients with muscular dystrophy, the isometric strength remains constant or even diminishes as a child grows larger (deLateur & Giaconi, 1979; Fowler & Gardner, 1967; Hosking, Bhat, Dubowitz, & Edwards, 1976; Sockolov, Irwin, Dressendorfer, & Bernauer, 1977; Vignos & Watkins, 1966; see Table 5.16). Thus, the dystrophic individual becomes progressively weaker relative to body mass. Function may further be impaired by a drop in peripheral nerve conduction velocity (Chrétien, Simard, & Dorion, 1987). With Duchenne's dystrophy, the peak force that can be developed is often at less than the 5th percentile of scores for a healthy individual (Hosking et al., 1976). Probably because the residual muscle of the dystrophic person must contract at a large fraction of its maximal force, muscular endurance is greatly reduced relative to normal individuals (Hosking et al., 1976).

On the Wingate all-out cycle ergometer test of anaerobic power and capacity, the peak (5 s) power output is much less in the dystrophic patient than in normal individuals. The power produced over the entire 30 seconds is also much reduced, although if the "drop-off" is calculated in percentage terms, it is similar to that for a healthy individual (a 40% decrease from the initial rate of working, Bar-Or, 1983).

Cardiovascular Performance

Logan et al. (1981) studied the cardiovascular performance of female multiple sclerotic patients. They noted a resting diastolic volume, stroke volume, and cardiac contractility within the normal range. However, 42% of the subjects had a mitral valve prolapse, and the mean ventricular volume–muscle ratio was 49% greater than that of able-bodied females, both of these findings suggesting "extreme functional deconditioning" secondary to a very sedentary lifestyle.

Table 5.16 Isometric Muscle Strength of Able-Bodied Boys and Boys With Duchenne's Dystrophy, Expressed in Newtons

Variable	Age 5-6 years		Age 9-10 years		Age 15-16 years	
	Able-bodied	Duchenne	Able-bodied	Duchenne	Able-bodied	Duchenne
R handgrip	85	45	152	71	433	62
R elbow flexion	71	22	138	27	294	13
extension	54	18	98	22	192	13
Shoulder abduction	58	18	174	27	375	18
R hip flexion	67	22	161	58	491	31
R knee flexion	45	13	112	13	187	27
extension	89	31	214	40	602	18
Trunk flexion	71	22	143	54	508	9
extension	129	40	161	58	549	36

Note. Based on data from "Quantitative Strength Measurements in Muscular Dystrophy" by W.M. Fowler and G.W. Gardner, 1967, Archives of Physical Medicine and Rehabilitation, 48, pp. 629-644.

Habitual Activity

Many factors exacerbate the impact of muscle weakness upon the functional mobility of a dystrophic patient. Asymmetry of the muscular deficit often leads to the development of contractures (particularly about the knee joint). The patient becomes anxious about falling, and actual falls lead to enforced bed rest with a further loss of muscle strength and aerobic power plus a worsening of any contractures (Bowker & Halpin, 1978).

The mechanical efficiency during submaximal exercise shows surprisingly little change in the dystrophic patient (Carroll et al., 1979), but peak aerobic power and maximum oxygen intake are poor (Carroll, Hagberg, Brooke, & Shumate, 1979; Sockolov et al., 1977). The limitation of oxygen transport reflects not only the loss of functioning lean tissue with resultant difficulty in perfusing the active muscle (Kay & Shephard, 1969), but also a deterioration of ventilatory function (Inkley, Oldenburg, & Vignos, 1974), and in some instances, a tendency to cardiac failure (Gailani, Danowski, & Fisher, 1958).

Fitness and Scoliosis

Scoliosis usually begins as a single curvature of the spine, but there is often a secondary deviation in the opposite direction. The functional consequences depend greatly upon severity. This is graded in terms of the primary curvature, 15 to 35° being regarded as mild, 35 to 75° as moderate, and 75 to 150° as severe scoliosis. Mild or moderate scoliosis is quite common, particularly in individuals with cerebral palsy (Robson, 1968), in les autres, and in the elderly (Robin, Span, Steinberg, Makin, & Menczel, 1982). Robson (1968) noted that 33% of adolescents and young adults with cerebral palsy had a postural scoliosis, and a further 15% had a structural scoliosis; however, the lesion was severe (here defined as an angulation of more than 60°) in only 4% of subjects. By itself, a moderate spinal curvature seems compatible with a relatively normal level of fitness, but severe scoliosis leads to a substantial restriction of aerobic power, the primary impact upon ventilatory function being compounded by inactivity and detraining.

Respiratory Function Changes

Many of the adverse effects of scoliosis can be traced to an associated deformity of the chest. This causes a decrease of static and dynamic lung volumes (sometimes to only 40-50% of age-, height-, and sex-specific normal values), with a stiffening of the rib cage and an increase in the work of breathing (Bergofsky, Turino, & Fishman, 1959; Bjure, Grimby, & Nachemson, 1969; Stoboy, 1978, 1985; Stoboy & Speierer, 1968).

A rapid and shallow pattern of breathing is adopted, leading to a poor distribution of inspired gas; the physiological dead space and the alveolar-arterial oxygen tension gradient are enlarged (Bar-Or, 1983) and the pulmonary arterial blood pressure is high (Shneerson, 1978). The pulmonary hypertension is attributable not only to hypoxic pulmonary vasoconstriction but also to a narrowing of the pulmonary arterioles by a medial proliferation within the vessel walls (Stoboy, 1985).

Habitual Activity

A combination of an awkward gait and an increased respiratory work load leads to a high energy cost of ambulation in subjects severely affected by scoliosis. Partly because of these physical problems and partly because of embarrassment at personal appearance, the level of habitual activity in such individuals tends to be low, exacerbating poor inherent fitness levels.

Aerobic Power

The peak power output is about 40% less than normal in severe cases of scoliosis. Some authors have found a maximum oxygen intake as low as 11 to 25 ml/kg • min in scoliotic patients (Bjure et al., 1969; Shneerson & Edgar, 1979; Shneerson & Madgwick, 1979), although a recent report from Stoboy (1985) cites figures of 30 to 32 ml/kg • min, a 40% reduction over healthy normals.

Fitness and Mental Retardation

The bulk of mentally retarded individuals show no obvious inheritance of the disorder or physical cause. In some cases, sensory deprivation (severe defects of sight and hearing) or neglect may be responsible for much of both physical and mental impairment. Some 10% of those who are institutionalized for mental retardation have an underlying chromosomal abnormality, Down's syndrome being the most common of such conditions, and a further 17% have congenital defects of the cerebrum and cranium. Other potential causes include fetal hypoxia or intoxication, premature birth, endocrine and nutritional disorders, postnatal disease of the brain, and the sequelae of some psychiatric disorders. Given this quite varied etiology, a case could be made for discussing the fitness and training responses for each category separately, and indeed a trend has developed to distinguish Down's syndrome from physically less-recognizable forms of mental retardation.

A review of physical fitness and mental retardation (Moon & Renzaglia, 1982) concluded that relatively little information was available on this topic. Unfortunately, much of the existing empiric data is flawed by failure to describe carefully the severity of the retardation (mild, moderate, severe, or profound). The nature and degree of disability inevitably influence both assessment and performance.

Children with subnormal intelligence commonly show deficiencies of static balance, muscle force, and coordination (Cooke, 1984; Drouin, Simard, & Cloutier, 1981), scoring badly on both motor performance tests (a retardation of 2-4 years) and on measures of physical fitness (Kerr & Hughes, 1987; Rarick, 1980a, b). However, the basic factor structure of the common fitness test variables is similar in normals and in the educable mentally retarded (Rarick, 1980b).

Particularly low scores are observed for items that require learning and neuromuscular coordination (Francis & Rarick, 1959; Howe, 1959; Kasch & Zasueta, 1971; Keogh & Oliver, 1968; Sengstock, 1966; Sloan, 1951). The time for a visual search is prolonged (Eason, Smith, & Stamps, 1981), and a low level of cerebral arousal as shown by anticipatory heart rates (Stamps, Eason, & Smith,

1983) has negative effects upon both the learning process and the immediate rapidity of response to signals (Karrer, 1985; de Potter, 1981; Snaith, 1974; Welford, 1962).

Body Size and Physical Performance

Many of the early studies of physical performance compared normal and mentally retarded students in terms of their calendar ages, but this approach can be misleading. Adult mentally retarded individuals may have normal anthropometric characteristics including height and body mass (Nordgren, 1971), but unusual distribution of body mass occurs in Down's syndrome (DePauw, 1984). Mental deficiency may also be associated with slow processes of both growth and maturation (Abernathy, 1936; Jochheim, 1971; Sengstock, 1966; Zasueta & Kasch, 1973), so that mentally retarded children are small for their age.

The development of motor skills is often retarded. Although some authors have found no difference between those with Down's syndrome and those with other types of mental retardation, Connolly and Michael (1986) found that Down's syndrome students were particularly disadvantaged with respect to running speed, balance, strength, visual motor control, and composite scores for fine and gross motor skills.

Studies in normal individuals (Cumming & Keynes, 1967; Drake, Jones, Brown, & Shephard, 1968) emphasize that scores on physical performance tests are strongly influenced by body size. Much of the poor performance of mentally retarded students on the Kraus-Weber, American Alliance of Health, Physical Education and Recreation (AAHPER), and other performance test batteries (Connolly & Michael, 1986; Dobbins, Garron, & Rarick, 1981; Kasch & Zasueta, 1971; Ulrich, 1983) could thus be attributed to small body size. As adult size is relatively normal, this is a less convincing explanation of the poor physical performance observed in mentally retarded adolescents and adults (Beasley, 1982; J. Brown, 1967; R.S. Coleman & Whitman, 1984; Corder, 1966; Fernhall & Tymeson, 1988; Giles, 1968). A second cause of poor performance at all ages may be a lack of opportunity to develop the required motor skills (Londeree & Johnson, 1974; Speakman, 1977). Thus Stein (1965) found normal AAHPER test scores among pupils who had been integrated into the normal school program.

However, Jochheim (1971) suggested that even if appropriate allowances are made for factors of size and specific test experience, the performance of the mentally retarded student remains poor due to muscle weakness, lack of coordination, a general underdevelopment of movement patterns, difficulty in understanding abstract concepts such as competing against a clock (Fernhall, Tymeson, & Webster, 1988; Tomporowski & Ellis, 1984), and a poor endurance. Both Londeree and Johnson (1974) and Rarick, Widdop, and Broadhead (1970) found that educable mentally retarded subjects performed better than did the trainable mentally retarded subjects in times for a 300-yd run. Attempts to teach better methods of carrying out selected activities are hampered by impulsiveness and a lack of concentration on the part of the mentally retarded subjects. Performance of motor tests is adversely affected by the complexity of the required procedures, below average motivation, and use of a number of trials prior to the definitive test which is inadequate relative to the child's learning rate (Johnson & Londeree, 1976; Speakman, 1977). In a competitive situation, the mentally retarded quickly become discouraged, and they perform best when competing against themselves with repeated positive feedback (Snaith, 1974).

W.E. Davis (1987) suggested that the mentally retarded are affected by a deficiency of muscle activation. The time from stimulus to the appearance of muscle fiber activity is prolonged, and there is difficulty in sustaining contractile activity, particularly in children affected by Down's syndrome. There is also a slowing of reaction times. Both premotor and movement times are affected. Coleman (1973) found that these changes may be related to a cerebral deficiency of serotonin, but Pueschel (1984) disagreed. Levarlet-Joye and Ribauville (1981) noted that mentally retarded students had poor scores relative to normal Belgians with respect to handgrip force, standing broad jump, 25-m run, ball throwing, and trunk flexion tests. W.E. Davis (1987) also noted inaccuracy and a low velocity in ball-throwing tests. Sengstock (1966) further demonstrated that in terms of performance on the AAHPER test battery, educable mentally retarded boys achieved scores midway between those of comparable chronological age and those of comparable mental age.

Body Composition

Bar-Or et al. (1971) found a relatively normal body density (and by inference, a normal percentage of body fat in children with an IQ of less than 90; density readings ranged from 1.027 to 1.042 in the girls and from 1.054 to 1.057 in the boys. Reid et al. (1985) examined 185 mentally handicapped adults; the males had some excess fat, and the females were clearly obese. Nordgren (1970), Kreze, Zelinda, Julias, and Gargara (1974), Polednak and Auliffe (1976), and R. Fox and Rotatori (1982) all commented on the prevalence of excess body mass or obesity among the mentally retarded, and Skrobak-Kaczynski and Vavik (1980) found that young men with Down's syndrome had 80% more body fat than controls.

Kelly, Rimmer, and Ness (1986) made skinfold estimates of body fat in 553 institutionalized, mentally retarded adults. Some 45% of the men and 51% of the women were obese (more than 20% fat in males, 30% fat in females), the problem being more prevalent in moderate and severe than in profound mental impairment. The authors noted their disagreement with a previous, smaller study by Polednak and Auliffe (1976). They hypothesized that the profoundly retarded were likely to be assigned physical work and physical recreation within the institution. In contrast, those with less severe impairment tended to have sedentary employment and sedentary pastimes. Moreover, because of wage earning they were able to purchase additional food items such as candy and soft drinks.

Muscle Strength

Several reports suggest that the muscular strength of the mentally retarded is less than normal; such suggestions must be interpreted with caution because muscle force varies approximately as height 2.9, and, at least in children, the mentally retarded have a disadvantage of stature.

Asmussen and Heebøll-Nielsen (1956) found that even after matching for height, boys with an IQ of 70 to 90 had lower maximum inspiratory and expiratory forces than those with an IQ of over 95. Reid et al. (1985) also reported a poor muscle strength and endurance in mentally retarded adults. Howe (1959) and Kasch and Zasueta (1971) both reported a normal grip strength and throwing accuracy in educable mentally retarded children, but in adults Nordgren (1970, 1971, 1972; Nordgren & Backstrom, 1971), Arvidsson, Dencker, and Grimby (1970), Morgan (1974), Skrobak-Kaczynski and Vavik (1980), and Malkia, Joukamaa, Maatela, Aromaa, and Heliovaara (1987) all found a significant limitation of muscular performance or maximal isometric strength, this being more obvious in the non-educable than in the educable mentally retarded. Nordgren commented that the functional loss affected not only large muscles but also the small muscles responsible for fine movements of the fingers; thus muscle weakness could have contributed to a limitation of industrial performance in tasks involving fine motor skills.

A limitation of maximum voluntary isometric force thus seems fairly well documented. However, we cannot be certain that differences of test comprehension and motivation have not had an adverse effect upon test scores in the severely retarded.

Aerobic Fitness

Aerobic power is another variable that is strongly influenced by stature. The reported maximum oxygen intake or cardiovascular fitness of the mentally retarded is generally lower than in the nonhandicapped population, although values reported have ranged quite widely from normal to markedly impaired (Andrew, Reid, Beck, & McDonald, 1979; Beasley, 1982; Björke, Hagen, Lie, & Klieve, 1978; Burkett & Ewing, 1984; Coleman, Ayoub, & Friedrich, 1976; Fernhall & Tymeson, 1988; Maksud & Hamilton, 1974; Millar, 1984; Nordgren, 1970; Rarick, Dobbins, & Broadhead, 1976; Rarick, Widdop, & Broadhead, 1970; Reid et al., 1985; Schurrer, Weltman, & Brammerl, 1985; Yoshizawa, Ishizaki, & Honda, 1975). In some studies (Maksud & Hamilton, 1974) low maximal heart rates suggest poor motivation, but in others there is no reason to doubt the authenticity of scores that are 8 to 12% below those for able-bodied individuals of the same age. Presumably, much depends on the individual's comprehension of the test requirements (Lavay, Giese, Bussen, & Dart, 1987) and opportunities for active leisure (Dresen, Groot, Brandt Corstius, Krediet, & Meijer, 1982; Dresen, Vermeulen, Netelenbos, & Krot, 1982), although there has also been some speculation about a lesser release of catecholamines.

Hayden (1968) found a correlation of 0.25 to 0.30 between IQ and the performance of such endurance activities as a 300-yd run and a 10-minute run-walk. Some later authors have questioned the existence of a direct relationship to intelligence and have further challenged the use of 300-yd times as a predictor of aerobic fitness in the mentally retarded, due to the dominant influence of body size

(Fernhall & Tymeson, 1988). Lavay et al. (1987) also stressed the difficulty that many mentally retarded subjects have in facing a run-walk.

Nordgren (1971) claimed a relatively normal physical working capacity at a heart rate of 170 beats/min (PWC_{170}) in mentally retarded adults, although a significant proportion of subjects unable to complete the required cycle ergometer test were excluded from his average, and those who did complete the evaluation demonstrated a considerable range of performance. Reid et al. (1985) made step test predictions of maximal working capacity in 184 employees of sheltered workshops. Fitness levels in this sample were very low, although this may have reflected in part difficulties in comprehending and performing the step test.

Part of the problem is an inadequate level of habitual activity, a combined response to sedatives, protective restrictions on movement, and the mental condition itself (Bar-Or et al., 1971; Burkett & Ewing, 1984; Coleman et al., 1976; Dresen, Groot, et al., 1982; Dresen, Vermeulen, et al., 1982; Fernhall et al., 1988; Malkia et al., 1987; Yoshizawa et al., 1975). Mechanical efficiency tends to be poor (Dresen, Groot, et al., 1982; Dresen, Vermeulen, et al., 1982). Bar-Or et al. (1971) commented that although the maximum oxygen intake of retarded subjects was less than in that of their control group, the figures observed for the mentally retarded sample were essentially similar to other data for normal students as found in the literature (an average of 50.3 ml/kg • min in boys aged 8.4 years and 43.9 ml/kg • min in girls aged 8.0 years). Kasch and Zasueta (1971) reported rather lower maximum oxygen intake figures than Bar-Or et al. (1971) in six mentally retarded boys of unspecified height and age (average score 45.4 ml/kg • min). The figures of 25 to 28 ml/kg • min observed in mentally retarded young adults (Fernhill & Tymeson, 1988; Schurrer et al., 1985) are much lower than would be anticipated in normal individuals.

Fitness of Autistic Individuals

Several early authors (Alderton, 1966; Kanner, 1943; Rimland, 1964; Wing, 1966) suggested that motor performance developed normally in autistic individuals. More recent reports question this view (DeMyer, 1976; Geddes, 1977; Lotter, 1966; Ornitz, Guthrie, & Farley, 1977; Wing, 1976). Reid, Collier, and Morin (1983) demonstrated poor scores for flexibility (sit-and-reach test), catching, throwing, and balance tasks in autistic students.

The learning of motor skills in the autistic individual is hampered by excessive selectivity in responding to sensory cues. Autistic learners tend to have a sensory preference, some responding best to auditory and others to visual cues (Kolko, Anderson, & Campbell, 1980; Rincover, Cook, Peoples, & Packard, 1979). Cues which take the individual physically through the required movements seem to provide the best basis for skill acquisition in this type of disability (Collier & Reid, 1987; Frith & Hermelin, 1969; Prior & Chen, 1975).

Key Ideas

1. Body composition of the wheelchair disabled is affected by wasting of muscles and osteoporosis in paralyzed limbs. Inactive individuals may also accumulate substantial amounts of body fat.

2. Resting oxygen consumption and cardiac output may be reduced by limb paralysis. High-level lesions create additional problems because of venous pooling and impaired respiratory mechanics.

3. Mechanical efficiency may not differ greatly between experienced and inexperienced wheelchair users.

4. In spinally injured tetraplegics, the increase of heart rate with exercise is smaller and occurs later than that seen in able-bodied individuals.

5. Regular participation in wheelchair sport is associated with an increase of cardiac stroke volume and correction of a "hypokinetic" response of the heart to exercise. Depending on the extent of training of the arm muscles, arteriovenous oxygen differences during vigorous exercise may be normal or increased.

6. Handgrip force is not substantially increased by wheelchair confinement, but the strength of shoulder and elbow muscles is greater than in the able-bodied; the extent of such differences reflects habitual activity patterns and the type of sport in which the more active wheelchair-confined individuals are involved.

7. Biopsies show substantial hypertrophy of both Type I and Type II muscle fibers in the arms of many wheelchair-confined subjects.

8. Although some wheelchair-confined subjects have a very limited aerobic power, others can develop a larger maximum oxygen intake than a sedentary able-bodied person. Scores for the wheelchair athletes are higher among those involved in track and swimming events than in those who compete in strength events.

9. Maximum oxygen intake is much more limited in spinally injured tetraplegics than in paraplegics.

10. Normal wheelchair ambulation demands anywhere from 9 to 55% of maximum oxygen intake, depending upon the age and the fitness of the wheelchair user. For young and well-conditioned individuals, daily wheelchair activity does not provide an adequate training stimulus.

11. The fitness level of amputees depends on age, the reason for surgery (e.g., trauma vs. peripheral vascular disease), and the extent of other clinical problems (e.g., diabetes, cerebrovascular disease, or blindness). Many elderly amputees lack the aerobic power to master the use of a prosthesis.

12. Blind children are sometimes shorter than those with normal vision. However, they have a normal level of aerobic fitness provided that they receive an adequate program of physical education.

13. Deaf children may have problems of balance. However, early reports that they developed a high level of aerobic fitness due to compensatory hyperactivity have not been confirmed.

14. Children with mental retardation show problems of balance and coordination. Both strength and aerobic power are below normal, but it is difficult to be certain to what extent the deficit is due to problems of motivating test candidates to all-out effort.

15. Performance of the person with cerebral palsy may be limited by muscle spasm, athetoid movements, and lack of coordination, with limitations of strength and fine motor skills. Aerobic power may also appear low, but this is due to an increase of cell water and a reduced body mass.

16. Muscular dystrophies limit strength, and because of lack of habitual physical activity aerobic power may also be small.

17. Mild scoliosis has little influence upon fitness. Severe scoliosis restricts ventilatory function, with secondary inactivity and progressive detraining of the affected individual.

Practical Applications

1. What physiological mechanisms permit an increase of cardiac output when a high-level paraplegic engages in vigorous exercise?

2. Define hypokinetic circulation. Why might the circulation be hypokinetic in a paraplegic?

3. What factors might influence the mechanical efficiency of arm work in a paraplegic?

4. What are the determinants of arteriovenous oxygen difference during vigorous exercise? What changes, if any, would you anticipate in a wheelchair-confined person?

5. Has the extensive study of grip strength in the wheelchair disabled been worthwhile? Why was handgrip tested so frequently? What lessons would you draw for future research?

6. What technical factors influence the results obtained by isokinetic dynamometry? How would you like to see muscle performance reported?

7. Has muscle biopsy advanced our understanding of the pathophysiology of wheelchair confinement to date? How might it do so in the future?

8. Some authors equate fitness with maximum oxygen intake. What is your attitude to this stance?

9. Why does maximum oxygen intake decrease with age? Would you expect a similar rate of aging in able-bodied and disabled individuals?

10. What factors modify the energy cost of wheelchair ambulation?

11. What clinical abnormalities frequently accompany a need for amputation? How do these conditions influence rehabilitation?

12. What are the main obstacles to maintenance of personal fitness in a blind child?

13. By what mechanisms does deafness modify physical performance?

14. What is the impact of mental retardation on physical fitness?

15. How do other disorders such as cerebral palsy, muscular dystrophy, and scoliosis influence fitness?

Chapter 6

Training Programs

Hoffman (1986) presented a well organized review of responses to training after spinal cord injury. In this chapter we look first at the relative merits of cross-sectional versus longitudinal study and then consider in more detail the evidence obtained by each of these approaches both in the spinally injured and in those with other types of disability.

Cross-Sectional Versus Longitudinal Study

Researchers generally agree that an appropriate training regimen can induce significant gains in both muscle strength and peak oxygen intake during rehabilitation of such varied groups as paraplegics (Chawla et al., 1977; G.M. Davis et al., 1984a; DiCarlo, Supp, & Taylor, 1983), the blind (Shephard et al., 1987), the cerebral palsied (Bar-Or et al., 1976), and the mentally retarded (Schurrer et al., 1985). Moreover, training-induced gains of physical condition can be further developed if individuals continue a graded program of enhanced activity after discharge from the hospital. As in able-bodied individuals, the disabled person's response to training can be inferred from cross-sectional comparisons of elite disabled athletes with inactive individuals and from longitudinal observations as a selected sample of subjects undergo either normal seasonal training or deliberate, controlled conditioning in the laboratory.

The main advantage that can be claimed for a modern cross-sectional study is that the training undertaken by the current generation of disabled athletes has been both rigorous and prolonged. There are thus no fears that a larger benefit of training might have been demonstrated if a better motivated sample had been followed for a longer time. On the other hand, it is difficult to obtain quantitative information concerning the frequency, duration, and intensity of training that has been undertaken by disabled athletes as part of their normal training program.

The Issue of Constitutional Advantage

A further problem among the able-bodied (Bouchard et al., 1986; Shephard, 1978a, b) is that at least half of the functional difference between an average person and an outstanding athlete is inherited. Such constitutional factors are perhaps less important for the disabled than for the able-bodied individual, as selection pressures remain less intense for adapted competitions than for the able-bodied Olympics. Nevertheless, some suspicion remains that the elite disabled athlete begins training with a constitutional advantage that predisposes him or her to an outstanding ultimate performance (Gandee et al., 1980, 1981). Certainly, a constitutional selection exists for some events, whether of height (an advantage for the wheelchair basketball or table tennis player) or of body mass (important in throwing and lifting events). Data from disabled competitors can thus provide only limited guidance on either likely training responses or the minimum exercise prescription needed for the cardiorespiratory health of an average disabled patient.

A further variable influencing physical capacity is lifestyle. For a person with an acquired disability, exercise and nutritional habits prior to onset of the disorder are important, whereas for those with congenital disability, the lifestyle of the family members and their attitudes toward the child are critical. Any training-induced advantage of aerobic power is quickly lost if the disability requires a period of hospitalization, but regression of skeletal and cardiac muscle occurs more slowly. Some advantage may persist from vigorous exercise undertaken before hospital admission. The physiological characteristics and athletic performance of outstanding competitors may thus reflect not the impact of postmorbid training, which has been carefully quantitated by the investigator, but rather the more general influence of an active lifestyle in earlier years.

Potential of the Inactive Individual

Because of the confounding influences of a possible constitutional advantage or an earlier interest in vigorous physical activity, one must accept with caution suggestions by some researchers (Guttmann, 1976b; Jochheim & Strohkendl, 1973; Spira, 1967a, 1967b) that observations on the elite wheelchair performer provide a measure of the ultimate adaptation that a disabled person who is inactive could achieve, given sufficiently rigorous athletic preparation.

In our recent experiments, 24 weeks of rigorous training took initially inactive spinally disabled subjects no more than halfway toward the peak cardiac output and aerobic power scores seen in top-level wheelchair athletes (G.M. Davis & Shephard, 1988). Although some of the residual disadvantage might have been made good by more prolonged conditioning, it seems unlikely that this would have abolished all of the discrepancy.

Advantages of a Longitudinal Training Experiment

The typical longitudinal training experiment takes a group of relatively untrained subjects and follows changes in their physical condition over either a normal season of athletic training or a comparable 3- to 6-month period of regular exercise in the laboratory. Motivation is generally greater for normal athletic participation, but it is more difficult to quantitate the amount of training undertaken. Laboratory training makes heavy demands on equipment, space, and personnel, so that periods of observation are sometimes as short as 8 to 10 weeks; this is probably sufficient time for the regulatory changes of training to develop (e.g., increases in venous tone), but it is unlikely to allow substantial hypertrophy of either cardiac or skeletal muscle.

The main advantage of laboratory training (e.g., using a forearm ergometer) is that one can obtain a very precise measure of the frequency, intensity, and duration of exercise that is undertaken, together with a clear assessment of the total work performed. In the able-bodied person, controlled laboratory experiments have demonstrated that the two main determinants of aerobic training response are the intensity of effort and the initial fitness of the individual (Shephard, 1969b); nevertheless, in older individuals a training response is eventually achieved with the regular practice of low-intensity exercise (Sidney & Shephard, 1978).

The main difficulty when organizing a longitudinal study is to develop and sustain the motivation of participants. Repeated visits to a laboratory can be boring and may also present those who are wheelchair confined with considerable problems in arranging the necessary transportation. It is thus difficult to recruit a sizable study population, and once the required number of subjects has been recruited, much effort must be expended in sustaining their interest and reducing the dropout rate.

The Spinally Injured

The previous chapter briefly discussed much of the data pertaining to cross-sectional comparisons between spinally injured athletes and their inactive peers. However, we may make some additional comments on the basis of observations on both able-bodied and disabled groups.

Cardiorespiratory Fitness

In able-bodied normal individuals, the endurance competitor demonstrates a somewhat lower maximum heart rate (5-10 beats/min), a 20 to 30% advantage of peak power and oxygen intake (sometimes a larger difference in top competitors), and an increased tolerance of submaximal effort (Shephard, 1977).

In cross-sectional comparisons among a disabled sample, G.M. Davis and Shephard (1988) found no differences of arm ergometer peak heart rates between wheelchair athletes and inactive individuals; however, the athletes had a 57% larger maximum power output, a 34% longer endurance time, a 44% greater peak oxygen intake, and a 53% larger maximum respiratory minute volume than the inactive group (see Table 6.1). At each of the selected submaximum steady-state heart rates, the wheelchair athletes also showed a 38 to 44% larger cardiac stroke volume than the inactive subjects and a correspondingly smaller arteriovenous oxygen difference (see Table 6.2). There was also a suggestion ($p < 0.1$) of greater mechanical efficiency in the active group.

Some authors have attempted to establish five-category norms of aerobic fitness for the able-bodied population (Åstrand & Rodahl, 1977; K.H. Cooper, 1968b). Kofsky et al. (1986) proposed similar tables for the wheelchair disabled. She collected data on a broadly recruited sample of 163 male and 97 female paraplegics and divided scores for the predicted peak oxygen intake of both athletes and inactive subjects into five categories based on their distribution relative to the population means (poor, -3.0 to -1.8 SD; below average, -1.8 to -0.6 SD; average -0.6 to $+0.6$ SD; above average, $+0.6$ to $+1.8$ SD; and excellent, $+1.8$ to

Table 6.1 Physiological Responses to Maximal Forearm Ergometer Exercise in Wheelchair-Disabled Males With Highly Active and Less Active Lifestyle Patterns

Physiological response	Highly active group (n = 15)		Less active group (n = 15)	
Peak power output* (W)	97.1	± 6.3	61.7	± 5.2
Endurance time* (min)	13.3	± 0.8	9.9	± 0.5
Peak heart rate (b/min)	181.7	± 4	183.0	± 3
Peak oxygen intake* (L/min STPD)	2.24	± 0.41	1.56	± 0.09
Peak respiratory minute volume* (L/min BTPS)	105.6	± 5.6	68.8	± 4.1
Peak tidal volume* (ml/breath)	1830	± 116	1361	± 96

Note. Based on data from *Cardiovascular Fitness and Muscle Strength in Lower Limb Disabled Males* by G.M. Davis, 1985, Doctoral dissertation, University of Toronto and "Cardio-respiratory Fitness in Highly Active Versus Less Active Paraplegics" by G.M. Davis and R.J. Shephard, 1988, *Medicine and Science in Sports and Exercise*, **20**, 463-468.

Values are means ± *SE.* *$p < .05$ highly active vs. less active.

Table 6.2 Physiological Responses to Submaximal Arm Ergometer Exercise in Wheelchair-Disabled Males With Highly Active and Less Active Lifestyle Patterns

Submaximal power output	Highly active group (n = 15)	Less active group (n = 15)
Power output I (mean heart rate = 115 b/min)		
Loading (W)	42.9 ± 5.2	21.9 ± 4.1
Oxygen intake (L/min STPD)	1.03 ± 0.07	0.69 ± 0.06
Stroke volume (ml)	79 ± 4	55 ± 3
Cardiac output (L/min)	9.1 ± 0.4	6.3 ± 0.3
Arteriovenous O_2 extraction (ml/L)	113 ± 7	108 ± 6
Power output II (mean heart rate = 132 b/min)		
Loading (W)	62.7 ± 5.6	35.9 ± 3.6
Oxygen intake (L/min STPD)	1.30 ± 0.11	0.88 ± 0.06
Stroke volume (ml)	80 ± 4	56 ± 2
Cardiac output (L/min)	10.3 ± 0.5	7.4 ± 0.3
Arteriovenous O_2 extraction (ml/L)	126 ± 7	119 ± 5
Power output III (mean heart rate = 152 b/min)		
Loading (W)	78.4 ± 6.0	50.5 ± 3.6
Oxygen intake (L/min)	1.54 ± 0.11	1.10 ± 0.06
Stroke volume (ml)	76 ± 3	55 ± 3
Cardiac output (L/min)	11.2 ± 0.5	8.4 ± 0.4
Arteriovenous O_2 extraction (ml/L)	137 ± 6	131 ± 4

Note. Based on data from Davis, 1985 and Davis and Shephard, 1988 (see note to Table 6.1).

$*p < .05$ highly active vs. less active.

Table 6.3   Normative Values for Maximum Oxygen Intake (ml/kg • min) in the Wheelchair Disabled

Fitness level (SD)	Females	Elite males	General male population
Poor (−3.0 to −1.8)	<5.4	<17.2	<10.5
Below average (−1.8 to −0.6)	5.4 − 16.2	17.2 − 31.5	10.5 − 21.9
Average (−0.6 to +0.6)	16.3 − 27.1	31.6 − 45.9	22.0 − 33.4
Above average (+0.6 to +1.8)	27.2 − 38.0	46.0 − 60.3	33.5 − 44.9
Excellent (+1.8 to +3.0)	>38.0	>60.3	>44.9

Note. Based on data from "Fitness Classification Tables for Lower-Limb Disabled Individuals" by P.R. Kofsky, R.J. Shephard, G.M. Davis, and R.W. Jackson, 1986, in C. Sherrill (Ed.), *Sport and Disabled Athletes* (pp. 147-156). Champaign, IL: Human Kinetics.

+3.0 *SD*). In general, the men had a 28% advantage of relative aerobic power over the women (see Table 6.3). Moreover, the male elite performers had a significant 14% advantage over their recreationally active counterparts, but in women the elite and recreational performers did not differ significantly.

As the advantage of the elite men over the recreational group was seen throughout the respective distribution curves for the two categories of individual, the researchers thought it reflected mainly the influence of athletic selection, a factor currently more important among the men than among the women. The residual difference (between inactive subjects and the recreationally active group) provides a fairer measure of the usual training response. This amounted to an average of 34% in men and 44% in women—a figure not dissimilar to that seen in comparisons between the recreationally active and very sedentary able-bodied subjects (Shephard, 1977).

Muscular Fitness

Although able-bodied subjects can induce a considerable development of both isometric and isokinetic force through participation in specific muscle-strengthening programs, the response of the skeletal muscles to endurance training is usually more modest; indeed, endurance training that involves largely the legs can lead to some weakening of the arm muscles (Hellerstein, 1977), possibly because of a high daily energy expenditure and the protein needs of developing leg muscles.

A larger relative difference of arm strength between active and inactive individuals might be anticipated among the wheelchair disabled than among the able-bodied, as many wheelchair sports competitions involve rapid and forceful movements of the trunk and upper limbs rather than sustained bouts of endurance work. Both isokinetic and isometric data confirm this anticipation. Relative to inactive controls, the active disabled subjects show advantages of peak moment, peak power, average power, and work per contraction during isokinetic testing, although in percentage terms the endurance dropoff score with repeated submaximal contractions does not differ from that seen in inactive individuals (Davis et al., 1986).

Kofsky et al. (1986) categorized the total upper body isometric strength (N/kg) of the disabled separately for females, elite male competitors, and the general male population. The men were 35% stronger than the women on this index of muscular development. Elite performers had an advantage of isometric upper body strength over the general disabled population of the same sex, 23% in men and 17% in women.

Longitudinal Training

The following discussion examines specificity of training; the threshold intensity of activity inducing a response; the efficacy of wheelchair, arm ergometer, swimming, and other training programs; and resultant physiological changes, including gains of stroke volume, cardiac output, peripheral blood flow, muscle strength, balance, and agility. Studies of the able-bodied show a considerable specificity of training response. For example, only 50% of the gains from leg ergometer training are transferable to the performance of arm work, whereas arm ergometer training has almost no influence on the subsequent response to leg work (Clausen et al., 1973). Likewise, gains of muscle force induced by isometric training tend to be specific to the joint angle at which training has been undertaken.

When considering the conditioning of the disabled, authors have discussed the relative merits of specific (wheelchairlike) training versus less specific forms of cardiorespiratory stimulation. Those concerned with increasing the mobility of the spinally injured note important differences of limb position, mechanical efficiency, and patterns of neuromuscular recruitment between wheelchair propulsion and such alternative forms of activity as forearm cranking, swimming, or weight training (Coutts, Rhodes, & McKenzie, 1983; Getman, Greninger, & Molnar, 1968; Glaser et al., 1979, 1981; Marwick, 1984; McCafferty & Horvath, 1977; Rhodes et al., 1981; Steadward, 1980); they have thus argued that exercise in a wheelchair provides the best form of conditioning.

On the other hand, there does seem some generalization of response from forearm cranking to wheelchair performance. In practice, much depends on the motivation and skill of the wheelchair user. Normal wheelchair ambulation provides little training stimulus for the cardiovascular system, but high-speed road work and participation in vigorous basketball games plainly provide an excellent form of conditioning. The main obstacles to novel forms of training include fear of unusual activities, technical difficulties (e.g., poor balance, difficulty of flotation in water, lack of vision or hearing, or poor comprehension), venous pooling, and associated disorders (e.g., blindness or peripheral vascular disease).

The forearm ergometer can serve as an effective means of cardiac conditioning in young, well-muscled, and well-motivated able-bodied subjects (Simmons & Shephard, 1971a). However, its use with paraplegics has been criticized on the basis that gains of fitness are inconsistent (Hjeltnes, 1980; McDonnell, Brassard,

& Taylor, 1980), a very limited response being observed in patients with a major restriction upon usable muscle mass (Huang, McEachran, Kuhlmeier, DeVivo, & Fine, 1983; Stoboy & Wilson-Rich, 1971). Typical training responses to the various possible forms of exercise are summarized in Tables 6.4 and 6.5.

Training Threshold

Many researchers have discussed the optimum of frequency, intensity, and duration of exercise needed to induce a training response in able-bodied individuals (Crews & Roberts, 1976; C.T.M. Davies & Knibbs, 1971; Fox, Bartels, Billings, O'Brien, Bason, & Matthews, 1975; Pollock, 1973; Shephard, 1969b). A common and effective recommendation to improve the cardiorespiratory condition of an average sedentary person is that the individual undertake four or five 30-minute sessions of exercise per week at 60 to 70% of his or her personal maximum oxygen intake. If participation is less frequent or of shorter duration, the training response is less, significantly less if the subject participates in fewer than three sessions per week or cuts the length of sessions to less than 20 minutes. However, if training is serious and is pursued to the point where muscle glycogen depletion or subclinical injury may be anticipated, a strong case can be made for alternating heavy and light training days in order to allow replenishment of carbohydrate reserves and repair of microtraumata (Shephard, 1977, 1982b).

Remarkably few guidelines are available for designing an effective program for the lower-limb disabled. However, as the arm muscles are much smaller than those in the legs, the margin between an intensity that provides an effective cardiorespiratory stimulus and that which causes signs of local overtraining is probably smaller than in an able-bodied person who uses the lower limbs as the main source of conditioning.

The threshold intensity of activity needed to initiate an endurance training response does not seem to be substantially changed because the exercise is performed with the arms rather than the legs. Nevertheless, in able-bodied individuals the oxygen cost per unit of external work is 25 to 33% greater for arm ergometry than for leg ergometry (Bevegard et al., 1966; Fardy, Webb, & Hellerstein, 1976; Franklin et al., 1983; Shephard et al., 1988; Stenberg et al., 1967); this is due mainly to the added energy cost of stabilizing the trunk during arm exercise. Thus, the same training stimulus is derived from a lower ergometer power output when using the arms. On the other hand, the heart rate needed to induce cardiorespiratory training in the able-bodied (70-80% of the maximum heart rate, corresponding to 60-70% of maximum oxygen intake) is much the same for arm and for leg exercise (Fardy, Webb, & Hellerstein, 1977; Franklin et al., 1983; Vander et al., 1984).

The training threshold for a disabled person remains more controversial. Some authors argue that disabled subjects can tolerate a greater intensity of arm exercise than the able-bodied, partly because the disabled are accustomed to performing work with the arms (and thus have a high mechanical efficiency) and partly because they have learned to distribute the oxygen cost of activity more widely than in an able-bodied person (additional effort is expended to stabilize the trunk and a wider range of the available arm muscles contribute to propulsive movements). Both a high work rate and a high heart rate might thus be essential to augment the training of a disabled athlete.

Other authors, probably working with a less active sample of the disabled population, have found a training response when subjects have used only 50 to 60% of the heart rate reserve that separates resting from maximal heart rate (Jochheim & Strohkendl, 1973); participants in these latter studies were previously almost totally inactive, so that exercise at even 50% of the heart rate reserve was a new experience for them. Such grossly detrained persons tolerate effort poorly and have corresponding difficulty initiating the prolonged and repeated exercise sessions needed for effective rehabilitation. Voight and Bahn (1969) suggested that in individuals with high-level lesions, the effective muscle mass was very limited, and it became fatigued too quickly to allow any effective training response.

The Efficacy of Training

In the able-bodied, normal daily activity is probably an important determinant of physical condition. Among large population samples, differences in maximum oxygen intake of as much as 30% have been demonstrated between the most active and the least active quintiles of the community (Bailey, Shephard, & Mirwald, 1976).

Wheelchair Training

Are there similar, activity-related differences among the disabled? Although no formal measurements are available, the wheelchair marathon competitor who moves at 25 km/hr probably develops an oxygen consumption of at least 3 L/min. On the other hand, most wheelchair users move very slowly (3-5 km/hr); despite a lower mechanical efficiency than the marathoner, they thus derive little stimulus from habitual daily activity (Greenway et al., 1970; Grimby, 1980; Nilsson et al., 1975). Stoboy, Rich, and Lee (1971) found an average energy expenditure of 43 ± 5 watts during normal ambulation, this corresponding to an oxygen consumption of 800 ml/min. Possible factors that influence the impact of wheelchair ambulation upon physical condition include not only the usual speed of operation, but also age, initial fitness level, skill in operation of the wheelchair, and any added energy costs due to the "wasted" movements of spasticity or clonus (Gordon & Vanderwalle, 1956).

Endurance Training

Engel and Hildebrandt (1973) suggested that ordinary wheelchair ambulation not only failed to improve physical condition but in many instances was not even of sufficient vigor to maintain it. Nevertheless, the same authors showed that deliberate vigorous wheelchair activity could have a beneficial effect upon physical condition. They noted a 14 to 16% reduction of heart rate during submaximal exercise among 13 paraplegic men who undertook a planned regimen of vigorous

Table 6.4 Exercise Training of Physically Disabled Subjects: Submaximal Cardiorespiratory Responses

Authors (year)	Group (n)		Type of training (weeks)	Power output	Heart rate initial (b/min)	% Change	Oxygen intake initial (L/min)	% Change
Ekblöm & Lundberg[b] (1968)	CP	(8)	WERG, CAL	15.3	153	nc	0.76	nc
	P	(10)	WERG, CAL	26.0	157	-11	0.70	-10
Engel & Hildebrandt[c] (1973)	P	(13)	WERG @ 2 km/h	0°	118	-14		
				1°	130	-15		
				2°	146	-16		
Knuttsson et al. (1973)	P	(10)	ARC	40.2[a]	170	nc		
Pollock et al. (1974)[j]	AB	(11)	ARC	50 – 130	118	-6		
	P	(8)	ARC	50 – 130	165	-16		
Bar-Or et al.[b] (1976)	CP	(17)	CAL & sports games	24.5	121	-10		
	P	(17)		24.5	127	nc		
Hjeltnes[c] (1980)	CP	(8)	WT, ARC, sports games, & swimming	low	100	-10	0.65	nc
				heavy	112	nc	0.81	nc
	P	(14)		low	135	-19	0.88	nc
				heavy	175	-14	1.18	nc

Study			Program						
Glaser et al.[cd]	AB	(6)	Interval WERG	(5)	4.9	98	-10	0.42	-17
					9.8	106	-13	0.51	-16
					14.7	115	-15	0.57	-10
					19.6	125	-14	0.70	-12
					24.5	141	-16	0.85	-13
Miles et al. (1982)	P	(8)	Interval WERG at 3.5 km/h	(6)	10.0			0.58	nc
					20.0			0.75	nc
					30.0			0.91	nc

Note. Based on data from Davis, 1985 (see note to Table 6.1). Values are for male subjects unless otherwise noted. P = paraplegia, CP = cerebral palsy, AB = able-bodied, CAL = mixed calisthenics, ARC = forearm cranking, WERG = wheelchair ergometry, WT = weight training, nc = no change. [a]Increased by 41 W after training. [b]Subjects were male and female students aged 14-24 years. [c]Values estimated from figures. [d]Subjects were female.

Table 6.5　Exercise Training of Physically Disabled Subjects: Maximal Cardiorespiratory Responses

Authors (year)	Group (n)	Type of training	(weeks)	Peak power Initial (W)	Gain %	Peak O$_2$ intake Initial (L/min)	Gain %	Peak respiratory minute volume Initial (L/min)	Gain %
Ekblöm & Lundberg[a] (1968)	P (7)	WERG, CAL	(6)	53.5	+21	1.09	nc		
Pollock et al. (1974)	AB (11)	ARC	(20)			1.93	+37	97.0	+28
	P (8)	ARC	(20)			1.88	+19	96.7	+22
Nilsson et al.[b] (1975)	P (7)	ARC & WT	(7)	100	+31	1.88	+11		
Bar-Or et al.[b] (1976)	CP (17)	CAL & sports games	(52)			1.42	+8	45.8	nc
	P (17)					1.09	nc	35.4	nc
Hjeltnes (1980)	TP (8)	WT, ARC & Swimming	(12)	30.0	+33	0.84	nc	35.0	nc
	P (14)			80.0	+50	1.32	+30	68.0	+18
Miles et al. (1982)	P (8)	Interval WERG	(8)	78.3	+31	2.19	+26	99.6	+32
DiCarlo et al. (1983)	TP (4)	ARC	(5)	68.6	+55	0.90	+67		
Ornstein et al. (1983)	Mixed (6)	Swimming	(8)			1.32	nc		
Hjeltnes[c] (1984)	TP (7)	ARC	(16)	20.8	nc	0.70	+24	38.1	nc
	T$_1$-T$_6$ (9)	ARC	(16)	45.9	+56	1.01	+32	49.5	+15
	T$_7$-L$_2$ (23)	ARC	(16)	71.8	+46	1.34	+33	62.9	+11
	L$_2$-S$_2$ (7)	ARC	(16)	79.4	+50	1.49	+26	63.6	+23

Note. Based on data from Davis, 1985 (see note to Table 6.1). Values are for male subjects unless otherwise noted. P = paraplegia, TP = tetraplegia, CP = cerebral palsy, AB = able-bodied, CAL = mixed calisthenics, ARC = forearm cranking, WERG = wheelchair ergometry, WT = weight training, nc = no change. [a,b]Subjects were male and female students aged 14-24 years. [a]Subjects aged 14-24 years. [b]Values estimated from figures. [c]Values estimated from figures.

daily wheelchair exercise. After 14 weeks of such training, the subjects also demonstrated a 9 to 15% decrease in the oxygen cost of operating the wheelchair on the treadmill, suggesting an improvement of mechanical efficiency.

Wheelchair basketball offers a more effective training stimulus than normal ambulation, both the intensity and the duration of activity required by this sport falling within the generally accepted training zone. Burke et al. (1985) suggested that a typical game demanded an average energy expenditure of 36 kJ/min, 77% of peak oxygen intake for their sample of subjects.

Dreisinger (1978) prescribed a more controlled program of endurance training for a group of paraplegics, using a wheelchair ergometer. Sessions were at what might be judged a minimum effective frequency and duration for a conditioning response (20 minutes, 3 times per week). Nevertheless, Dreisinger demonstrated an increase of peak power output and peak oxygen intake over 8 weeks of such activity, compared with a small decrease of aerobic performance in a control group of disabled individuals who were followed for a similar period.

Interval Training

Interval training can be used to develop both aerobic and anaerobic performance. A typical plan is that of Miles, Sawka, Wilde, Durbin, Gotshall, & Glaser (1982): Aerobic sessions comprised two 10-minute bouts of wheelchair ergometry at 80% of the individual's heart rate reserve, with an intervening 5-minute rest period to allow clearance of anaerobic metabolites. Anaerobic sessions consisted of four 2-minute exercise bouts at 95% of heart rate reserve, separated by 2-minute recovery intervals.

Glaser et al. (1978a) applied a similar wheelchair ergometer interval training protocol for 5 weeks. Initially inactive subjects showed a 20% increase of power output with a decrease of heart rate during submaximal exercise, but much of these two changes was apparently due to an improvement of mechanical efficiency, as the researchers observed a parallel decrease of oxygen intake at any given intensity of submaximum effort. A second investigation (Glaser et al., 1981) used female subjects. Again, there were parallel reductions in the oxygen cost and heart rate response to fixed work rates over 5 weeks of training, which suggested that much of the observed gain in performance was due to an improvement of mechanical efficiency rather than of cardiorespiratory conditioning.

However, a greater mechanical efficiency is not always the explanation for improved physical performance. For instance, Miles et al. (1982) carried out a program of interval training on a group of eight initially active wheelchair basketball players. In this group, there was no change in the response to submaximum exercise over the period of conditioning, and one must thus conclude that the mechanical efficiency of ergometer operation remained unchanged. Nevertheless, the peak oxygen intake and the peak respiratory minute volume increased by 26% and 32%, respectively, over the course of an 8-week training program that was at the threshold of effectiveness in terms of the frequency of exercise (three sessions per week).

We must thus accept that although some of the improved wheelchair performance that follows endurance or interval training is due to mechanically more efficient patterns of movement, if the intensity, frequency, and duration of wheel-chair activity are appropriate, it is also possible to induce a true cardiorespiratory training effect.

Forearm Ergometer Training: Advantages of Ergometer

The cycle ergometer has several advantages as a laboratory training tool. The task is well standardized and easily understood by most subjects, the rate of limb movement can be controlled, and the amount of work performed in any one training session is easy to quantitate. Moreover, most people have ridden a bicycle before. There is thus little anxiety or test learning when operating a laboratory cycle ergometer. Finally, the equipment is relatively compact, and it can be transported to a patient's place of residence (Hook, 1971; Marincek & Valencic, 1978).

The advantages become less clear-cut when an able-bodied individual is required to perform arm work. The forearm ergometer is plainly not as specific a method of training as is vigorous wheelchair operation (Getman et al., 1968). The task of arm cranking is initially unfamiliar, and the mechanical efficiency of movement may increase with test learning. Moreover, the relationship between oxygen consumption and power output is relatively complex when the arms are used to operate the machine, as the volume of active muscle increases progressively with ergometer loading. Finally, researchers are uncertain as to how far any observed training responses reflect local muscular conditioning rather than a true cardiorespiratory training effect (Clausen et al., 1973), particularly if the same device is used to induce training and to measure the body's response. When arm crank ergometer training has been applied to able-bodied subjects, the performance of arm work has improved, but there has often been little generalization of this response to cardiorespiratory function and thus the performance of leg exercise (for example, in the studies of Clausen, Trap-Jensen, & Lassen, 1970; Clausen et al., 1973; Magel et al., 1975; but not in those of Tahamont et al., 1986).

Possible explanations of the localized, limb-specific nature of the arm training response include (a) involvement of a smaller muscle mass than in leg work, (b) a limitation of arm work by peripheral factors such as local muscle strength and a resultant local limitation of perfusion rather than by the pumping ability of the heart, (c) poorer initial motor unit recruitment patterns (with a correspondingly greater scope for improvement), or (d) lower initial concentrations of aerobic enzymes in the arm muscles (Brooks & Fahey, 1984; Magel et al., 1975). These various factors allow more peripheral adaptation in the active tissues than would be likely with a comparable intensity of leg training. Nevertheless, there is some possibility of a generalization of training response within the working limbs, in that arm ergometer training can condition the upper limbs for wheelchair activity.

Gains of Oxygen Transport and Power Output

Aerobic conditioning is demonstrated most convincingly by an increase in the directly measured peak oxygen intake. However, if we are to accept this measure of training, we must critically evaluate whether a central, cardiovascular limitation of oxygen transport has been achieved. This is harder to demonstrate for arm than for leg work. Accepted criteria for a central limitation of leg exercise include an oxygen consumption plateau (an increased oxygen consumption of less than 2 ml/kg • min for a further small increase of work rate), a peak heart rate that is close to the age-related maximum value, a respiratory gas exchange ratio of 1.10 or more, and a peak arterial blood lactate concentration of 10 to 11 mmol/L observed 2 to 4 minutes after the end of peak effort.

Except in athletes who have used their arms a great deal (e.g., swimmers or kayakers), peak arm effort tends to show the characteristics of peripheral, muscular limitation rather than central, cardiovascular limitation, with complaints of local weakness and muscular fatigue rather than breathlessness, faintness, and poor coordination. An oxygen plateau is difficult to demonstrate during all-out arm work. The peak heart rate may also be much less than for leg work, and because of the small volume of active muscle in the arms, increases of respiratory gas exchange ratio and blood lactate concentration are relatively small. Improved aerobic performance after a period of arm conditioning could thus reflect a strengthening of the arm and shoulder muscles and a lessening of the various peripheral constraints upon performance, rather than a true cardiovascular conditioning (Shephard, 1977, 1982b).

Whether the subject performs arm or leg exercise, a second indication of cardiorespiratory training is provided by a decrease of heart rate during submaximal exercise, with an increase of both the physical working capacity at a heart rate of 170 beats/min (PWC_{170}) and the maximum oxygen intake as predicted by the Åstrand nomogram. However, if we estimate oxygen consumption from the power output rather than measure it directly, we can misinterpret a gain of mechanical efficiency as an increase of aerobic power. Likewise, if the subject is anxious during the initial evaluation, habituation to the laboratory environment may give a decrease of heart rate during submaximal exercise and a misleading impression of the extent of aerobic conditioning (Shephard, 1969a).

Knuttson et al. (1973) reported that the PWC_{170} of wheelchair-confined subjects increased by 16.5 watts (41%) after 6 weeks of forearm ergometer interval training at heart rates of 140 to 180 beats/min. However, the researchers did not measure oxygen consumption in these experiments, and an unknown portion of the apparent gain in aerobic power could thus represent an improvement of mechanical efficiency.

Pollock et al. (1974) found that experienced users of wheelchairs increased their directly measured peak oxygen intake by 19% over 20 weeks of forearm ergometer training. Although this was a gratifying response, with considerable implications for the quality of daily life, it was nevertheless less than the 37% gain shown by a control sample of able-bodied peers who undertook a similar training program. Pollock et al. (1974) suggested that the able-bodied group showed a greater aerobic conditioning response than the disabled subjects for three main reasons: (a) the able-bodied subjects were able to use their leg and trunk muscles to a greater extent when stabilizing the body and thus had a greater potential to increase the involvement of accessory muscles at the second test, (b) because they were initially unfamiliar with techniques for vigorous use of the forearms, the able-bodied subjects had greater opportunity to learn new trick movements to maximize effort, and (c) the able-bodied began training with a lesser peripheral oxygen extraction than their disabled peers (many of whom were accustomed to vigorous arm activity and had above-average initial development of their upper limbs).

In a further study focusing primarily on cellular changes, Taylor, McDonnell, & Brassard (1986) had five active male paraplegics undertake 8 weeks of arm ergometer training (30 minutes 5 times per week at 80% of maximum heart rate). The researchers observed gains of both peak oxygen consumption and peak work rate; moreover, postexercise blood lactate levels remained unchanged, showing that the improved performance reflected an improvement of cardiorespiratory performance rather than an increase of motivation with more willingness to accept an oxygen debt.

Although some spinally injured athletes have put great effort into maximizing the potential working capacity of their residual muscles, other people with similar injuries have been content to live very sheltered and dependent lives. Resultant interindividual differences in initial fitness levels greatly complicate the interpretation of training experiments. Perhaps because the subjects concerned started from a relatively low fitness baseline or learned for the first time ways of developing vigorous arm effort, some studies of the spinally injured have reported substantial gains of oxygen intake after quite short periods of training. Nilsson et al. (1975) found a 12% increase of peak oxygen intake and a 31% gain of physical work capacity over 7 weeks of combined forearm conditioning and weight training, and DiCarlo et al. (1983) found a 67% increase of peak oxygen intake and a 55% increase of peak power in four tetraplegics over only 5 weeks of forearm cranking (30-minute sessions at 60-80% of maximal heart rate).

The intensity of effort relative to the subject's initial level of fitness seems to be the immediate determinant of training response (Shephard, 1969b, 1977). However, if a certain minimum intensity of training is achieved repeatedly over a substantial period of weeks, the crucial factor in developing maximum oxygen intake ultimately becomes the total quantity of work that has been performed, rather than the intensity of effort (American College of Sports Medicine, 1978).

G.M. Davis (1985) attempted to compare the effectiveness of different intensities and durations of exercise in a small sample of paraplegics who were followed over 24 weeks of forearm ergometer training. Three exercise sessions of 20 (S) or 40 (L) minutes duration were undertaken each week at 50% (L) or 70% (H) of the individual's peak oxygen intake. It was thought that the lower intensity of exercise would lie below the training threshold, and the higher intensity would be above it (Davies & Knibbs, 1971; Hollmann & Venrath, 1962; Karvonen, Kentala, & Mustala, 1957; Shephard, 1977). The duration of the individual training sessions was based on common prescribing practices for the able-bodied (E.L. Fox, 1984). Unfortunately, G.M. Davis was somewhat limited in his conclusions by a small initial sample size and a substantial number of dropouts over the 24 weeks of training. Nevertheless, the HL group showed a progressive improvement of endurance time (increases of 31%, 45%, and 57% at 8, 16, and 24 weeks, respectively).

Moreover, the HL, HS, and LL groups all showed significant gains of peak oxygen intake (see Table 6.6); these were first apparent after 8 weeks of training, and after 24 weeks the gains had increased to an average of 0.32 L/min, or 21%. Changes in the HL and LL groups were significantly greater than in LS or control subjects, but by 16 and 24 weeks all four exercised groups had higher scores than the control subjects. Moreover, as in cross-sectional studies (Engel &

Table 6.6 Changes in Physiological Response of Paraplegic Subjects to Maximal Forearm Ergometer Exercise Over 24 Weeks of Arm Ergometer Training

Physiological response	Duration of training			
	0 Weeks	8 Weeks	16 Weeks	24 Weeks
Endurance time (min)				
C	9.8 ± 0.4	12.0 ± 0.8	11.0 ± 0.8	11.0 ± 0.7
HL	9.7 ± 1.3	12.7 ± 0.7	14.1 ± 1.0	15.2 ± 0.7
HS	8.5 ± 1.5	11.0 ± 0.7	—	12.3 ± 0.7
LL	12.6 ± 0.9	13.7 ± 1.1	14.0 ± 1.2	14.7 ± 1.7
LS	8.0 ± 0.1	10.3 ± 0.9	—	—
Peak oxygen intake (L/min STPD)				
C	1.66 ± 0.15	1.71 ± 0.12	1.48 ± 0.11	1.54 ± 0.17
HL	1.61 ± 0.07	1.87 ± 0.10	1.91 ± 0.06	1.85 ± 0.05
HS	1.35 ± 1.00	1.57 ± 0.04	—	1.54 ± 0.11
LL	1.51 ± 0.11	1.82 ± 0.13	1.95 ± 0.21	2.03 ± 0.35
LS	1.20 ± 0.10	1.29 ± 0.16	—	—
Peak respiratory minute volume (L/min BTPS)				
C	84.4 ± 10.2	93.6 ± 10.4	81.2 ± 11.6	86.7 ± 15.4
HL	94.4 ± 7.0	110.6 ± 9.4	106.4 ± 8.3	111.3 ± 8.7
HS	66.5 ± 7.8	75.1 ± 2.7	—	73.3 ± 1.6
LL	91.4 ± 8.9	106.2 ± 7.6	106.5 ± 10.1	105.9 ± 11.7
LS	72.5 ± 14.9	79.1 ± 13.0	—	—

Note. Subjects conformed to one of 5 regimens: control (C), high intensity/prolonged (HL), high intensity-short (HS), low intensity/prolonged (LL), or low intensity/short (LS) training. Based on data from Davis, 1985 and Davis and Shephard, in press (see note to Table 6.1).

Hildebrandt, 1973; Glaser et al., 1981; Zwiren & Bar-Or, 1975) and other longitudinal observations (DiCarlo et al., 1983; Hjeltnes, 1980; Pollock et al., 1974), training increased the power output at each of the three submaximum heart rates in groups HL, LL, and HS but left it unchanged in LS or control.

A further important variable in arm cranking is the rate of arm movement. Some authors have used quite slow rates (40-50 rpm) as might be adopted in leg ergometry, but this requires the relatively weak arm muscles to develop a very large force, resulting in early fatigue. G.M. Davis (1985) adopted a crank rate of 80 rpm in order to minimize this problem. Hardison, Israel, and Somes (1987) also argued for a cranking rate of 70 rpm on the basis that this minimized the perceived exertion for a given oxygen consumption, thus encouraging adherence to the training program.

Swimming

Swimming has traditionally been a popular sport for the lower-limb disabled, as satisfactory propulsion can be achieved in the absence of any major contribution from the lower limbs (N. Croucher, 1976; Rathbone & Lucas, 1970). DiRocco (1986) also commended tethered swimming, arguing that those unable to exercise to an adequate training intensity on land might nevertheless accomplish effective training with the buoyancy support and greater cardiovascular efficiency of the horizontal posture.

Pachalski and Mekarski (1980) claimed dramatic improvements in a fitness index based on resting heart rate, vital capacity, and apnea index when 60 paraplegics became involved in a 3-year swimming program. In contrast, Ornstein, Skrinar, and Garrett (1983) saw no gains of peak oxygen intake as measured on a forearm ergometer when six previously inactive disabled men undertook 8 weeks of aerobic swimming. As with other types of conditioning, much presumably depends on the intensity of effort and the period for which the program is sustained.

Other Types of Training

A final conditioning option is to encourage participation in such activities as upper-body calisthenics and weight training, along with sports like tennis, basketball, and adapted downhill skiing. These various pursuits have the merit of increasing local kinesthesis; they also appeal to the participant because of their variety, challenge, and perceived relevance to daily life (Marwick, 1984). However, sports participation is less satisfactory from an experimental point of view, as it is difficult to be certain how much training a subject has undertaken. Moreover, because of the need for equipment, facilities, and other participants, it is often difficult to ensure that a disabled person undertakes the minimum frequency of exercise needed to develop a cardiorespiratory conditioning response.

Ekblöm and Lundberg (1968) arranged twice-weekly sessions of calisthenics and wheelchair training for 10 spinally injured paraplegics and eight patients with cerebral palsy. After 6 weeks on this regimen, the sample of paraplegic youths demonstrated an increase of mechanical efficiency on the ergometer, with a 10%

average decrease in the oxygen consumed at a fixed power output; in contrast (and perhaps because they had more difficulty in undertaking sustained training), the cerebral palsy victims showed no improvement of mechanical efficiency. The paraplegic subjects also showed a substantial increase of peak power output (21%), but (in contrast to some of the ergometer studies) no significant gain of peak oxygen intake.

Provided that lesions were below the level of the sixth thoracic vertebra, Knuttson et al. (1973) found a 50% increase in the forearm physical work capacity of spinally injured paraplegics in response to a 6-week conditioning regimen that combined weight training (pulley exercises), calisthenics, and forearm ergometry; however, the researchers observed little or no improvement of cardiorespiratory condition in those patients with spinal lesions above the T6 level.

Bar-Or et al. (1976) obtained somewhat conflicting results on the effectiveness of other types of training. After a year of biweekly sports (low organizational games) and calisthenics that strengthened the arm muscles, 34 subjects with spastic cerebral palsy showed a decreased oxygen cost of submaximum exercise and an average 8% increase of peak oxygen intake. However, a group of poliomyelitic paraplegics who initially were more active showed no response to this pattern of training.

Hjeltnes (1980) applied a combination of daily calisthenics, swimming, weight training, and forearm cranking to 14 spinally injured paraplegic and eight tetraplegic patients, beginning the program 8 to 10 weeks after spinal cord trauma. Over the first 12 weeks of such therapy, peak power output showed a 33% increase in the tetraplegics and a 50% increase in the paraplegics; the latter group also showed a 30% increase of peak oxygen intake and parallel increases of stroke volume. Although the arteriovenous oxygen difference was unchanged by training, blood lactate levels decreased during both light and heavy submaximal exertion, suggesting some improvement of local muscular perfusion. The main criticism of this research is that it is difficult to dissociate the training response from the normal recovery process that might have been anticipated in the first few months following spinal cord injury. A second experiment by the same author (Hjeltnes, 1984) followed a larger sample of 48 lower-limb disabled. Routine physiotherapy was supplemented by daily forearm cranking and wheelchair sports over the first 16 weeks of rehabilitation. Among the paraplegic subjects, age apparently had little influence on the training response, but the author found larger gains of oxygen intake in those who were free of drug, alcohol, and family problems (34%) than in those with such difficulties (19%). The response of the tetraplegic subjects was smaller than that of the paraplegics, even when expressed in percentage terms (a gain of 24%).

We may conclude that other types of training can produce an aerobic response in the wheelchair disabled, provided that the lesion level is not too high, the necessary equipment and facilities are available, and participation is sufficiently vigorous. Relative to regular periods of exercise on a laboratory ergometer, such initiatives seem more likely to sustain long-term motivation and are thus recommended provided the subjects have easy access to the necessary facilities.

Physiological Responses to Training

The prime determinant of maximum oxygen intake is peak cardiac output. We now review methods of measuring cardiac output and discuss the basis of gains in stroke volume in terms of increased preloading of the ventricle, improved contractility, hypertrophy, and reduced afterloading.

Available Technology

Substantial practical difficulties exist in examining changes of peak cardiac output and stroke volume over the course of training. We cannot justify invasive measurements of cardiac output, except in occasional cases in which this information is required for clinical purposes. Most of the noninvasive methods of determining cardiac output have only a limited accuracy and are difficult to apply during exercise. Moreover, one can imagine reasons (such as pooling in the inactive lower limbs) why errors (both random and systematic) might be increased in the disabled relative to an able-bodied group. Two of the more widely used approaches are CO_2 rebreathing and M-mode echocardiography, as discussed next; unfortunately, the latter can only be applied at rest and during isometric effort.

Stroke Volume and Cardiac Output

G.M. Davis et al. (1987) used the CO_2 rebreathing principle to measure cardiac output. In essence, the Fick principle is applied to the elimination of carbon dioxide; the arterial CO_2 content (Ca,co_2) is estimated from expired CO_2, assuming a ventilation dependent spiratory dead space, and the pulmonary venous CO_2 pressure ($C\bar{v},co_2$) is determined from the equilibrium "plateau" established during the rapid rebreathing of a 10 to 15% mixture of CO_2 in oxygen:

$$\text{Cardiac output (L/min)} = \frac{CO_2 \text{ output (ml/min)}}{(C\bar{v},co_2 - Ca,co_2) \text{ (ml/L)}}$$

G.M. Davis et al. (1987) noted that during exercise, the pretraining cardiac output of spinally injured subjects was 1 to 2 L/min less than in able-bodied individuals. Comparing responses before and after training, the researchers found that subjects who followed a high intensity–prolonged or high intensity–short duration training regimen boosted their cardiac outputs by 0.6 to 1.5 L/min at the higher work intensities (heart rates of 132 and 147 beats/min); this response was due mainly to a 6 to 12 ml increase of stroke volume relative to pretraining values (see Figures 6.1 and 6.2).

The average response to conditioning was of a similar order to the 8% gain of stroke volume, cardiac output, and peak oxygen intake described by Simmons and Shephard (1971a) when healthy young men undertook 4 weeks of forearm ergometer training. Because the able-bodied subjects developed a larger stroke volume and larger cardiac output during leg ergometry than during arm work, Simmons and Shephard (1971a, 1971b) argued that during vigorous arm exercise there was initially a substantial limitation of oxygen intake by either inadequate

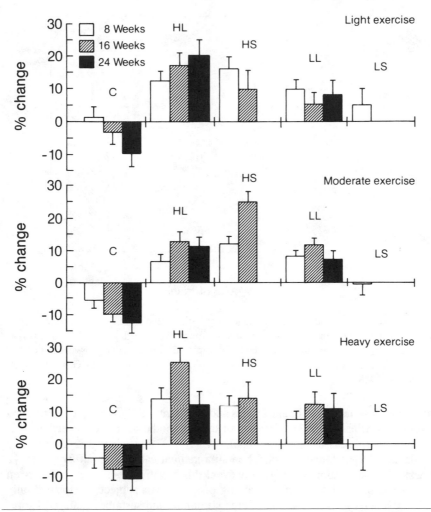

Figure 6.1.   Percent change of stroke volume in control (C), HL, HS, LL, and LS groups after 8, 16, and 24 weeks of training. Top, middle, and lower panels are responses to light (heart rate 115-125 beats/min), moderate (130-140 beats/min), and heavy submaximal (145-155 beats/min) forearm ergometry. Values are mean percent change from initial scores ± *SE*. Based on data of G.M. Davis, 1985 and G.M. Davis & Shephard, 1988.

preloading or excessive afterloading of the ventricles. If blood accumulated in the veins of the legs, this reduced venous return and thus diastolic filling of the ventricles (a reduction of maximum cardiac output due to inadequate preloading). But if the left ventricle had difficulty in expelling blood because the active muscles were contracting at a high percentage of their maximum voluntary force and thus compressing intramuscular blood vessels, the problem would be one of excessive afterloading. Whether a problem of preloading or afterloading, the difficulty was

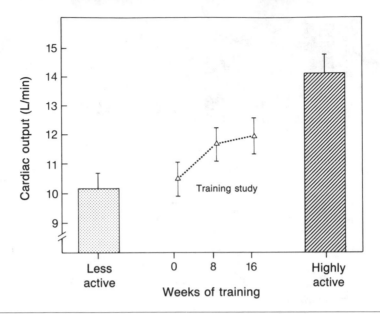

Figure 6.2. Theoretical maximal cardiac output calculated from measured peak oxygen intake and assumed stroke volume as in submaximum effort. Data for highly active versus less active disabled males and for a group of paraplegics followed over 16 weeks of endurance training. Mean ± *SE*. Based on data of G.M. Davis, 1985 and G.M. Davis & Shephard, 1988.

apparently lessened by training. Davies and Sargeant (1974) subsequently reached a similar conclusion. The application of these hypotheses to the wheelchair disabled is next discussed in more detail.

Hjeltnes (1980) found no change in submaximal cardiac output over 6 to 12 weeks of rehabilitation therapy. However, this negative result may have arisen because he used a low intensity training program. His subjects performed only mild calisthenics, as compared with the strenuous and sustained pattern of forearm training adopted by G.M. Davis et al. (1987). Like other investigators, Hjeltnes (1980) observed an increase of stroke volume, although in his experiments this was accompanied by a decrease of exercise heart rate. Other reports confirm increases in stroke volume after the training of disabled individuals (Heigenhauser et al., 1976; Hjeltnes, 1984).

Improved Myocardial Function

Among possible explanations for the improved cardiac performance during vigorous exercise, we may note increased preloading, improved myocardial contractility, ventricular hypertrophy, and decreased afterloading of the left ventricle.

Increased Preloading of the Left Ventricle. According to this scenario, training augments cardiac output through an increase of end-diastolic volume (the classical

Frank-Starling mechanism whereby distention of the ventricle increases the force of contraction and thus the stroke volume of the heart). If venous return were to improve and thus increase end-diastolic volume after training, this would likely represent the combined effects of an increased use of the lower part of the body during movement (a "muscle pump"), a general improvement of venous tone, and a reduction of pooling in the veins of the lower extremities. Evidence to support the hypothesis that training increases preloading of the ventricles has been obtained from tilt-table studies (Corbett et al., 1975; Wolf & Magora, 1976) and experiments in which venous return has been modified by exposing the lower part of the body to varying external counterpressures (Hjeltnes, 1980). In subjects with paralysis of the lower limbs, no change of muscle pumping could be envisaged from paralyzed regions of the body, but an increase of venous tone after training certainly remains possible.

G.M. Davis et al. (1987) had their subjects complete up to 24 weeks of forearm ergometer training. Data were analyzed by M-mode echocardiography; in essence, this technique displays images of the ventricular walls and cavities formed by an oscillating ultrasound generator applied over the heart in the fourth intercostal space. The researchers found no evidence of a training-induced increase of ventricular diameters or end-diastolic volumes either at rest or during isometric exercise (a sustained handgrip at 30% of the individual's maximal grip force). Such data argue somewhat against an increase of venous return, yet the supine or semi-supine position needed to record good quality echocardiograms in itself limits the possibility of demonstrating any improvement of venous tone with training.

Development of a Greater Contractile Force by the Heart Muscle (Increased Myocardial Contractility) or Structural Thickening (Hypertrophy) of the Left Ventricular Wall.   Cross-sectional comparisons in able-bodied subjects show greater end-diastolic ventricular dimensions in trained athletes than in sedentary controls (Gilbert et al., 1977; Morganroth, Maron, Henry, & Epstein, 1975; Zoneraich, Rhee, Zoneraich, Jordon, & Appel, 1977). Longitudinal research clarifies that the increase in heart size and improvement of cardiac function are largely due to training rather than to a constitutional advantage enjoyed by the active individuals (DeMaria, Neumann, Lee, Fowler, & Mason, 1978; Stein, Michielli, Fox, & Krasnow, 1978).

Ehsani, Health, Hagberg, and Schechtman (1981) demonstrated increases of left ventricular diastolic volume and left ventricular mass in able-bodied subjects after only 9 weeks of conditioning, with reversal of these changes over only 3 weeks of deconditioning. Others have argued that improvements of myocardial function occur much more slowly (Wolfe, Cunningham, Rechnitzer, & Nichol, 1979) in response to prolonged and strenuous training (Adams et al., 1981; Frick, Sjogren, Perasalo, & Pajunen, 1970; Perreault et al., 1978).

G.M. Davis et al. (1987) applied the technique of M-mode echocardiography to trained and control spinally injured subjects at rest and during supine isometric exertion. Certain limitations of their echocardiographic technique should immediately be stressed, particularly the assumptions that the interior dimensions of the ventricles as seen in the plane of the echocardiogram can be cubed to provide an estimate of their volumes (Krause, 1981; J.L. Weiss, 1980) and that cardiac fibers contract at the same time and rate not only where observed (at the minor equator of the heart) but at all other points in the ventricle (Bhatt, Isabel-Jones, Villoria, Lendriem, & Harris, 1978; R.H. Cooper, O'Rourke, Karliner, Peterson, & Leopold, 1972; Ruschhaupt, Sodt, Hutcheon, & Arcilla, 1983).

G.M. Davis et al. (1987) noted that over 16 weeks of endurance conditioning the trained group developed a 31% increase in directly measured peak oxygen intake. The final tests also showed a substantially smaller increment of heart rate (9 beats/min) during the sustained isometric handgrip contractions, with a slight reduction of the corresponding diastolic pressure and a marked decrease of the corresponding rate-pressure product (heart rate × systolic blood pressure, a simple estimate of cardiac work rate). However, there were no changes in the echocardiographic diameter or the corresponding estimates of ventricular volumes either at rest or during isometric contraction. Yet the trained group showed a decreased heart rate (and thus an increased stroke volume) for a given cardiac output during the isometric contractions.

Over the 4 months of training, G.M. Davis et al. (1987) saw no substantial evidence of a change in myocardial contractility, based on their measurements at the minor equator of the heart. However, this does not rule out the possibility that such a change would have been demonstrated had it been possible to substitute vigorous ergometer exercise for the handgrip contraction (see Table 6.7). The researchers observed a small and insignificant increase in the mean velocity of circumferential fiber shortening, but fractional shortening and the fraction of the ventricular contents ejected per beat remained unaltered. Thus, there was little evidence of any improvement in myocardial performance. However, given also the substantial decrease of the heart rate-blood pressure product, it seems likely that at any given external power output, the efficiency of the heart's action (the ratio of pumping work to pressure work) was improved by training.

Reduced Impedance to Cardiac Ejection (Afterload). The impedance to perfusion of an actively contracting muscle varies with the percentage of maximal force that is exerted (Kay & Shephard, 1969; Royce, 1958); a local restriction of blood flow sometimes begins with deployment of as little as 15% of muscle force, and occlusion of the intramuscular vessels becomes complete at about 70% of maximal force. We could thus envisage easier perfusion of the active muscles and a reduced cardiac afterload if the arms were strengthened as a result of training. Measurements of isokinetic strength support this hypothesis. The data of G.M. Davis et al. (1987) further show that after participation in the training program, subjects develop a lesser increase of blood pressure at fixed intensities of isometric handgrip contraction, a finding that supports the cardiac afterload hypothesis.

Do arteriovenous oxygen differences provide further evidence that an initial high-impedance afterload is reduced by training? A reduction of impedance and thus a greater limb flow during vigorous submaximal work should allow the same power output to be sustained with a smaller arteriovenous oxygen difference.

The precise effect of training upon the arteriovenous oxygen difference depends on the relative impact of the conditioning program upon the various factors increasing peripheral oxygen extraction; these factors include an increase in the concentration of aerobic enzymes within the mitochondria, a decrease in the average

Table 6.7   M-mode Echocardiographic Variables in Paraplegic Subjects Over 16 Weeks of Arm Ergometer Training

Variable	Duration of training		
	0 Weeks	8 Weeks	16 Weeks
Left ventricular end-diastolic diameter (mm)			
Control	47 ± 3	47 ± 3	46 ± 3
Experimental	45 ± 2	46 ± 1	46 ± 2
Left ventricular end-systolic diameter (mm)			
Control	32 ± 2	33 ± 3	30 ± 2
Experimental	28 ± 2	30 ± 2	28 ± 1
Left ventricular end-diastolic volume (ml)			
Control	109 ± 20	108 ± 19	105 ± 21
Experimental	95 ± 10	99 ± 10	96 ± 10
Left ventricular end-systolic volume (ml)			
Control	36 ± 7	39 ± 8	29 ± 6
Experimental	23 ± 5	28 ± 5	24 ± 4
Stroke volume (ml)			
Control	73 ± 13	74 ± 11	76 ± 16
Experimental	71 ± 5	70 ± 6	73 ± 7

Note. Based on data from "Cardiac Effects of Short-Term Arm Crank Training in Paraplegics: Echocardiographic Evidence" by G.M. Davis, R.J. Shephard, and F.H.H. Leenen, 1987, *European Journal of Applied Physiology, 56*, pp. 90-96. Data obtained during handgrip exertion at 30% of maximum isometric force ($M \pm SE$).

diffusion distance from capillary to muscle fiber (Brooks & Fahey, 1984; Douglas & Becklake, 1968; Shephard, 1982b), and a more ready overall perfusion of strengthened muscles that contract at a smaller fraction of their maximum force.

These several influences have a variable overall effect upon arteriovenous oxygen differences in able-bodied subjects. Simmons and Shephard (1971a) described a slight narrowing of the arteriovenous oxygen difference with arm ergometer training, whereas Clausen et al. (1973) described some widening of the gradient in response to their training regimen. The initial pretraining arteriovenous oxygen differences of the spinally injured are high relative to able-bodied norms for either the upper limb (Hjeltnes, 1977, 1980) or the lower limb (Shephard, 1982b). But neither cross-sectional nor longitudinal studies of the disabled have demonstrated any substantial changes in peak arteriovenous differences with upper limb training (G.M. Davis et al., 1987; G.M. Davis & Shephard, 1988; Hjeltnes, 1980). We must conclude that if there is indeed an effect from a strengthening of muscles and reduced cardiac afterload, the subjects immediately counter this by exercising to a higher peak power output, thus reaching the same peak arteriovenous oxygen difference as before training.

A training-induced increase of stroke volume arising from one of the three mechanisms discussed previously would normally be associated with a slow resting heart rate (bradycardia). Some authors (Hullemann et al., 1975; Pollock et al., 1974) suggest that variations in resting heart rate are sufficiently large to obscure any resting bradycardia that might result from a training-induced improvement of cardiovascular performance. G.M. Davis et al. (1987) attempted to obtain waking pulse rates on each of their spinal cord–disabled subjects, but nevertheless only those who were taking intensive and prolonged exercise developed a significant bradycardia.

The study of G.M. Davis et al. (1987) may be compared with earlier research on elderly subjects (Sidney & Shephard, 1978), which showed that although immediate benefit was largely confined to those undertaking frequent high-intensity exercise training sessions, a training response did ultimately develop in response to alternative patterns of conditioning (infrequent high-intensity or frequent low-intensity sessions). Whether spinally injured subjects respond in similar fashion to the elderly depends in part upon their initial physical condition; however, there is reason to suspect that those who have previously been very inactive will show an eventual cardiovascular training response to even a low-intensity training regimen.

Although the available data suggest that a decreased cardiac afterload is the main explanation of the training-induced gains of stroke volume, care is needed in extrapolating conclusions drawn from either resting data or isometric activity to the problems of dynamic exercise. In particular, the supine posture (which is essential for high-quality M-mode echocardiographic studies) eliminates gravitational effects; this in turn minimizes the influence upon cardiac performance of any training-induced changes in lower-limb pooling and thus cardiac preloading (Ruch & Patton, 1966).

Peripheral Effects of Training

A number of authors have suggested that much of the response to arm-ergometer training is peripheral and limb specific, reflecting either alterations in the impedance to local blood flow (as discussed previously) or changes in the activity of aerobic enzymes (Clausen et al., 1970; Davies & Sargeant, 1975; Henriksson & Reitman, 1977; Klausen, Rasmussen, Clausen, & Trap-Jensen, 1974; Knuttsson et al., 1973; Lewis et al., 1980; McKenzie, Fox, & Cohen, 1978; Rasmussen, Klausen, Clausen, & Trap-Jensen, 1975; Saltin ct al., 1976; Stamford, Cuddihee, Moffatt, & Rowland, 1978). In consequence, some have queried how far training effects can be transferred from the muscles involved in arm cranking to those used in wheelchair operation, although some authors (D. Sedlock, personal communication) have seen a good transfer.

Given that some spinally injured paraplegic and tetraplegic subjects initially show both an impairment of stroke volume and a rapid exercise heart rate (tachycardia), peripheral training responses such as an augmentation of blood volume (Holmgren, 1967; Sjöstrand, 1967), a redistribution of blood flow (Rowell, 1974), ultrastructural changes within the muscle fibers (Howald, 1975), and changes in mitochondrial enzyme concentrations (Holloszy & Booth, 1976) may be of even greater importance to the disabled than to able-bodied individuals (Bruin & Binkhorst, 1984; Glaser, Fichtenbaum, Simsen-Harold, Petrofsky, & Surprayasad, 1982; Hjeltnes, 1977; Siefert, Lob, Stoephasium, Probst, & Brendel, 1972). However, there have been few formal studies of this question.

Wakim et al. (1949) attempted to examine peripheral factors by measuring the limb blood flow immediately after exercise (Berry, Baldes, Essex, & Wakim, 1948). Data were collected before and after several weeks of posttraumatic rehabilitation. In response to a similar amount of upper-limb exercise (shoulder and elbow flexion and extension, using free weights), the upper-limb blood flow increased 190% over the baseline values with training, whereas flow to the lower limb increased by only 17%. The authors considered the observed hyperemia to be a beneficial response to exercise per se, although as the measurements were made after rather than during the exercise bouts, the data could also be interpreted as reflecting an increased ability of the subjects to develop and subsequently repay an oxygen debt. In support of the latter explanation, both Nilsson et al. (1975) and Ornstein et al. (1983) observed increases in maximal lactate concentration after periods of arm crank and swim training, respectively. Interestingly, Wakim et al. (1949) observed that changes in postexercise hyperemia were much greater in subjects whose exercise training had been supervised than in those individuals who had been unsupervised, emphasizing the difficulty of ensuring exercise compliance in a disabled population.

Ekblöm and Lundberg (1968) remarked that during submaximal exercise, accumulations of blood lactate in paraplegic adolescents were reduced after training; in contrast, the authors saw no training-induced changes in subjects affected by cerebral palsy. Hjeltnes (1980) equally noted a 50% decrease in blood lactate levels during submaximal exercise after six paraplegics had undergone 12 weeks of rehabilitation; these changes were associated with an increase of stroke volume. Nevertheless, the interpretation of such findings remains uncertain. One possible explanation would be that a strengthening of the active muscles allows a greater local perfusion of the working limbs. Among other alternative explanations, muscle perfusion might be improved by an increase of cardiac preloading or an improvement of myocardial contractility.

Muscle Strength

Muscle strength can be increased through an increased or better coordinated recruitment of functional motor units, a growth of existing muscle fibers (hypertrophy), or formation of new fibers (hyperplasia), although only limited evidence exists that training can activate this last mechanism in humans (D.H. Clarke, 1973; Edgerton, 1978; E.L. Fox, 1984; Gonyea, 1980). Indeed, even in animal experiments, hyperplastic changes have only been seen following bouts of heavy resistance exercise sufficient to cause substantial hypertrophy of fast twitch glycolytic (Type IIb) muscle fibers (Edgerton, 1978; Goldspink, 1970; Ho et al., 1980). Muscle hypertrophy is itself a relatively slow process, and much of the increase of muscle strength observed over the first few weeks of training must be attributed to altered patterns of fiber recruitment.

Few studies have specifically examined the changes of muscular strength and endurance that occur during training of the disabled. Thus, almost nothing is known about an appropriate frequency, intensity, and duration of training to recommend in order to maximize skeletal muscle function. Strength training programs in general have developed rather empirically from plans that have proved success-ful in conditioning able-bodied subjects (Gairdner, 1983). However, in some cases account has also been taken of biomechanical data for wheelchair users (Walsh & Steadward, 1984).

As Hickson (1980) stressed, the development of cardiorespiratory and muscular fitness tend to be diametrically opposed objectives. Attempts to increase both cardiorespiratory and muscular fitness through a common exercise program have often had a negative effect upon one or other aspect of function. Given a harsh choice between the two goals, most physicians opt for cardiorespiratory rather than muscular training.

Unfortunately, ordinary wheelchair ambulation does not provide an adequate stimulus to either cardiorespiratory or muscle development. Thus Gersten et al. (1963) could find no difference of triceps performance between those who had been spinally injured in the previous 2 to 4 months and those who had been using a wheelchair regularly for 3 to 5 years.

Anthropometric Evidence

In some cases, inferences of muscle hypertrophy have been drawn from increases of limb circumference. However, even if we make due allowance for changes in the amount of overlying subcutaneous fat, there is often a lack of parallelism between the increase in maximum muscle force and gain of limb dimensions during a rehabilitation program (Fried & Shephard, 1970).

Pollock et al. (1974) found a 1 mm (3%) increase in the forearm and upper arm girth of disabled subjects after 20 weeks of rehabilitation; as the researchers also observed a 5% decrease in skinfold readings, the logical inference was that there had been some local muscle hypertrophy. On the other hand, Bar-Or et al. (1976) were unable to demonstrate any increase in the lean mass of cerebral palsied or paralytic adolescents after 1 year of training. Likewise, Nilsson et al. (1975) found that the upper arm girth remained unchanged after forearm ergometer train-ing despite increases in dynamic strength and endurance of 19 and 80%, respec-tively (as judged by the lifting of free weights).

G.M. Davis et al. (1984a) and Davis et al. (1986) found no strong evidence of an increase in muscle dimensions after 8 to 16 weeks of training, yet their subjects reported lesser fatigue during normal wheelchair ambulation. Such obser-vations are most easily explained in terms of training-induced alterations in the patterns of neural firing or muscle fiber recruitment.

Isometric Force

As noted, Gersten et al. (1963) found that the maximum isometric forces recorded from the biceps and the triceps were almost identical in recently injured paraplegics and in those who had been ambulatory for 3 to 4 years. However, both groups showed comparable gains of strength in response to 7 weeks of deliberate, vigorous isometric training; biceps force increased by 55% and triceps force by 37%, with an associated 20% improvement of muscular endurance in both muscle groups. On the other hand, perhaps because their subjects were enrolled in physically less demanding classes, Bar-Or, Inbar, and Spira (1976) saw no increase of grip strength when youths with cerebral palsy or poliomyelitis underwent a mixed training program.

Isotonic Strength

Nilsson et al. (1975) examined isotonic strength (the lifting of free weights after 7 weeks of combined weight training and ergometry). The maximal lift of the disabled subjects increased by 19% (from 626 N to 743 N) over 7 weeks of training, and the endurance of repeated submaximal lifting (tested at 85% of maximal lift) increased by 80%.

Isokinetic Force

Davis, Shephard, and Ward (1984b) demonstrated some increases of isokinetic performance in response to 8 weeks of forearm cranking (three sessions per week). Although their training program had been devised primarily to improve cardiovascular condition, 11 previously inactive disabled men also developed increases of peak torque, peak power, and average power for several arm and shoulder movements. Comparing these three indices of isokinetic performance, the researchers observed the best discrimination of the muscular training response using average isokinetic power (possibly because the type of training used in their study, forearm ergometry, emphasized steady rather than explosive movements of the arm). The isokinetic training response was most obvious for the movement of elbow extension—10 to 20% increase of average power over joint velocities of 2.09 to 4.19 rads/s (see Figure 6.3), with the greatest response being observed at the higher angular velocities of elbow movement. The subjects also showed significant training-induced gains of average power for elbow flexion and shoulder flexion. This pattern of response is a little different from that seen in the cross-sectional studies mentioned previously, suggesting a specific training of the elbow muscles in response to forearm cranking.

The isokinetic force data have some practical importance, as shoulder flexion and elbow extension are the primary movements in wheelchair ambulation. The data imply that endurance training can increase the power of the pectoralis and triceps muscles. Further analysis of the data shows (as might be expected) that changes were greatest in subjects following the high intensity, long-duration pattern of training (see Figures 6.4 and 6.5). In contrast to some earlier reports, dynamic endurance was unchanged, perhaps because the assessment technique (isokinetic power drop-off) was somewhat different from the training method (forearm cranking).

In studies that based training on the use of crutches, walking frames, or wheelchairs, gains of dynamic power have not always led to gains of forearm static strength. Indeed, subjects who have pursued their training at high limb velocities

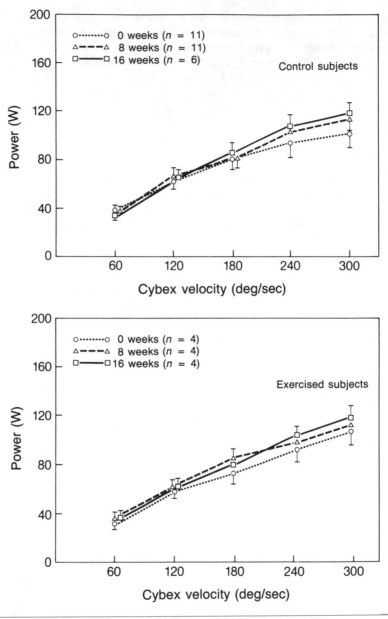

Figure 6.3.   The relationship between Cybex angular velocity and average power of iso-kinetic elbow extension. Based on data of G.M. Davis, 1985 and G.M. Davis et al., 1984 for control and exercised subjects after 0, 8, and 16 weeks of training. Values are means ± *SE* of data.

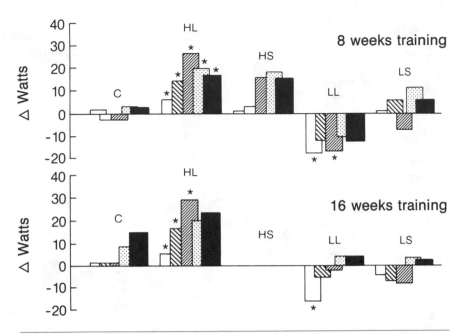

Figure 6.4. Change of average isokinetic elbow extension power over 8 and 16 weeks of endurance training on arm ergometer. Mean change from initial scores $\pm$ *SE*. Bar clusters denote angular velocities of 1.05 (open), 2.09 (right diagonal), 3.14 (left diagonal), 4.19 (screen), and 5.24 (solid) rad/s. * indicates significant differences from 0 weeks ($p < 0.02$). Based on data of G.M. Davis, 1985 and G.M. Davis et al., 1984 for control (C), high intensity prolonged (HL), high intensity short (HS), low intensity prolonged (LL), and low intensity short (LS) training programs.

have not shown increases of moment, work, or power scores at the lower speeds of joint rotation (Caiozzo, Perrine, & Edgerton, 1981; Kanehisa & Miyashita, 1983b; Smith & Melton, 1981). We may conclude that although a potential conflict exists between muscular and cardiovascular training, an appropriate regimen can develop both functions with considerable advantage to the quality of life in the disabled.

Cellular Changes

The relative proportions of fast and slow twitch fibers remain substantially unchanged in the arm muscles of well-trained wheelchair athletes. However, such individuals show considerable hypertrophy of both slow and fast twitch fibers with little change of intracellular enzyme levels (A.W. Taylor et al., 1979; A.W. Taylor, 1981). In contrast, 8 weeks of arm ergometer training induces a hypertrophy only of the slow twitch muscles (A.W. Taylor et al., 1986); this presumably reflects the steadier rhythm of movement on the ergometer.

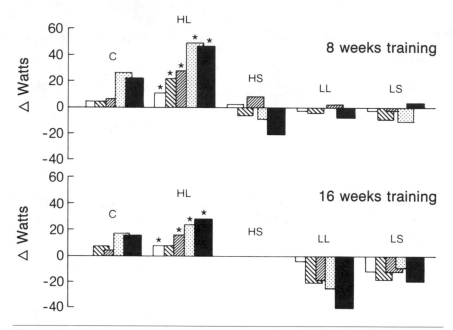

Figure 6.5. Change of average isokinetic shoulder flexion power over 8 and 16 weeks of endurance training on arm ergometer. Mean change from initial scores $\pm$ *SE*. Bar clusters denote angular velocities of 1.05 (open), 2.09 (right diagonal), 3.14 (left diagonal), 4.19 (screen), and 5.24 (solid) rad/s. * indicates significant differences from 0 weeks ($p < .02$). Based on data of G.M. Davis, 1985 and G.M. Davis et al., 1984 for control (C), high intensity prolonged (HL), high intensity short (HS), low intensity prolonged (LL), and low intensity short (LS) training programs.

Balance and Agility

Spira (1967a, b) examined the responses of 131 previously inactive poliomyelitic youth aged 10 to 21 years to a twice-weekly program of wheelchair basketball, swimming, javelin throwing, and table tennis. The subjects, particularly the more disabled subjects, demonstrated a progressive increase in the speed of walking and stair climbing, with improved scores for beam balancing over the course of 6 months' participation in the program.

Other Types of Disability

Amputations

Much of the research with amputees has been geared to improve performance by better assistive devices rather than by specific training (Michael, 1986). Head pointers give impetus to a ball, fins boost the performance of a recreational swimmer, a handle attached to a ball helps the bowler, or a Velcro strap fixes a sporting implement to a limb. Detailed rules govern the use of prostheses and orthoses in international competition. Volleyball players may use lower-limb but not upper-limb devices. Archers can use a prosthesis or orthosis to assist in drawing the bow, and Class A6, A8, and A9 athletes may also use a releasing aid. Lawn bowlers in Classes A5 and A7 may also use a prosthesis or orthosis. However, such devices are not allowed in swimming, table tennis, or shooting contests.

In those with a congenital limb deficiency or amputation in early childhood, performance in many events may be close to that of the able-bodied. The main item that needs greater attention during training is the development of balance.

Older subjects who receive an amputation for peripheral vascular disease may have had very limited activity or even bed rest for some months prior to operation and subsequently may have too little cardiovascular capacity to allow ambulation other than by wheelchair. Bruderman, Najenson, Gelbard, Serepka, and Solsi (1971) examined the possibility of rehabilitating such a group by upper arm exercises, including light weight lifting, wheelchair push-ups, and wheelchair racing. Four 2-hour sessions were held each week for 5 weeks. This led to a progressive and substantial increase of speed when operating a wheelchair, with a lesser increase of heart rate and blood pressure at any given work rate. Mechanical efficiency improved by 15%, the respiratory dead space–tidal volume ratio decreased during exercise, and the arterial oxygen pressure increased slightly during exercise.

Kabsch (1973) argued that the sequence of movements involved in skiing was particularly helpful to restoration of normal gait in those using a prosthesis. Such training allowed the amputee to reduce the amplitude of head and trunk oscillations and to walk on a narrower, more normal base; in consequence, the energy cost of ambulation decreased from 160 to 130% of that for an able-bodied person. Others have found the review of movement patterns by high-speed cinematography helpful in correcting abnormalities of gait (Eberhart, Elftman, & Inman, 1954).

Blindness

In recent years great advances have been made in athletic records at competitions sponsored by IBSA, the USABA, and the Canada Blind Sports. At the 7th Annual USABA Games, approximately 38% of competitors were legally blind (Class B3), 30% could perceive only hand movements (Class B2), and 32% were totally blind (Class B1); in 61% of the sample the disability was congenital (Rainbolt & Sherrill, 1987). Performances in such events as the 10,000-m run testify to the seriousness of training (C. Buell, 1987), with types of training including jogging (48%), practice of specific skills (29%), weight training (12%), other activities (6%), and practice in game play (5%) (Rainbolt & Sherrill, 1987).

Nevertheless, the level of fitness in too many blind individuals remains poor. Training programs for the blind attempt to counter both the physical weakness and the lack of spatial orientation that limit independence (Dawson, 1981; Dordel, 1971), particularly through the development of other sensory receptors. The extent of participation in physical activity and thus the extent of the training response are influenced by the completeness of visual impairment, gender, age, available types of activity, the normal method of ambulation, and parental attitudes (Winnick, 1985).

Rather than focusing on the handicap, coaches for the blind use the techniques of normal sport to develop not only the cardiorespiratory and muscular systems, but also coordination, an appreciation of the shape of movement, and a sense of achievement in a risk-free environment. In a school environment, those with residual vision can sometimes serve as guides to those who are completely blind. It is necessary to stress the danger points in a facility, supplementing this information by guide ropes (e.g., at the extremities of a pool) or texturing of the floor (e.g., the placement of carpet strips in a bowling alley; Stanley & Kindig, 1986). Where special equipment such as a treadmill, cycle ergometer, or universal gym is used, coaches must take much time to identify the various parts of the equipment in terms of shape, texture, size, and weight.

Those with some residual function are helped if features of a facility are painted in brightly contrasting colors. Technical manuals for a sport can be reproduced in braille, but this is very costly and leads to a bulky volume. For most purposes, an audio-cassette is a more practical solution.

It is also important to teach safe forms of recreation that the blind person can perform alone or with a minimum of supervision, for example, swimming and dancing (C. Buell, 1982). Several schools have now introduced walking, jogging, and cross-country running programs for blind students (C. Buell, 1984; Laughlin, 1975; Sonka & Bina, 1978); empirical observations suggest the value of endurance training programs (DePauw, 1981; Stamford, 1975), with improvements in treadmill scores and decreases of resting heart rate (George & Patton, 1975). Shephard, Ward, and Lee (1987) induced an increase of lean tissue and peak power output with a decrease of body fat in blind students who undertook a special program of adapted exercises in a residential school. But most of these gains were dissipated over a summer vacation (DiNatale, Lee, Ward, & Shephard, 1985), when access to the teaching program and special facilities was no longer available. Hamill et al. (1985) noted that orientation and mobility training made visually impaired adults less hesitant, more consistent in movement patterns, and mechanically more efficient.

Deafness

The improvement of equilibrium is a substantial element in teaching deaf children. The students are encouraged to broaden their standing base and exercise within it. Special activities are devised to enhance both vision and proprioceptive sensitivity; dancing, karate, and T'ai Chi are all helpful in improving kinesthesis. Specific activities to improve balance are more controversial; damage to the vestibular apparatus is permanent, but substantial compensation is nevertheless possible through an increased use of visual and proprioceptive cues (Myklebust, 1964).

If the hearing loss is severe, gait may need attention; children with normal hearing learn much of the normal movement of heel and toe from the sound of the footsteps, and those with impaired hearing may be helped by augmented auditory feedback (Flordmark, 1986). It is undesirable to encourage a child to watch his or her feet while walking, but walking patterns can be improved by use of mirrors or a videotape monitor. Black (1983) suggested that an outdoor residential program provides a more effective basis of training than traditional physical education classes, perhaps because of the novelty of the experience.

Most of the available empirical studies suggest that the balance of deaf children can be improved by an appropriate training program. For example, Effgen (1981) found that a 10-day program of static balance activities increased the length of time deaf children were able to stand on one leg. Lewis, Higham, and Cherry (1985) also noted an improvement of both static and dynamic balance in profoundly hearing-impaired children, although this was only significant at the .10 level of probability.

Cerebral Palsy

A variety of specific therapeutic programs have been devised for the spastic child (B.L. Robertson, 1980; Sherrill, 1986a). Before the age of 7 years, the emphasis is upon inhibition of abnormal reflex activity, normalizing muscle tone, and developing reactions to increase equilibrium. At this stage, the attempt is to avoid inducing primitive reflexes that the physiotherapist has been working to suppress. For example, a ball should be struck with the open hand, as normal throwing could stimulate the primitive grasp reflex, and instruction should be given at eye level to minimize the extensor thrust. If the child exercises from a chair, strapping may be needed both to inhibit reflexes and also to prevent falls from exaggerated extensor movements. Muscle tone is normalized by passive movements of the limbs, supplemented where possible by pursuits that encourage reciprocal active movements of the limbs (e.g., swimming), while balance is developed by work on boards. The design of games and exercises must take due account of associated perceptual defects.

In older children, the emphasis shifts to development of the range of motion and strength, with less concern about provoking unwanted reflexes (Bleck & Nagel, 1982); if such reflexes persist, an attempt is made to build them into an individualized approach to task performance. One important obstacle to group training is that individual subjects differ substantially in their type and level of disability (Best, 1971). In general, responses to conditioning are similar to those observed in the able-bodied (Bar-Or et al., 1976; Berg, 1970; Ekblöm & Lundberg, 1968; Jones, 1984; Lundberg et al., 1967; Rieckert et al., 1977). The spastic muscles have a subnormal exercise blood flow (Landin et al., 1977), but flow is increased with training. Conditioning also leads to some decrease in the ratio of the H-reflex to the direct motor action potential (Spira, 1967a, b; 1974); the H-reflex serves as a measure of spasticity, while the direct motor action potential represents all of the active motor neurons. There have been suggestions of a favorable response (increased strength and flexibility) to progressive resistance exercises, although some authors still advocate caution since resistance can increase abnormal flexion and muscle tone (Bobath, 1971; Horvat, 1987). McCubbin and Shasby (1985) noted improvements in movement time and peak torque in response to isokinetic training, gains being much as anticipated in the nonhandicapped population.

Rotzinger and Stoboy (1974) commented on improvements in gait and other skills with training, but they were unable to demonstrate a clear-cut reduction in the integrated EMG potential. Sommer (1971) noted that wheelchair-bound cerebral paralytics initially reacted more slowly and showed poorer skills than some other classes of subject. Their training program developed skills in operating a wheelchair (acceleration, braking, passing through narrow gaps, avoidance of collisions), in addition to wheelchair roadwork. At the end of 26 such sessions, there was a substantial improvement in scores for various wheelchair skills, and the exercise heart rate was less at a given level of exercise stress (Sommer, 1973). Others, also, have commented on gains of motor function and increases of walking speed (Berg, 1970; Rotzinger & Stoboy, 1974). One somewhat negative report is from Lundberg (1973). He trained young men and women with cerebral palsy 5 days per week for 14 to 27 months; the program intensity was moderate, with no training over school vacations and, perhaps for this reason, the end result was a disappointingly small gain of physical work capacity.

Muscular Dystrophies and Multiple Sclerosis

Both active and passive movements are prescribed for people with muscular dystrophy or multiple sclerosis, the intent being to improve coordination and neuromuscular function (Caillet, 1980; Chrétien et al., 1987; Robertson, 1977). Specific aims are to decrease unwanted movements while inhibiting those that would increase contractures. Eickelberg et al. (1976) applied passive movements to the lower limbs of 12 students with muscular dystrophy on the basis that the legs were first affected by muscular dystrophy and were most likely to become immobilized. A stimulation of ventilatory and cardiac function was noted, together with an immediate increase of associative learning. The authors speculated that cardiorespiratory stimulation caused a transient increase of arterial oxygen pressure, thus improving cerebral function.

An appropriate program of dynamic exercises can be helpful in both muscular dystrophy and mutliple sclerosis, increasing muscular strength (particularly in the early stages of the condition) and reducing the complications of inactivity (Russell, 1976), including obesity. Such programs maximize residual function, although no evidence exists that they affect progress of the disease.

Running and jogging may not be well tolerated because of problems of endurance and balance; in such individuals, the buoyancy of an aquatic fitness program is helpful. Gehlsen, Grigsby, and Winant (1984) noted gains of isokinetic strength and endurance when 40-year-old adults were given a 10-week program of this type. Training sessions of 60 minutes duration 3 times per week at 60 to 75% of maximal heart rate improved isokinetic force (46-85%), work (41-177%), and power (59-205%) of the upper limbs over the course of 10 weeks. Gains were greatest at the highest speeds of limb rotation; however, knee flexion and extension were not improved by training. Vignos and Watkins (1966) prescribed a graduated home program of weight training for 14 children with Duchenne muscular dystrophy and 10 with other types of dystrophy. Gains in the weight lifters appeared over the first 4 months of the program, amounting to over 50% of initial readings for stronger muscles and less for those muscles that were already weakened. Over the next 8 months gains apparently plateaued, and as the increments of strength did not translate into greater functional ability, a learning of technique may have contributed to the initial improvement. Researchers Delateur and Giaconi (1979) used a Cybex isokinetic dynamometer to exercise four children with muscular dystrophy. Over a period of 6 months, the peak torque in the exercised limbs improved by about 30%, and contrary to some earlier reports no adverse effects of training were seen in a 30-month follow-up.

Scoliosis

The objectives of training in the scoliotic patient are (a) to slow down, and if possible to reverse, the development of spinal curvature and (b) to increase pulmonary function and physical work capacity. However, any training-induced correction of spinal curvature is somewhat equivocal relative to the progress of a control group (Stone, Beeckman, Hall, Guess, & Brooks, 1979). Training generally increases both aerobic power and the ventilatory equivalent for oxygen, although the extent of this response decreases in those with more severe scoliosis; in patients who have developed pulmonary hypertension, vigorous training is probably inadvisable (Shneerson, 1978).

Mentally Retarded

When designing exercise programs for the mentally retarded, trainers must take due account of the nature and type of disability. Although initially mildly retarded students often have a poor motor performance (Rarick, 1980a, 1980b; see chapter 5), the aim should be to encourage incorporation into normal school and community sport and fitness programs as rapidly as possible. Trainers must assign activities for moderately retarded students according to mental rather than chronological age. The former is typically in the range 2 to 7 years; the student thus needs a play approach supplemented by much physical and verbal encouragement, with manual demonstration of movement techniques. Early attempts to train the mentally retarded used music and rhythm of the types proposed by Jaques-Dalcroze and Orff (Decker, 1973; Josef, 1967; Kiphard, 1973; Maurer-Keller [cited in Jochheim, 1971], Tauscher, 1969). Case reports have suggested the value of this approach, but it remains difficult to separate a true physiological response from the impact of increased personal attention and enhancement of self-image (Cratty, 1973).

A number of studies of mentally retarded children suggest that if an adequate physical activity program is provided, physical performance can be substantially improved to the point where test scores do not differ significantly from those observed in a normal population of the same age (Bar-Or et al., 1976; Berg, 1970; Björke et al., 1978; J. Campbell, 1972, 1978; Chasey, 1970; Corder, 1966; Funk, 1971; Lundberg, Ovenfors, & Saltin, 1967; Nordgren, 1971; Skrobak-Kaczynski & Vavik, 1980). However, few investigators included appropriate controls.

In the profoundly retarded, the prime emphasis of the physical educator has naturally been upon the development of motor skills. Nevertheless, there is some evidence that the frequent repetition of gross motor activities can have a favorable influence upon the cardiovascular performance of such individuals (Mulholland & McNeill, 1985). J. Campbell (1978) found gains in 300-yard run scores among institutionalized mentally retarded, the response being larger with the Royal Canadian Air Force physical fitness program than with a physical education program. Kasch and Zasueta (1971) reported improvements of times on both a 300-yd and a 600-yd run after training, but scores were unchanged for a simple 3-minute step test. In adolescents, as in children, gains have apparently been seen in field tests (Corder, 1966; Giles, 1968) but not in laboratory measurements of PWC_{170} (Bundschuh & Cureton, 1982) or treadmill testing (Millar, 1984).

In adults, Beasley (1982) found an improvement of 12-minute walk-run distances after 8 weeks training of educable and trainable mentally retarded, but Coleman and Whitman (1984) found no change of 300-yard times in response to an unspecified training program. Andrew et al. (1979) noted that young educable retarded adults improved their score on the Canadian Association for Health, Physical Education and Recreation (CAHPER) fitness test battery after 12 weeks of training, although there was no change of PWC_{170}; likewise, Montgomery, Reid, and Seidl (in press) reported gains on the Canadian Standard Test of Fitness. It is thus arguable that the improved performance test scores in this experiment reflected practice of the required procedures rather than a true training response. Nordgren (1971) claimed that training induced a 30% increase of PWC_{130} in males but not in females. Likewise, Tomporowski and Ellis (1984, 1985) found significant gains of PWC_{150} after 7 months of varied endurance exercise that included jogging, games, calisthenics, and circuit training. Andrew et al. (1979) and Schurrer et al. (1985) made direct measurements of maximum oxygen intake; the former reported an 8% increase of $\dot{V}O_2$max after 12 weeks of training, whereas the controls sustained a 12% decrease over this same interval. Schurrer et al. (1985) did not include a control group but claimed a 36 to 43% increase of $\dot{V}O_2$max in five mentally retarded adults who participated in a 23-week walk-jog program at an intermediate care facility; a decrease of body mass and a high level of motivation contributed to this unusually favorable response.

Brown (1967) and Skrobak-Kaczynski and Vavik (1980) further stressed that specific benefit is obtained from muscle strengthening exercises. Favorable changes in physical condition are often associated with gains in body image (Chasey, Swartz, & Chasey, 1974; Kinney, 1979), personal development, social acceptance, and academic achievement (Anthony, 1979; Cross, 1980).

Skrobak-Kaczynski and Vavik (1980) noted reductions of body weight and skinfold thicknesses with training. Dresen (1985) also observed decreases of skinfold thicknesses, improvements of mechanical efficiency, and gains of classroom attention in response to training, although in their study the heart rate at a given oxygen consumption remained unchanged. Rieckert et al. (1977) saw improvements of mechanical efficiency in children, although others found no change in adolescents (Bar-Or et al., 1976; Lundberg & Pernow, 1970).

McCubbin and Jansma (1987) compared the response of mentally retarded adults to four fitness training sessions, four hygiene sessions, or two fitness and two hygiene sessions per week. In terms of running speed, muscular strength, muscular endurance, and flexibility, the largest gains were registered by the fitness-trained group, although relative to control none of the three groups showed significant differences of score on the Adaptive Behavior Scale (a tool used in the deinstitutionalization process). Others, also, found that training had disappointingly little influence on absenteeism from work (Beasley, 1982), IQ, or general behavior (Tomporowski & Ellis, 1984, 1985).

Hartley (1986) reviewed specific information on the child with Down's syndrome. Although he observed delay in all areas of development, he noticed such children had particular difficulty in mastering advanced cognitive strategies and processes. He thus found it important to avoid complicated sequences of instructions and situations that require the child to choose between alternative solutions to a problem. Chapter 7 details abnormalities of gait (Parker, Bronks, & Snyder, 1986), although it is worth noting here that many features of gait in Down's syndrome speak to a total body instability. Kerr and Blais (1985) studied motor learning patterns on a pursuit tracking task. Relative to other mentally retarded children, individuals with Down's syndrome apparently opted for accuracy of pursuit at the expense of speed.

Autistic Individuals

The problems of the autistic individual in learning specific skills (see chapter 4) are a handicap to any training program for individuals with this type of disability (Collier & Reid, 1987). Schover and Newsom (1976) suggested that frequent repetition of a task (overtraining) gradually broadens the range of cues to which the autistic person will respond. Others have suggested that autistic individuals respond particularly well to swimming programs (Killian, Joyce-Petrovich, Menna, & Arena, 1984).

Clark, Wade, Massey, and Van Dyke (1973) and Stamford (1973) applied moderate-intensity exercise to elderly subjects with psychiatric impairment. Although treadmill scores showed substantial physiological gains (Stamford, 1973), Clark et al. (1973) found only slight improvements in such measures as activity level, physical tolerance, attitude, and capacity for self-care.

Key Ideas

1. Most studies of training in the disabled have made cross-sectional comparisons of athletes and nonathletes. This avoids difficulties of recruitment and retention of volunteers and ensures prolonged training. However, it leaves largely unanswered the question as to how far the advantage of the athletes reflects selection rather than training.

2. Wheelchair athletes show a substantial advantage of peak oxygen intake and peak power output relative to their inactive peers; these findings are accompanied by a greater stroke volume and a narrower arteriovenous oxygen difference in submaximal exercise.

3. Both isometric and isokinetic muscle force data show higher values in wheelchair athletes, particularly in the muscles used in ambulation.

4. Normal-speed propulsion of a wheelchair does not provide an adequate training stimulus for the young wheelchair athlete. However, the training threshold varies widely with age and habitual activity.

5. A variety of wheelchair and arm ergometers can be used as sources of training, as well as muscle training programs, calisthenics, swimming, and participation in individual or team sports.

6. Longitudinal training experiments confirm the cross-sectional data in showing a gain of maximum oxygen intake, due largely to an increase of cardiac stroke volume.

7. At least some of the gains in performance with training may reflect peripheral changes—either an increase of muscle enzyme activity or an increase of blood flow to the working muscles.

8. Gains of muscle strength apparently reflect a substantial hypertrophy of both Type I and Type II muscle fibers. Improvements of score have been demonstrated in isometric, isotonic, and isokinetic tests.

9. Balance and agility are also improved by training, with significant benefit to the performance of everyday activities.

10. Amputees have often been weakened by prolonged bed rest prior to operation. In such instances, exercises to strengthen the arm muscles can improve wheelchair performance.

11. Blind subjects can be brought to normal fitness levels if they are given an adequate program of habitual activity. The condition of children may deteriorate over a summer vacation, when the encouragement of teachers and special facilities are lacking.

12. Deaf students are difficult to motivate because of communication problems. A disturbance of balance may also impair performance of some tests.

13. Trainers of the cerebral palsied must attempt to improve skills yet take care not to provoke inappropriate movements; progress is often disappointing.

14. In multiple sclerosis, carefully designed training can reduce both the likelihood of contractures and the general complications of inactivity.

15. With patience, educators can bring the physical performance of the mentally retarded to normal levels; however, instructions must be explained slowly, and account taken of a limited attention span.

Practical Applications

1. How would you determine the relative contributions of selection and training in the development of a wheelchair athlete?

2. What are some of the practical difficulties one might encounter when attempting a longitudinal training experiment with disabled subjects?

3. How important do you think the specificity of training is when preparing a wheelchair athlete?

4. What difficulties are likely in using maximum oxygen intake as a measure of training response in the wheelchair disabled?

5. If a wheelchair patient becomes fatigued or develops musculoskeletal problems with a low intensity of training, what course of action would you recommend?

6. What possible reasons could you envisage for a training-induced increase of maximum cardiac output in the wheelchair disabled?

7. What potential ''peripheral'' training responses could you envisage? Which do you judge as being important in the paraplegic subject?

8. Would you be disappointed if you found no change of arm circumference after 8 weeks of arm training in a wheelchair-confined population? Justify your answer.

9. What would be special obstacles to an effective training program in (a) blindness, (b) deafness, (c) cerebral palsy, (d) multiple sclerosis, and (e) mental retardation?

Chapter 7

Biomechanical Factors, Wheelchair Design, and Injury Prevention

In this chapter, we discuss various definitions of mechanical efficiency and apply these concepts to the performance of leg work by various classes of ambulatory disabled, including amputees, those with muscle spasm or weakness, and those with mental retardation. The chapter also notes special problems of walking and running encountered by the blind and reviews mechanical characteristics peculiar to the performance of arm work. Finally, the text applies these principles to issues of wheelchair design, wheelchair operation, the prevention of athletic injuries in the disabled, and the design of buildings and athletic facilities for the disabled.

Mechanical Efficiency

The mechanical efficiency of an individual provides a measure of that person's ability to translate the energy of ingested food into usable external work. It is particularly important to examine the mechanical efficiency of the disabled, as obesity, reduced sensory input, spasticity, clonus, and attempts to carry out activities from a reduced base of functioning muscle all diminish mechanical efficiency (Gordon & Vanderwalde, 1956), thus placing a correspondingly heavier metabolic burden on the cardiac, respiratory, and neuromuscular systems when the individual attempts to carry out any predetermined task (Jankowski & Evans, 1981). A large amount of muscle spasm and abnormal reflex activity also increases intrasubject variation of energy costs (Skrotsky, 1983). Sawka (1986) discussed possible indices of mechanical efficiency, including calculations of gross, net, work, and delta efficiencies.

Gross Mechanical Efficiency

Gross mechanical efficiency relates the total energy expenditure of the subject to the observed external power output (e.g., the rate of working on a cycle ergometer). The efficiency figure that is thus calculated depends not only on the

173

metabolic cost of the activity itself but also upon the resting energy expenditure of the individual. The resting metabolism of a disabled person may be decreased (and the gross efficiency at any given power output may thus be increased) if a limb has been amputated or paralyzed, or if diseased tissue has become atrophied or replaced by tissue such as fat (which has a lower level of energy expenditure per kilogram than resting muscle). On the other hand, if the resting oxygen consumption is increased by involuntary muscle spasm or athetoid movements, the gross efficiency of the individual at a given external power output will be low.

As external power output is increased, the resting energy expenditure accounts for a decreasing proportion of total metabolism. Gross efficiency thus tends to increase at higher work rates. However, if a disabled subject has a low peak power output, he or she will show a correspondingly low peak gross efficiency of effort.

Net Mechanical Efficiency

The net mechanical efficiency is based upon the gross metabolic cost of a given activity (as estimated from the oxygen consumption), minus either the resting or the basal energy expenditure (also estimated from oxygen consumption as measured after either a standard rest period, or the basal condition of a good night's rest with no food, exercise, or metabolic stimulant for 12 to 14 hours). Because true basal values demand considerable cooperation from a subject, a standard resting oxygen consumption of 3.5 ml/kg • min is sometimes assumed. However, there are problems when making such an assumption in disabled subjects. If the resting oxygen consumption is not measured, it may fail to conform to the assumed figure; the tissue atrophy seen after spinal injury decreases resting metabolism (Mollinger et al., 1985), but muscle spasm or athetoid movements increase it. Moreover, problems of stabilizing body posture may increase the paraplegic subject's baseline metabolic cost of performing a given task such as sitting on an ergometer or balancing in a wheelchair, before any "useful," external work has been undertaken.

Work and Delta Efficiency

The work efficiency calculation overcomes some of the difficulties noted previously. It measures the added cost of external work relative to a realistic baseline, such as the loadless pedaling of a cycle or an arm ergometer. The loadless condition takes account not only of resting metabolism but also of energy costs incurred by sitting in a working posture, rotating the limbs, and moving the mechanical parts of the ergometer. The main limitations to the work efficiency index are that postural work, cardiorespiratory work, and ergometer energy losses all increase as power output rises; the baseline for loadless pedaling is thus inaccurate for high work rates.

Delta efficiency (the slope of the oxygen cost–power output line) bears some similarity to work efficiency. Delta efficiency also excludes from the efficiency calculation the costs of torso stabilization and, if the rate of limb movement is kept constant, energy losses incurred in moving the limbs (Gaesser & Brooks, 1975; Glaser et al., 1984; Kofsky et al., 1983a, 1983b; Powers et al., 1984; Whipp & Wasserman, 1969).

Mechanical Efficiency of Leg Work

Although many of the disabled require a wheelchair for ambulation, some are able to use their legs. Nevertheless, the mechanical efficiency of leg work is decreased by a number of the disabilities discussed in this volume. Specific problems associated with blindness are discussed later in this chapter. Deafness, also, can impair mechanical efficiency, particularly if the individual's sense of balance is disturbed (Brunt & Broadhead, 1982; Effgen, 1981). The following section discusses specific problems of amputees, spastic individuals, patients with postural deformities, and those who experience difficulty in learning efficient movement patterns due to mental retardation.

Amputees. Under resting conditions, an able-bodied person minimizes the energy costs of sitting and standing by a careful alignment of body segments to minimize postural work. However, the disabled person has much greater difficulty in assuring such an alignment of body parts. Thus, when an amputee who has been fitted with a prosthesis sits on a chair, the center of gravity of his or her body passes through the hip on the unaffected side, because the prosthesis is effectively longer and lighter than the normal limb. As a consequence of the asymmetry there is a small (2-5%) increase of resting heart rate and oxygen consumption relative to sitting values for able-bodied subjects (Ganguli, Datta Chatterjee, & Roy, 1974a, 1974b; Ghosh, 1980). A somewhat similar disturbance of posture develops if a unilateral amputee sits without wearing a prosthesis. Subjects with poliomyelitis may also show an increase of energy cost while sitting due to poor body alignment associated with (a) soft tissue contractures, with paralytic dislocation or deformation of the hip, or (b) paralysis of the anterior thigh muscles, with deformities such as knock-knee and genu recurvatum (a backward curvature of the knee). However, in poliomyelitis such effects are offset by a loss of oxygen consumption in the paralyzed muscles.

When an amputee is standing, differences of mass between the normal limb and that fitted with a prosthesis again shift the center of mass of the body as a whole, leading to an increase of energy expenditure relative to the able-bodied (Ganguli et al., 1974a, b; Ghosh, Tibarewala, Mukherjee, Chakraborty, & Ganguli, 1979; Ghosh, 1980; Stott, Hutton, & Stokes, 1973). Whereas the able-bodied person increases oxygen consumption by about 26% on standing, the increment is about 42% for those with an above-knee prosthesis and as high as 46% for those with a below-knee prosthesis. Noting this problem, Hannah, Morrison, and Chapman (1984) used electrogoniometers to make a three-dimensional analysis of limb motion, seeking to teach the users of prostheses how to reimpart symmetry to their leg movements.

Possibilities for Ambulation. The patient who has undergone a lower-limb amputation has three options for ambulation—the use of crutches, a prosthesis, or some type of wheelchair. A young person can learn to move quite rapidly on crutches, but these become difficult and dangerous when crossing an icy surface. Crutch length is critical for the growing child (McGill & Dainty, 1984). Amputees and other disabled persons with long leg braces use axillary crutches; in terms of oxygen consumption, they may be more economical than an above-knee prosthesis, but if used in track events they may put pressure in the brachial fossa (armpit) and cause nerve injury. Forearm (Lofstrand, or Canadian) crutches are used by individuals with low-level spinal injuries, cerebral palsy, and les autres. Body mass is supported by the hands, and movement is costly. Although crutches provide a simple means of ambulation, there are obvious practical and psychological advantages to the fitting of a prosthetic limb that looks real, functions in a fairly normal manner, and leaves the arms unencumbered.

There are at least five possible techniques of crutch use (Bromley, 1981; Sherrill, 1986c; Sorenson & Ulrich, 1977)—four point, two point, three point, step to, and step through. The safest and most stable method, used by those severely affected by spinal injury, poliomyelitis, or cerebral palsy, is a four-point gait (Zhuo, 1985). One crutch is advanced, then the opposite foot, followed by the second crutch and then the trailing limb. The possible speed of movement is quite slow with this technique, but as the subject has three points of contact with the ground at all times, equilibrium is stable and the risk of injury is low. In subjects with the same disabilities but better preserved muscle function, a faster but less stable two-point gait becomes technically possible; this method of ambulation is more like normal running, a crutch and the opposite limb being moved forward in unison.

When first relearning ambulation after the fitting of a prosthesis, an amputee might use four-point and then two-point gait. However, the experienced amputee prefers a three-point technique; both crutches are advanced, then the prosthesis, and finally the normal leg.

The step-to gait is used by those who are very severely disabled. The crutches are moved forward, and then the body weight is taken by the arms while the legs are swung or dragged forward to the new position. The step-through gait is popular with those temporarily disabled; the person brings the crutches forward and then swings his or her body through the crutches to land on the normal limb.

If a prosthesis is provided, it is important that the subject learn to walk without excessive effort, without loss of stability, and with a natural appearance. The greater the amount of tissue that has been replaced by the prosthesis, the greater the disturbance of normal locomotor mechanisms and the greater the increase in the energy cost of ambulation.

Influence of Age on the Success of Prosthesis Use. A young adult can learn to walk effectively on an artificial leg after as little as 3 weeks of training. Although the initial cost of prosthetic ambulation may be 3 or 4 times greater than that of normal walking at a comparable pace, energy expenditures are kept within reasonable bounds by adopting a slower pace than an able-bodied subject.

An older individual learns the use of a prosthesis much more slowly. Residual proprioceptors are less sensitive than in a young person, new automatic movements are less readily learned, and residual muscles in the limb stump have become weaker. Furthermore, problems can arise from associated illnesses. Thus, the amputation may have been undertaken to treat gangrene, which in turn is secondary to diabetes and peripheral vascular disease. In such a patient, stump healing tends to be slow and incomplete. Cerebral ischemia or blindness may further hamper the learning of new movement patterns in the elderly, and coronary atherosclerosis may preclude development of the increased energy expenditures that are needed when walking with an artificial limb. DuBow, Witt, Kadaba, Reyes, and Cochrane

(1983) compared the oxygen cost per meter traversed of ambulation in a wheelchair (0.090 ml/m/kg) versus use of a bilateral below-knee prosthesis (0.232 ml/m/kg). Given such a stark difference, permanent use of a wheelchair may become the preferred therapeutic option (Kavanagh & Shephard, 1973). Nevertheless, age per se is not a contraindication to prosthesis use, and one recent survey (Steinberg, Sunwoo, & Roettger, 1985) found 73% of below-knee amputees over the age of 65 years were using their prostheses successfully.

Mechanical Characteristics of Prosthesis.   Whereas a normal lower limb weighs 8 to 10 kg, a typical stump plus artificial limb is much lighter (about 4 kg depending on body size, the level of amputation, and the extent of local muscular development). It is sometimes difficult to maneuver a prosthesis because of its limited inertia. Moreover, the reduced mass of stump plus prosthesis distorts the proprioceptive feedback from the residual muscle and joint tendon receptors, and the affected individual tends to lift the prosthesis too high when walking. The resonant frequency of the prosthesis limits the maximum speed of ambulation (Corcoran, 1971).

There have been various suggestions for augmenting proprioceptive feedback after amputation. Thus, lower-limb prostheses have been equipped with pressure sensors in the sole that transmit an electrical signal to the skin of the thigh, whereas upper-limb prostheses have been fitted with a piezoelectric crystal in the prehensile part in order to strike a suitable balance between slippage and the crushing of a delicate object (Salisbury & Colman, 1969).

For people of all ages, the main locomotor problem presented by an artificial knee joint is its uniplanar pattern of movement; this causes considerable difficulty when the subject walks over rough ground. The typical prosthesis is arranged to jackknife when weight is applied to the front of the foot, and locking is achieved when weight is applied to the heel. The amputee must therefore learn to place the foot on the ground with unusual care. Hydraulic devices that limit the rate of collapse of knee and ankle joints have been devised, but these have not been universally popular because they increase the mass to be supported and displaced by a limited volume of residual muscle in the leg stump. Nevertheless, Radcliffe and Ralston (cited in Corcoran, 1971) claimed that at fast speeds of walking, a hydraulic knee unit is 10% more efficient than a constant friction device, and more recently Murray, Mollinger, Sepic, Gardner, and Linder (1983) claimed that the hydraulic type of device allows a wider range of walking speeds, a greater equality of successive swing and stance phases, and a greater uniformity of forward progression.

Technique and Mechanical Efficiency.   A number of recent reports examined energy expenditures and the net mechanical efficiency of walking and running in amputees (Enoka, Miller, & Burgess, 1982; Kegel, Burgess, Starr, & Daly, 1981; D.I. Miller, 1981; Suzuki, Takahama, Mizutani, Arai, & Iwai, 1983) and in paraplegics (Merkel, Miller, Westbrook, & Merritt, 1984). The energy cost of ambulation is increased by such factors as a heavy prosthesis, a more distal center of gravity, or a decrease in the alignment stability of the limb (Peizer, 1961). When the prosthesis is first fitted, the amputee also tends to allocate an increased swing phase to the amputated limb and an increased stance phase for the normal leg (Kabsch, 1973). Training at a ski camp is one method to correct these defects; particularly in younger subjects, it leads to a more normal, better balanced, and more economical gait (Kabsch, 1973).

Enoka et al. (1982) found that 6 of 10 young below-knee amputees were able to run after a suitable training program. This observation is of current interest because of international controversy over standing and running competition by amputees. At the 1984 New York Games, the amputees played a demonstration basketball game from a standing position, and the USAAA would like this to become an official international event. Likewise, Class A-4 amputees wear their prostheses and use both limbs in running. However, European physicians argue that running by amputees places an excessive strain on the normal leg, predisposing it to injury or osteoarthritis. Given the long-term nature of this potential complication, we have no epidemiological data about it; inferences must be drawn from a study of current gait using cinematography, video cameras, and other more recent techniques of motion analysis.

The stride length and frequency in several of the amputees studied by Enoka et al. (1982) became much like that in able-bodied subjects. However, three of the runners showed an abnormally straight knee joint during a portion of the support phase of the gait cycle on the side of their bodies where the prostheses had been fitted. Possibly, those individuals who develop an abnormal gait are at an increased risk of osteoarthritis, but so are many able-bodied athletes, particularly those involved in contact sports. The issue thus becomes one of protective paternalism versus free personal choice; given the need to encourage independence in the disabled, my vote is for free choice. Lewallen, Quanbury, Ross, and Letts (1985) commented that many amputated subjects tended to use their prostheses mainly as a passive support. Moreover, in most amputees the intact limb was apparently unable to develop compensatory increases of force, because the overall walking speed was slowed, stride length was shortened, and the double-support phase of the gait cycle was increased.

Ghosh (1980) commented that whereas subjects with poliomyelitis tended to adopt a normal walking cadence with a shortened stride, below-knee amputees generally had a normal stride length with a decrease in cadence of 6% (see Table 7.1). In above-knee amputees, the decrease in cadence amounted to an average of 18%. Crutch users also showed some slowing of cadence. The oxygen consumption of able-bodied subjects at their voluntarily selected walking pace averaged 10.6 ml/kg • min STPD (i.e., standard temperature and pressure, dry gas—the usual reference condition for oxygen consumption measurement) compared with 14.6 ml/kg • min for below-knee amputees, 18.8 ml/kg • min for above-knee amputees, 14.4 ml/kg • min for crutch users, and 17.8 ml/kg • min for victims of poliomyelitis.

Merkel et al. (1984) measured the energy cost of paraplegic subjects who used crutches or a walker with bilateral knee-ankle-foot orthoses; the cost per meter traversed was 5.0 to 7.7 times normal for crutches and 8.8 to 12.8 times normal for a walker. Ambulation without a wheelchair is thus only practical for those with quite low-level lesions.

Other data on oxygen consumption for various types of disability were summarized by Fisher and Gullickson (1978; see Table 7.2). Results depend very

Table 7.1   Relationship of Cadence (f, steps/min) to Speed (v, km/hr) in Various Classes of Subject

Class of subject	Equation
Normal	$f = 34.2\ v^{0.81}$
Patellar-bearing prosthesis	
Well adapted	$f = 45.2\ v^{0.57}$
Limited training	$f = 47.8\ v^{0.45}$
Above-knee quadriceps socket	$f = 36.0\ v^{0.63}$
Crutch users	$f = 45.9\ v^{0.56}$
Unilateral poliomyelitis	$f = 48.9\ v^{0.66}$

Note. Based on data from *Selection of Clinically Suitable Tests/Methods for Ergonomic/ Physiological Evaluation of Lower Extremity Handicapped Persons* by A.K. Ghosh, 1980, Doctoral dissertation, University of Calcutta, India.

much on the pace at which comparisons are made—in general, the disabled slow down, so that their energy consumption per minute remains similar to that of the able-bodied. However, if the individual's concept of "fast walking" is requested, differences of cadence relative to the able-bodied are increased. The majority of data have been collected on level surfaces, but differences in energy cost per meter traversed are greatly enhanced by architectural barriers (N.E. Miller, Merritt, Merkel, & Westbrook, 1984); turns, stairs, and ramps can increase the cost 15-fold over that for able-bodied individuals.

The relationship of energy consumption to walking speed is a function of walking speed, both in normal subjects and those fitted with prostheses or crutches (Inman & Ralston, 1962). Ganguli et al. (1974c) set the oxygen cost at $[3.6\ (V) - 4.2]$ ml/kg • min in normal subjects and $[4.0\ (V) - 1.0]$ ml/kg • min in below-knee amputees, where V is the walking velocity in kilometers per hour. Ghosh (1980) described his data for the walking of normal subjects over the speed range 2 to 4 km/hr by means of the equation $[0.4\ (V^2) + 1.4\ (V) + 2.2]$ ml/kg • min (see Figure 7.1).

Well trained users of below-knee prostheses with 5 to 8 years of experience had a somewhat similar curve—$[0.64\ (V^2) + 0.4\ (V) + 7.4]$ ml/kg • min—but the cost was much higher for those who had been using their prosthesis for 6 months or less $[2.42\ (V^2) - 10.6\ (V) + 29.3]$ ml/kg • min. Above-knee prostheses demanded an even higher oxygen consumption $[3.00\ (V^2) - 12.4\ (V) + 30.5]$ ml/kg • min. In North America, children and young adults are invariably fitted with prostheses following amputation, but in the Indian setting of Ghosh (1980), long-term crutch users were also found among those sustaining industrial injuries. The oxygen cost curves for users of crutches following amputation and poliomyelitis were, respectively, $[1.20\ (V^2) - 4.8\ (V) + 19.2]$ ml/kg • min and $[0.68\ (V^2) - 3.6\ (V) + 4.2]$ ml/kg • min.

Energy costs drop to a minimum after 4 to 6 weeks of training in a given type of ambulation, although this advantage is lost if the skill is not practiced for several

Table 7.2   Energy Cost of Ambulation

Source and type of disability	Speed (m/min)	Energy cost (J/kg/min)	Energy cost per unit distance (J/kg/m)
Normals			
Fisher & Gullickson (1978)	83	264	3.20
Below-knee prosthesis			
Ralston (1971)	49	230	4.69
Molen (1973)	50	251	5.02
Ganguli et al. (1973)	50	251	5.02
Gonzales et al. (1974)	64	260	4.06
Waters (1976)	45-71	230-310	4.23-5.23
Above-knee prosthesis			
Muller & Hettinger (1953)	70	222	3.18
Bard & Ralston (1959)	68	255	3.77
Erdman et al. (1960)	47	147	3.18
Inman et al. (1961)	62	273	4.40
Durnin & Passmore (1967)	60	280	4.69
James (1973)	51	255	4.98
Ganguli et al. (1974a)	50	368	7.37
Waters et al. (1976)	36-52	225-260	4.98-5.23
Normals with crutches			
McBeath et al. (1974)	55-58	314-332	5.40-5.86
Above-knee amputees with crutches			
Erdman et al. (1960)	47	174	3.43
Ganguli et al. (1974b)	50	268	5.36
Traugh et al. (1975)	39	193	4.90
Hemiplegics			
Bard (1963)	41	184	4.44
Corcoran et al. (1970)	42	260	6.24
Hemiplegics with brace			
Corcoran et al. (1970)	49	280	5.73
Paraplegics			
Clinkingbeard et al. (1964)	4-20	180-201	9.92-37.88
Gordon & Vanderwalde (1956)	27	360-377	9.71-10.21
Wheelchair ambulation			
Hildebrandt et al. (1970)	67	155	3.85
Glaser et al. (1975, normals)	53-83	197-297	3.31-3.73

Note. Based in part on data from "Energy Cost of Ambulation in Health and Disability: A Literature Review" by S.V. Fisher and G. Gullickson, 1978, *Archives of Physical Medicine and Rehabilitation*, **59**, pp. 124-132.

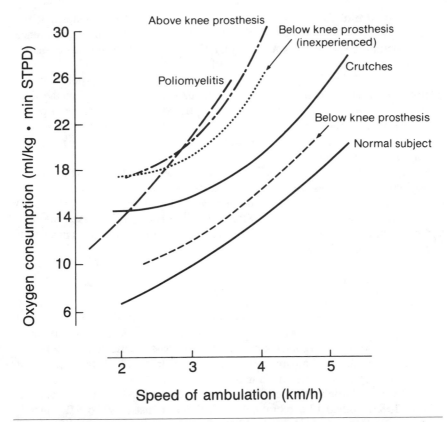

Figure 7.1.   The relationship between speed of ambulation and oxygen consumption in various classes of disabled individuals. Based on data of Ghosh (1980).

months (Clinkingbeard, Gersten, & Hoehn, 1964). We may conclude that although a pair of axillary crutches provides more economic immediate ambulation than a preliminary prosthesis (Cruts et al., 1985), once a definitive prosthesis has been fitted and the technique has been fully learned, a young adult can walk more economically with this prosthesis than with crutches (Ghosh, 1980); indeed, with developments in prosthetic technology, current energy costs of ambulation are likely to be even lower than those reported by Ghosh (1980).

If energy expenditures are related to the distance traversed (Fisher & Gullickson, 1978; see Table 7.2), the optimum speed of ambulation is found to be about 4 ml/hr for normal subjects (Ghosh, 1980), but it is substantially slower for the disabled (e.g., about 3.5 km/hr for below-knee amputees). The cost per unit distance at the optimum pace is higher in below-knee amputees than in the able-bodied, the increase ranging from 78% in those recently fitted to 17% in those who are well trained in the use of their prosthesis; Fisher and Gullickson (1978) noted an average 36% slowing of pace and a 41% increase of costs per meter traversed. For above-knee amputees, the optimum pace drops further, to 3.0 km/hr (Inman & Ralston, 1962) or 3.3 km/hr (Ghosh, 1980), with an increase in cost per unit distance of 89% (Fisher & Gullickson, 1978) or 100% (Ghosh, 1980) relative to able-bodied subjects. Crutch users with about 1 year of experience have an optimum speed of 4 km/hr (with a 37% increase over normal costs per meter).

Information on hemiplegia relates mainly to those affected by poliomyelitis (Ghosh, 1980). On average, this group chooses to walk 46% slower than the able-bodied, spending 63% more energy per meter traversed. For all cases of poliomyelitis (bilateral and dominantly unilateral), the most efficient walking speed is 3.5 km/hr; at this speed, there is an 88% increase over normal costs per meter traversed (Ghosh, 1980).

Much of the difference of mechanical efficiency between immediate and experienced use of a prosthesis reflects a progressive learning of techniques of walking, but part also is attributable to muscle hypertrophy. Thus, Kegel et al. (1981) commented that isometric muscle training and biofeedback increased the bulk of residual muscle in an amputated limb, with resultant improvements in suspension capability and the quality of gait.

Excessive Muscle Tone

Spasticity or uncontrolled athetoid movements of the limbs increases the energy cost of movement in patients with hemiplegia (Fisher & Gullickson, 1978) and cerebral palsy (Lundberg, 1975; 1976). In Lundberg's studies, the net mechanical efficiency of cycle ergometry was 12.1% in spastic patients and 16.6% in dyskinetic individuals, compared with 21.5% in controls. The extra energy cost attributable to spasm and dyskinesia may be exaggerated as a patient makes excessive movement at joints that are relatively unaffected by spasticity or weakness.

Pope (1985) studied 17 cerebral palsied sprinters (Classes VI to VIII) attending the ISOD Games in New York (1984). She found no significant differences of running pattern between disability classes but did observe a greater distortion of stride on the more involved side of the body. Relative to able-bodied athletes, she noted a shortening of stride, a slowing of horizontal velocity, and an increased ratio of support to nonsupport time, with other significant differences in trunk and hip angles, angle of touchdown, and stride time.

Stride frequency is comparable with that of able-bodied competitors. Stride length seems limited by forward leaning of the trunk, a limited range of hip motion, and a higher percentage of support time (Pope & Wilkerson, 1986).

A comparison between competitors with dominant and equal involvement of the two sides of the body (Pope, 1986) showed that those with equal involvement spent more time in support, developing more symmetrical angular displacements, with a slower movement of the limbs, a shorter step, and less vertical displacement. The center of gravity was also further forward than in those with a dominant unilateral involvement.

Postural Problems

In people with cerebral palsy, muscular dystrophies, and certain other disabilities that involve muscle weakness or contracture, mechanical efficiency may be reduced because the individual adopts a poor posture or attempts to supplement the action of weakened prime movers with accessory muscles that are poorly positioned to undertake the required task (Berg & Olsson, 1970). Thus Gehlsen et al. (1986) noted that subjects with multiple sclerosis had a shortened stride, a slower free walking rate, and a higher cadence than the able-bodied; the center of gravity of the body was also lifted less, and the trunk was allowed to lean at a greater angle to the vertical (Beuter & Garfinkel, 1985). Likewise Sanjak et al. (1987) found a 25% reduction in the efficiency of cycle ergometry in amyotrophic lateral sclerosis. In spastic children, problems may also arise from inappropriate mechanical damping of the limbs (Maki, Rosen, & Simon, 1985).

Any secondary deformity or joint immobilization interferes with the normal efficiency of gait (Aptekar, Ford, & Bleck, 1976; Saunders, Inman & Eberhart, 1953), although corrective tendon transplants can restore a more normal efficiency. If fixation of the knee or hip joint is unavoidable, the angle of immobilization should be selected carefully in order to minimize energy expenditures (Ralston, 1965; see Table 7.3). Severe scoliosis further augments the cost of moving (Lindh, 1978), in part because respiratory work is increased by a rapid breathing rate and by rigidity of the thoracic cage, whereas the primary deformity of the spine leads to postural problems (Stoboy, 1985).

In hemiplegia, the use of appropriate metal, plastic, or pneumatic braces substantially improves the mechanical efficiency of ambulation (Corcoran et al., 1970; Fisher & Gullickson, 1978; Ragnarsson, Sell, McGarrity, & Reuven, 1975). Subjects with low-level spinal injuries can sometimes walk (at a rather high energy cost) using braces and crutches, but with thoracic-level lesions the energy cost

Table 7.3 Effects of Various Types of Disability Upon the Energy Costs of Ambulation

Type of disability	Increase (%) of energy cost of ambulation
Body cast	10
Hip cast	
180°	20
150°	0-10
120°	30
Hip arthrodeses (150°)	
Slow walking	0-10
Fast walking	25
Knee cast	
150-180°	5-10
135°	25-35
Ankle cast	6
Bilateral ankle cast	9

Note. Based on data from "Energy Expenditure During Ambulation" by P.J. Corcoran, 1971, in J.A. Downey and R.C. Darling (Eds.), *Physiological Basis of Rehabilitation Medicine* (pp. 185-198). Philadelphia: W.B. Saunders.

of walking becomes too high for this to be a functional solution (Rosman & Spira, 1974). In cerebral palsy, braces may also be helpful in controlling spasticity, and there have also been attempts to produce a more symmetrical gait by the use of biofeedback (Seeger & Caudrey, 1983).

A rigid ankle brace allows more efficient walking than one that permits free dorsiflexion of the foot; the former arrangement reduces the required leg lift by 2 to 3 cm during the swing phase of walking. Lehmann, DeLateur, Warren, Simons, and Guy (1969) compared two designs of brace—a posterior ankle stop, which allowed free dorsiflexion of the ankle, and anterior and posterior ankle stops with a heavy sole plate extending to the metatarsal heads. Addition of the anterior stop allowed the subject to pivot on the ball of the foot when leaning forward on crutches. This effectively lengthened the leg and reduced the pathway for the center of gravity, with a lower energy cost of ambulation.

Mental Retardation

Among subjects with mental retardation, hyperkinesia, a poor attention span, and resultant difficulty in instruction allow uneconomic patterns of movement to persist from childhood into adolescence and adult life. The motor ability of such individuals is impaired at all ages (Levarlet-Joye, 1978), particular difficulty being encountered in execution of tasks that require both coordination and speed (Levarlet-Joye & Ribauville, 1981; Moran & Kalakian, 1977). However, special activity classes that emphasize development of an understanding of the body schema can ameliorate psychomotor performance (Chasey & Wyrick, 1971; Sherrill, 1986c).

Walking and Running Efficiency of the Blind

The walking habits of many visually impaired people are severely restricted. Indeed, about 30% do not venture outside of their homes (Clark-Carter, Heyes, & Howarth, 1986a; Gray & Todd, 1967). The lack of visual information creates tension when the person is moving (C. Buell, 1982); steps tend to be small and mechanical efficiency low. However, the impact of visual impairment varies with the severity of the handicap (Gorton & Gavron, 1987), and it is thus important to relate observations on walking patterns to some system of disability classification, either medical or athletic.

This population has traditionally used a lightweight cane to facilitate ambulation (Croce & Jacobson, 1986). The cane provides about a meter warning of obstacles immediately ahead of the individual, and if a typical, able-bodied walking speed of 80 m/min were adopted, a blind person would have only about a 0.8-second warning of approaching hazards (Clark-Carter et al., 1986a). It is thus hardly surprising that the usual walking pace of the blind is much slower than 80 m/min. Indeed, some have suggested that the voluntarily selected pace provides an index of the stress that a subject encounters while negotiating a particular route (Heyes, Armstrong, & Willans, 1976; Shingledecker, 1978); thus, visually impaired schoolchildren accelerate to the pace typical of their age when they enter a familiar school yard. Attempts to extend the range of preview have included devices that use pulsed ultrasound (L. Kay, 1973) and lasers (Benjamin cited by Clark-Carter et al., 1986b). Unfortunately, such instruments fail to detect some serious hazards such as holes in the sidewalk, and they must therefore be used in conjunction with a cane.

Tests both in sighted and blind subjects suggest that a preview distance of about 3 m increases both the safety and the efficiency of walking. Although not eliminating all difficulties at turning points (Armstrong, 1975; Jansson & Schenlemen cited by Clark-Carter et al., 1986b), technical aids giving such a preview distance allow the blind to move at a normal walking speed for much of a journey (Clark-Carter et al., 1986a, b). In running events, the hand of a partner, a handrail, or the voice of a caller may provide guidance. The relative mechanical efficiency achieved when using the last two techniques is currently under debate, but it is probable that the caller minimizes distortion of normal movement patterns over a short distance.

Congenital Versus Acquired Blindness

Various researchers have suggested that the blind not only move slowly but also tend to walk and run in a mechanically inefficient manner, irrespective of the method of guidance and the speed that they adopt (Hamill, Knutzen, & Bates, 1985). Dawson (1981) reported that adults who had been blind from birth walked with their heads tilted backward, using their forward legs as probes. In contrast, those with acquired forms of blindness leaned forward, as if focusing upon the ground immediately in front of them. MacGowan (1983, 1985) observed that relative to normal children, those who were congenitally blind walked more slowly, took shorter steps, and spent more time in the support phase of gait.

Pope, McGrain, and Arnhold (1986) studied 19 totally blind, 6 Class B2, and 23 Class B2 students, 44 of the 48 being congenitally disabled. These researchers commented that the running speed of the blind was correlated with stride length, hip range of motion, and upper extremity range of motion; they argued that the last characteristic was important to blind runners as a means of maintaining contact with guides, rails, or wires. They further noted a tendency of Class B1 sprinters to lean backward while running. Arnhold and McGrain (1985) filmed 27 students aged 9 to 16 years during a 50-m dash; all three categories of blindness were represented, with 25 of the 27 students having congenital disabilities. The investigators concluded that stride length was substantially shortened with visual impairment and that both stride and speed could be improved if the hip were extended more in the driving phase and flexed more in the recovery phase.

Gorton and Gavron (1987) drew attention to differences of running gait between B1 and B3 categories of athlete. They filmed 26 male competitors in the ISOD competitions of 1984, noting a general tendency of the blind group to tilt their heads forward, 5° at take-off and 10° at footstrike. At contact, the lead foot was also placed undesirably far ahead of the center of gravity, slowing the runner down. The forward tilt of the head was on average greater in Class B3 competitors ($+16.2°$) than in Class B1 competitors ($+3.8°$); on the other hand the trunk was tilted forward less in B3 ($+7.2°$) than in the B1 group ($+12.2°$). At takeoff, the B1 group also developed a backward lean ($-3.7°$) compared with a neutral or forward lean (0-16°) in the partially and normally sighted. Gorton and Gavron (1987) suggested that the blind group needed to increase hip and knee extension at takeoff; this would increase the force developed against the ground and thus the horizontal distance covered. From the mechanical viewpoint, it would also be an advantage to lean forward when running, as opposed to the backward-leaning tendency adopted by those who have been totally blind from birth; the latter technique inevitably leads to a poor mechanical efficiency.

Efficiency of Well-Trained Blind Individuals

Despite the adverse findings noted above, the blind do not inevitably move in an inefficient pattern. Lee et al. (1985) had physically well-trained totally blind students run around a familiar 110-m track for 12 minutes while holding onto a handrail. The researchers found that contrary to earlier reports, the AAHPER physical fitness norms for students of comparable age were actually exceeded by the blind children. Given that the directly measured cycle ergometer oxygen intake of the group was only in the high normal range, one must postulate that these particular blind students were able to run just as efficiently as those with normal vision, at least when covering familiar territory.

Mechanical Characteristics of Arm Work

A substantial proportion of the disabled population depends on the arms for ambulation. Unfortunately, the arm muscles are smaller than leg muscles (particularly in women; Tahamont et al., 1986), and the mechanical efficiency is less for upper- than for lower-limb activity. For example, when the legs are used to drive a cycle ergometer, the net efficiency is commonly about 23%, yet when the arms are used to crank an ergometer, the net efficiency drops to 10 to 16% (Bevegard et al., 1966; Fardy et al., 1977; Marincek & Valencic, 1978; Stenberg et al., 1967; Stoboy, Rich, & Lee, 1971). Moreover, most subjects can develop only about 70% of the leg maximum oxygen intake when undertaking maximal work with their arms (Åstrand & Saltin, 1961; Fardy et al., 1977; Franklin et al., 1983; Simmons & Shephard, 1971b; Stenberg et al., 1967). Thus, relative to lower-limb exercise, the heart rate and respiratory minute volume during arm work are greater at any given external power output, and the anaerobic threshold is reached at a lower absolute work rate. The one advantage of the wheelchair disabled is prolonged experience of arm exercise; this commonly gives them an advantage of mechanical efficiency over able-bodied individuals who also attempt an arm-cranking task (Tahamont et al., 1986).

Influence of Power Output on Mechanical Efficiency

Powers et al. (1984) examined the influence of increasing power output on the mechanical efficiency observed during arm work. The gross efficiency naturally increased with power output (as resting energy expenditure became a progressively smaller part of the total energy consumption). However, both work and delta efficiency decreased as the power output rose; this reflects in part an increasing need to use accessory muscles, which are less well positioned for activating the arm cranks, and in part a greater recruitment of fast twitch muscle fibers (which relative to slow twitch fibers offer a less efficient coupling of biochemical reactions to the contractile process, Wendt & Gibbs, 1973).

At any given power output, all efficiency indices decreased as the rate of cranking was increased. Again, this is due in part to a greater recruitment of fast twitch muscle fibers at rapid speeds of rotation. Some authors suggest that the arm muscles contain more fast twitch fibers than do the leg muscles (M.A. Johnson, Polgar, Weightman, & Appleton, 1973; Susheela & Walton, 1969) and that they are recruited earlier as loading is increased (Cerretelli et al., 1979). If so, this could contribute to a low mechanical efficiency during arm work.

Lesion Level and Delta Efficiency

Kofsky et al. (1983a, 1983b) calculated the slope and intercept for the oxygen consumption–power output line in a large group of paraplegics. The average values for subjects falling into ISMGF Classes II through VI were for men, $\dot{V}O_2 = 18$ (W) $+ 400$ ml/min ($r = .88$), and for women, $\dot{V}O_2 = 17$ (W) $+ 370$ ml/min ($r = .85$). The slopes are very similar to those described by Franklin et al. (1983) for able-bodied men, although perhaps because the disabled had difficulty in stabilizing their trunks, the able-bodied subjects had a smaller intercept (zero power output) on the oxygen consumption ordinate: $\dot{V}O_2 = 18.4$ (W) $+ 191$ ml/min.

In agreement with earlier observations by Wicks et al. (1977), an analysis of variance carried out by Kofsky et al. (1983a) showed no significant intercategory differences of delta efficiency between ISMGF Classes II through VI. However, Class I (the tetraplegics) showed a large zero intercept (due to the high cost of trunk stabilization), only small increments of oxygen intake with an increase of ergometer loading, and very low peak oxygen intake values. Although studies of able-bodied subjects show some increase of mechanical efficiency as they learn such unfamiliar tasks as wheelchair propulsion, Kofsky et al. (1983a) found that the arm ergometer efficiency of disabled individuals was not influenced by their patterns of habitual activity.

Swimming Technique

Swimming is a specific form of arm exercise open to the lower-limb disabled, although because of paralysis, spasticity, or loss of flexibility, mechanical efficiency may be much lower than that observed in an able-bodied competitive swimmer (Persyn, Surmont, Wouters, & De Maeyer, 1975; Persyn & Hoeven, 1981). The main problems of the disabled swimmer relate to balance in the three primary axes of the body. In the transverse axis, the head tends to be lifted out of the water, whereas the hand and forearm are positioned too horizontally and the trunk adopts an upwardly inclined position. In the sagittal axis, the head moves laterally, whereas the arms move laterally or even cross the midline. In the longitudinal axis, the swimmer may have difficulty in rolling the trunk, so that the head is wrongly placed with respect to the water surface when an inspiration becomes necessary.

Wheelchair Design

Historical Origins

According to some authors, the concept of a wheelchair for the lower-limb disabled originated with King Philip V of Spain, although Jayasuriya (1974) claimed that cripples in the Buddhist civilization of Sri Lanka were given wheelchairs in a much earlier era. The Spanish king had a wooden chair built for personal use around 1700; it featured wooden wheels and spokes, an adjustable leg rest, and a reclining back. The current type of folding medical chair was first marketed in the 1930s by H.A. Everest, who was himself a paraplegic (LaMere & Labonowich, 1984a, 1984b; Sherrill, 1986a). Much of the biomechanical evaluation to date has centered on issues of safety, durability, and ease of handling (Munaf & Boenick, 1984; Peizer, Wright, & Freiberger, 1964; Staros, 1981).

Power output varies with the total weight of the system, the distribution of this mass over the wheels of the chair, the specific features of the wheel (including rim diameter and tire pressure), and the nature of the tire and floor surfaces (Bennedik, Engel, & Hildebrandt, cited in Van der Woude, de Groot, Hollander, Van Ingen Schenau, & Rozendal, 1986; G,A, Wolfe et al., 1977). If the design incorporates a chain, transmission energy losses amount to about 1.5% of the total power output (Whitt & Wilson, 1979).

Racing Chair Design

The normal wheelchair weighs up to 20 kg. Racing chairs developed in the era following World War II, as wheelchair games became popular (Botvin Madorsky & Curtis, 1984; Higgs, 1983; Weege, 1985). In general, racing chairs are built to couple a low mass and a high level of maneuverability with a potential for rapid acceleration and quick turns (see Figure 7.2). They are also commonly collapsible to facilitate transport by road and air (see Figure 7.3). Comfort is sacrificed to performance; features such as arm rests and handles are usually eliminated, the frame is narrowed, and the chair back is greatly foreshortened. The seat is lowered and moved forward, and its base is usually set at an angle to the horizontal mainly to improve the balance of the competitors (see Tables 7.4, 7.5, and 7.6; Higgs, 1983, 1987); the linear velocity seems to be affected relatively little by changes in seat position (Walsh, Marchiori, & Steadward, 1986). The footrest is usually rigid, and the axle height can be modified to improve maneuverability for specific types of contest. A racing chair often has no brakes, but casters prevent backward tipping and a roll bar guards against folding of the chair in the event of a spill.

Hand rim sizes vary with different types of competition. For example, marathon racers choose chairs with a large driving wheel and a small push rim; this arrangement decreases the mechanical advantage of the athlete so that a greater force must be developed over a smaller linear distance in order to apply the same angular momentum and acceleration to the chair (Coutts, 1986). Some have suggested that in consequence, the contestant can increase the arc of active movement by supplementing the normal forward and downward propulsive thrust with an upward

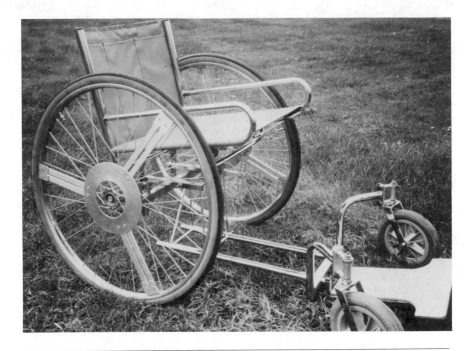

Figure 7.2. The classical wheelchair has undergone substantial modifications to facilitate high-performance sport.

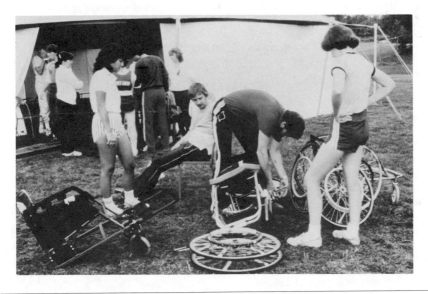

Figure 7.3. The modern wheelchair is rapidly dismantled when moving from one competitive site to another.

Table 7.4   Characteristics of the Wheelchair and Success in Track Events

Level of success	Mainwheel camber (degrees)	Push-rim diameter (cm)
1	7.2	35.7
2	7.0	34.2
3	5.1	39.7
4	6.3	39.3
4	3.2	43.2

Note. Based on data from "Analysis of Racing Wheelchairs Used at the 1980 Olympic Games for the Disabled" by C. Higgs, 1983, *Research Quarterly*, **54**, pp. 229-233.

Table 7.5   Relationship of Wheelchair Characteristics to Competitive Distance

Event	Mainwheel camber (degrees)	Push rim diameter (cm)
Sprint	5.6	39.3
Distance	6.8	35.3
Sprint + distance	6.4	37.4

Note. Based on data from "Analysis of Racing Wheelchairs Used at the 1980 Olympic Games for the Disabled" by C. Higgs, 1983, *Research Quarterly,* **54**, pp. 229-233.

Table 7.6   Typical Characteristics of Various Types of Wheelchairs

| Method of propulsion | Asynchronous | | Synchronous | |
	Crank	Lever	Standard push rim	Racing chair
Gearing ratio	1 : 1	1 : 1	1 : 1	1 : 1
Push rim diameter (m)	—	—	0.52	0.40
Rear wheel diameter (m)	0.615	0.615	0.615	0.615
Front wheel diameter (m)	0.615	0.615	0.10	0.20
Tire pressure				
Rear (Pa)	3×10^5	3×10^5	3×10^5	6×10^5
Front (Pa)	3×10^5	3×10^5	"Hard"	3×10^5
Wheel camber (degrees)	0	0	7.7	8.7
Mass (kg)	35.7	35.0	15.3	12.9

Note. Based in part on data from "Wheelchair Ergonomics and Physiological Testing of Prototypes" by L.H.V. Van der Woude, G. de Groot, A.P. Hollander, G.J. Van Ingen Schenau, and R.H. Rozendal, 1986, *Ergonomics*, **29**, pp. 1561-1573.

and forward pull (Coutts, 1986). NWAA/NWBA rules stipulate details of drive wheels, hand rims, seat heights, and methods to be used in securing the legs for various classes of competition.

The drive wheels of a racing chair have an inward camber, being further apart at the bottom than the top (Schuman, 1979); this arrangement improves the efficiency of pushing and reduces the danger of injuring the arm by bumping it against the wheel during rapid movements. Some athletes who compete in several types of event own a selection of sport-specific hand rims, and they adjust both rim dimensions and axle heights prior to participation in a particular type of competition. High performance distance racing chairs also use high-pressure tires that reduce the contact with the ground and thus the coefficient of rolling friction.

The seat of a racing chair is lower, with a rearward tilt; hip flexion is minimized, knee flexion is maximized, and air resistance is minimized by bending the trunk forward. Those with severe paralysis of the trunk cannot cope with the modern racing seat and still require a more traditional upright chair that offers them some spinal support.

Battery-Operated Chairs

Battery-driven chairs have a maximum speed of about 8 km/hr and can climb an incline of about 10°; as with other battery-driven devices, they become less efficient in cold weather, and both the battery and the supporting chair are inevitably quite heavy. The NASCP and its successor the USCPAA have arranged some contests in which participants can test their skill in maneuvering a motorized chair, but power-assisted devices are not allowed in international wheelchair basketball competitions.

Alternatives to Standard Wheelchairs

The fact that many disabled people find normal wheelchair ambulation very strenuous (Brattgard et al., 1970; Voight & Bahn, 1969) has prompted a search for vehicles that are mechanically more efficient (see Table 7.6; Glaser, 1987). Proposals have included the introduction of gears and levers (Engel & Hildebrandt, 1974; Glaser, Sawka, Young, & Surprayasad, 1980c; Kamenetz, 1969; Peizer et al., 1964) or an alteration of stroke mechanics to make maximal use of the available musculature (Gessaroli & Robertson, 1980c).

The conventional rim-operated chair is propelled with a gross mechanical efficiency of 10% or less (Brubaker, 1984; Brubaker & McLaurin, 1982). Improvements could be achieved either by optimizing the transfer of energy at the human–machine interface or by decreasing power losses from rolling friction, air resistance, and internal friction. Of these two possible tactics, the first is the more successful (Bennedik et al. cited in Van der Woude et al., 1986; Brubaker & McClay, 1983; Engel & Hildebrandt, 1971; Funk, 1971; Smith et al., 1983; Van der Woude et al., 1986). Designs using an arm crank or a lever are at least 2 to 3% more efficient than push-rim operation, although with all types of systems the wheelchair confined achieve a higher mechanical efficiency than their able-bodied counterparts (Van der Woude et al., 1986). Fink (cited by Van der Woude et al., 1986) further suggested that crank propulsion was more strenuous than use of an asynchronous lever.

Wheelchair Technique

Biomechanical aspects of wheelchair technique are attracting increasing attention (Cerquiglini, Figura, Marchetti, & Ricci, 1981; Sanderson & Sommer, 1985). Most of the published research relates to the spinally injured or able-bodied individuals, although a large number of wheelchair competitors are cerebral palsied. Such individuals have more difficulty in maintaining balance and adopt a more upright posture in the chair. Often, an extensor reflex tends to force them out of the chair; a high seat back, a greater seat angle, and strapping of the legs with or without a seat belt may all be required for the efficient functioning of such individuals (Sherrill, 1986c).

Brauer (1972) compared how normal and spinally injured subjects propel wheelchairs, both on hard, low-resistance surfaces such as a tiled floor and on high-resistance surfaces such as carpet or gravel. Disabled individuals have a lower "strike frequency" (the rate at which the rim of the driving wheel is grasped) than able-bodied subjects who propel the chair against the same submaximum resistance. Apparently the wheelchair confined can perform as much work as able-bodied subjects with fewer arm movements, because the disabled have learned to apply force with a greater torque during the strike phase. One trick that may contribute to this advantage is to apply part of the momentum generated by trunk movements—a technique used particularly in racing and maximum effort tests (Gessaroli & Robertson, 1980).

Higgs (1986) filmed the typical movement patterns adopted by spinally paralyzed wheelchair track competitors. He distinguished four phases of arm movement: initial contact with the hand rim, propulsion, disengagement, and the recovery movement (see Figure 7.4). In general, sprinters used a shuttle type of motion, whereas distance competitors adopted a more circular type of arm motion. However, Higgs found much interindividual variation, and many athletes made wasteful movements of their upper limbs. Higgs (1986) further noted that the velocity imparted to the chair was negatively correlated with the relative duration of nonpropulsive phases of the movement (contact, disengagement, and recovery).

Walsh et al. (1986), testing subjects with various disabilities, found that linear velocity increased as the hand time on the wheelchair rim was decreased. These reports run counter to earlier research (Schuman, 1979; Spooren, 1981; Steadward, 1980) and to biomechanical principles (Wells & Luttgens, 1976); researchers had earlier suggested that a racer could improve velocity by keeping his or her hand on the rim for a longer time and applying the force through as large an arc of arm movement as possible, provided that such a technique did not demand an excessive force relative to muscle strength. With modern, well-trained athletes, it seems that push frequency is a more important determinant of speed that the distance through which the push is applied.

Starting Movements

Particularly in wheelchair basketball and sprint events, performance depends more upon sudden acceleration of the wheelchair than on the ability to sustain high speeds. Success in initiating rapid movements depends upon the starting tech-

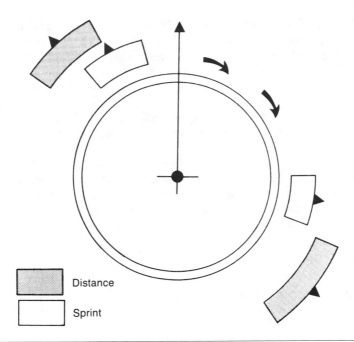

Figure 7.4. Typical hand position on wheel rim in distance and sprint wheelchair athletes. Based on data of C. Higgs, 1986. *Note.* Stroke rate = 102 ± 24/min (sprinters) and 92 ± 20/min (distance performers). Propulsion time = 34.5 ± 6.7% (sprinters), 38.7 ± 8.5% (distance).

nique that is chosen, the strength of the upper extremities, the stability of the trunk, and any other handicaps such as abnormal reflexes. The usual procedure adopted by the spinally injured is to grasp the wheel rim at its top, with the shoulders extended and the elbows flexed, pushing vigorously forward and downward to initiate a rotation of the driving wheels (Higgs, 1986). The velocity of forward motion depends on the net backward force exerted on the ground by the wheelchair and the rider, the time over which the force is applied, and the extent of frictional forces opposing forward movement.

Some sprint wheelchair athletes use a grab start similar to that adopted in normal daily ambulation, but others prefer a strike start. For the latter, the racer initially places the hands above and behind the top of the wheel rim; he or she then extends the arms forward and downward so that the palms of the hands strike the anterior superior surface of the rim. In order to increase the distance over which the driving force can be applied, the subject leans forward; this has the additional benefit that the center of mass is displaced forward, preventing the wheelchair from tipping backward.

Tupling et al. (1986) used a Kistler force plate to measure the ground reaction forces developed by spinally injured subjects during the two types of start. On average, the grab start transmitted 28% more backward impulse to the force plate than did the strike start, but the strike start produced 94% more impulse in the vertical direction (see Table 7.7). The grab start might thus seem the most appropriate technique for the amateur athlete. However, much depends on experience. Tupling et al. (1986) observed that two long-standing competitors (one a national caliber sprinter) who had used the striking technique regularly were able to produce a larger backward impulse in this fashion than by a grab start.

Ridgway, Hamilton, Hedrick, Nirse, and Adrian (1987) compared the first and second strokes of a racing start in eight elite participants in the 1986 U.S. national wheelchair athletic competitions. The researchers found differences with respect to point of first contact, speed, arc of propulsion, and trunk angle. Based on these observations, the authors recommended shortening the first stroke and commencing propulsion slightly forward of top dead center. Each individual showed a characteristic pattern for first, second, and typical sprint strokes, interindividual differences being related to classification, anthropometry, and personal technique (Ridgway, Morse, Hedrick, Adrian, & Hamilton, 1987).

Impulse Generation

Tupling et al. (1986) reported that the impulse generated by either a grab or a thrust starting movement was more closely correlated with habitual activity ($r = .74-.89$) than with lesion level ($r = .31-.86$) and thus trunk stability. The backward component of the overall impulse can be described by this equation:

$$BI = 33.8 \ (A) + 7.3 \ (E) - 2.14 \ (EP) - 30.2$$

where the backward impulse (BI) was measured in newton seconds, habitual activity A was grouped as 0 or 1, E was the average elbow power in watts, and EP was the peak elbow power in watts. The influence of elbow power upon impulse generation is further illustrated in Figure 7.5.

Although the backward impulse is plainly of paramount importance to a racing start and indeed to steady ambulation on level ground, the size of the vertical impulse may also be of significance in some of the activities of daily living (e.g.,

Table 7.7 **Mean Impulse (newton s) Generated in the X and Y Directions, Using Two Sprint-Start Techniques**

Group	Backward impulse		Vertical impulse	
	Grab start	Strike start	Grab start	Strike start
Highly active	174	142	22	49
Less active	132	97	42	74
Lesion above T-10	140	107	44	73
Lesion below T-10	162	129	23	54

Note. Based on force plate data from "Arm Strength and Impulse Generation: Initiation of Wheelchair Movement by the Physically Disabled" by S.J. Tupling, G.M. Davis, M.R. Pierrynowski, and R.J. Shephard, 1986, *Ergonomics, 29*, pp. 303-312.

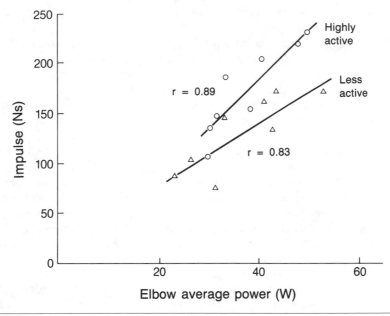

Figure 7.5. The influence of average elbow power (watts) on the impulse generated by a wheelchair start. Based on data of Tupling et al., 1986.

climbing a curb or a steep ramp). There thus remains scope to relate force plate information on both backward and vertical impulses to the success of the disabled individual in meeting the challenges of daily life. Propulsion by the feet (pulling or pushing) is allowed in Class 2 cerebral palsy. Backward propulsion is adopted when making a sprint start (R. Davis, 1985); the angle of the seat is reversed to maximize extensor power.

Injury Prevention

In the early days of sport for the disabled, many feared a substantial incidence of both injuries and illnesses. But in general the problems of competition in summer (Birrer, 1984) or in winter (McCormick, 1984, 1985) are no greater than for the able-bodied, and in physical education programs natural caution and the absence of contact sport give a low injury rate. Weakened muscles tire quickly, and in alpine skiing the likelihood of injury increases steeply over a long day on the slopes (McCormick, 1985).

In general, medical staff are kept busy treating such minor problems as sunburn, dehydration, gastroenteritis, and sprains rather than specific lesions related to the disability. Participants occasionally fracture paralyzed lower limbs, but given the absence of sensory nerves, the inconveniences are less than for an able-bodied athlete. For those with Down's syndrome, a specific concern is instability of the atlanto-axial joint; if undetected, this could lead to a cervical spinal injury.

Competitors with Down's syndrome should thus be excluded from diving, butterfly swimming, high-jumping, pentathlon, and soccer events until a careful clinical and radiological examination has excluded this possibility (Cooke, 1984). Precautions must be taken to ensure that blind competitors do not stray from the competitive area or collide with obstacles, and an appropriate choice of seats and cushions to increase thigh pressure will help to minimize pressure sores in both paraplegics and amputees (Seymour & Lacefield, 1985). The sports physician must finally be aware of the specific medications taken by many disabled competitors to counteract anxiety, seizures, hyperactivity, and excessive muscle tone and must understand the effects of such drugs upon both physical performance and environmental adaptation.

Jackson and Frederickson (1979) noted that 184 of 1,700 competitors in the Toronto Olympiad for the Disabled required treatment; they reported with a wide variety of minor injuries. Likewise, in a regional wheelchair competition, Curtis and Dillon (1986) treated 93 of 1,200 participants for 291 injuries (see Table 7.8). The highest risks of injury are for track, basketball, road racing, tennis, and field events (Bloomquist, 1986); low-risk sports include pool, bowling, archery, slalom, and table tennis. Many of the soft-tissue injuries and other accidents are inherent to the operation of a wheelchair at high speeds (Corcoran et al., 1980). Special features of wheelchair design that protect an athlete in the event that a chair is tipped over have been noted previously. There is international agreement that in order to minimize the risk of injury to the legs, footrests should be at a uniform height of 10 cm, with the seat no more than 51 cm above the ground.

Other injuries (sprains, strains, muscle pulls, tendinitis, bursitis, blisters, abrasions, lacerations, and hand weakness or numbness) might be thought indicative of overuse (Curtis & Dillon, 1986; Nichols, 1979), and in support of this view, the injury rate is highest for those competitors who train the greatest number of hours per week. For example, the constant compression of the heel of the hand on the push rim of a wheelchair can lead to carpal tunnel syndrome (a compression of the median nerve as it passes through the carpal tunnel, first noted as pain and tingling in the thumb and first two fingers; Curtis, 1984). Blisters reflect friction of the hands on the push rim and of the back on upholstery or the seat post; countermeasures include encouragement of callus formation and increased padding.

Abrasions and lacerations may arise from finger contact with the brake, arm rest, or push rim; scraping of the arms on the tires; or (in basketball) the trapping of the fingers between wheelchairs. Competitors should remove hazardous parts from their wheelchairs if possible and wear arm guards; the situation is also helped by a cambering of the wheels. Adequate cushioning, good skin hygiene, and use of clothing that absorbs sweat can reduce the likelihood of developing pressure sores on the buttocks and back (McFayden & Stoner, 1980; S.F. Stewart, Palmieri, & Cochran, 1980).

If environmental conditions are severe, lack of active muscle and problems of autonomic regulation (poor vasomotor activity and reduced sweating) increase the vulnerability of paraplegics to heat (Bloomquist, 1986; Totel, 1974; Totel, Johnson, Fay, Goldstein, & Schick, 1971) and cold stress (Claus-Walker, Halstead, Carter, & Campos, 1974; Corcoran et al., 1980; Downey, Darling,

Table 7.8 The Commonest Types of Injury in Wheelchair Athletes

Type of injury	Percent of total
Soft tissue (sprains, strains, pulls, tendinitis, and bursitis)	33
Blisters	18
Lacerations, abrasions, and cuts (including skin infections)	17
Pressure sores	7
Arthritis and joint disorders	5
Fractures	5
Hand weakness or numbness	5
Problems of temperature regulation	3
Head injury/concussion	1
Dental injury	1
Miscellaneous	4

Note. Based on data for 291 injuries reported by 93 disabled athletes from "Survey of Wheelchair Athletic Injuries—Common Patterns and Prevention" by K.A. Curtis and D.A. Dillon, 1986, in C.A. Sherrill (Ed.), *Sport and Disabled Athletes* (pp. 211-216). Champaign, IL: Human Kinetics.

& Chiodi, 1967). Racers should drink adequate fluids in the summer and wear appropriately insulating clothing in the winter, especially on inactive parts such as amputation stumps. During all seasons, the environmental limits between which competition is permitted must be more conservative than for able-bodied subjects; likewise, if hypothermia does develop, medical personnel must take care not to injure denervated parts during rewarming.

Ergonomic Considerations in Buildings and Athletic Facilities

Modifications are needed in stadia and other athletic facilities to allow free access for the disabled, both as athletes and as spectators. Desirable features include reserved parking areas near main entrances, replacement of stairs by shallow ramps, fitting of elevator controls at an appropriate height, installation of laboratories and bathrooms with doors at least 1 m wide, and the provision of hopper-type lockers. Floyd, Guttmann, Noble, Parkes, and Ward (1966) completed a detailed ergonomic study of the space requirements of wheelchair users. Zankel (1971) also provided detailed examples of structured modifications that facilitate the activities of daily living. Arguments continue on the merit of beautifully designed (but segregated) living quarters versus accommodation with other competitors. Specialized buildings can offer such amenities as broad passages, power-operated doors and windows, additional lighting (to minimize the need for stooping), and improved working surfaces to reduce the needs for reaching and stretching.

For wheelchair races, lane widths on the track or field must be increased to 1.5 to 2.0 m per competitor. Swimming events require a pool with a shallow ramp, allowing the athletes to enter the water at seat height. In other types of events, small adaptations to equipment facilitate the participation of the disabled; for example, cycles can be modified for hand operation (Axelson & McCormack, 1983; Slagle, 1982). The saddles of horses can offer greater support to the back (Hay, 1982), sailboats can be operated by radio-controlled devices splinted to the hands (Axelson, 1986), and even water sleds (Wilkinson, 1982) and downhill sleds (P. Taylor, 1983) can be devised to accommodate the disabled.

Blind competitors are helped by a readily recognizable texturing of the floor in a building. Wall signs, elevator controls, and swimming pool markings should be transcribed into braille. Insulation from extraneous noise must be sufficient to allow keen use of hearing, and excellent lighting will assist those with some residual vision.

Key Ideas

1. Whether efficiency is calculated as gross, net, or delta, the majority of disabled individuals have low values. Thus, their disability is compounded by difficulty in converting food energy into useful external work.

2. Although young amputees quickly adapt to use of a prosthesis, many older adults lack the mechanical efficiency and cardiorespiratory reserves to allow ambulation in this fashion.

3. Performance in other types of disability is impaired by fear of collision with obstacles (in the blind), poor balance, unusual posture, spasticity, athetoid movements, or difficulty in learning appropriate techniques of movement.

4. The arms operate with a lower mechanical efficiency than the legs, in part because effort is expended in stabilizing the trunk during arm work. Efficiency is particularly poor for individuals with high-level spinal cord injuries.

5. Over the past two decades, the wheelchairs used by disabled athletes have been progressively modified to improve competitive performance. The overall mass of the chair has been greatly decreased, the seat and back rest lowered, the wheels cambered, and the size of the push rims modified to suit the needs of individual events.

6. Habitual wheelchair users have a higher mechanical efficiency than the able-bodied when propelling any type of chair. However, crank- and lever-operated chairs appear more efficient than push rim designs, whether they are used by experienced or inexperienced operators.

7. The greatest velocities of ambulation are attained with rapid rather than long strokes on the push rims of a wheelchair.

8. The serious competitor must be protected against overuse injuries and extremes of heat and cold.

9. Adaptations of both facilities and equipment will be needed to realize the full potential of the disabled person, whether as a spectator or as a participant.

Practical Applications

1. What are some of the problems of calculating mechanical efficiency in the disabled?
2. What features of disability are likely to lead to a poor mechanical efficiency?
3. What practical measures could you suggest to extend the mobility of the blind?
4. How practical is it to use a prosthesis after amputation?
5. How does arm work differ from leg exercise? What are the implications for the performance of the lower-limb disabled?
6. How has the racing wheelchair evolved from the standard wheelchair? What further developments might increase competitive performance?

Chapter 8

Personality, Behavior, and Social Adjustment

In this chapter, we discuss the social difficulties faced by the disabled, the impact of these problems upon both lifestyle and various facets of personality, and the value of regular exercise in countering such handicaps. We review motivations to greater physical activity in the context of modern behavioral theory, and finally we examine factors influencing socialization into and via sport. Much of the available information on personality and behavior in the disabled (Sherrill, 1986b) relates to those with a neuromuscular handicap, although some information also concerns anxiety levels in the blind.

Social Problems of the Disabled

Whether a lesion be congenital or of recent origin, the disabled individual faces many discouragements during daily life. Schooling is hampered, employment prospects are poor, and the person faces much stigmatization and stereotyping.

Stigmatization

A physical handicap creates a visible stigma that tends to be socially discrediting, encouraging others to avoid the affected person (Aufsesser, 1982; Hunt, 1966); often, the handicapped are regarded as unproductive or socially deviant, and civilizations have considered them to be punished by the deity or a witch, or possessed by the devil (Adedoja, 1987; Goffman, 1963; Richardson & Green, 1971; Siller, 1982). Unfortunately, able-bodied children seem to develop negative stereotypes of the disabled at a very early age (A.B. Kennedy & Thurman, 1982). In general, sensory disabilities are the least stigmatized, physical handicaps rank next, and those with mental disorders are the most subject to ostracism (Aufsesser, 1982; Eisenberg, Griggens, & Duval, 1982; Tringo, 1970; see Table 8.1). The cause of the disability also influences perceptions (Table 8.2). Because the adverse stereotype is learned from significant others such as parents, it may be more rigid and difficult to overcome than beliefs formed from personal experience (Triandis, 1971). Surprisingly, the process can also occur among the disabled themselves,

Table 8.1   Rank Ordering for Choice of a Close Friend

Type of disability	Score	Type of disability	Score
Wheelchair	2.45	Stutterer	4.81
Blindness	3.09	Epilepsy	5.34
Amputee	3.63	Emotionally disturbed	6.68
Deafness	4.54	Mentally retarded	6.84
Harelip	4.65	Cerebral palsy	7.55

Note. Based on data from "Comparison of the Attitudes of Physical Education, Recreation and Special Education Majors Toward the Disabled" by P.M. Aufsesser, 1982, *American Corrective Therapy Journal, 36*, pp. 35-41. Factors influencing the choice include (a) the visibility of the affliction, (b) interference with communication, (c) social stigma, (d) reversibility, (e) degree of incapacitation, and (f) difficulties encountered in daily life. Other authors have ranked stigmatization as sensory < physical < mental. A low score indicates a favorable attitude.

Table 8.2   Evaluations of Disabled Subjects Made by a Class of Students, Based on the Viewing of a Videotaped Interview

Cause of injury	Score (high = favorable image)
War disability	151
Able-bodied	142
Car accident	74
Work accident	74
Poliomyelitis	70

Note. Based on data from "The Relationship Between Physical Disability, Social Perception and Psychological Stress" by S. Katz, E. Shurks, and V. Florian, 1978, *Scandinavian Journal of Rehabilitation Medicine, 10*, pp. 109-113.

those least affected by stigmatization disdaining those with a more heavily stigmatized type of handicap (Hunt, 1966; Sherrill, 1986b).

Stereotyping

Some of the more obvious stereotypes that affect the disabled are a perceived lack of physical attractiveness, intelligence, and ability. In many instances, the entire stereotype is inaccurate and inappropriate. Thus, the disabled are placed in special schools and sheltered workshops, when in fact they are well able to cope with normal education and employment opportunities.

It is particularly unfortunate that the existence of negative stereotypes has contributed to conflicts over the "ownership" of athletic contests. For example, some able-bodied runners have wished to exclude wheelchair athletes from events such as marathon races (see chapter 3). Such exclusion immediately has an adverse impact on a majority of the handicapped participants who wish to be judged on their overall competitive performance (i.e., as 42-km racers) rather than as "blind" or "paraplegic" patients.

As already noted, in certain instances individuals affected by one class of disability develop adverse stereotypes of those affected by other types of lesion. This phenomenon has possibly contributed to the spirit of exclusiveness and excessive rivalry that has arisen between disabled sports organizations, a process that has frequently threatened solidarity among the various categories of disabled sports participants (see chapter 2).

Lifestyle and Disability

The social problems faced by the disabled often cause a reactive depression, and this can lead in turn to acceptance of an adverse lifestyle. Particularly when a disabled individual sees no prospect of employment, he or she may show little concern for the maintenance of general health; the person may then make attempts to escape from boredom and despair through the abuse of tobacco, alcohol, and drugs (Nelipovich, 1983; Nelipovich & Parker, 1981).

Employment

Despite negative stereotypes that are too often held by potential employers, many supposed "cripples" are better motivated and more productive than their able-bodied peers. Studies of the employed blind have shown further that if they are given appropriate training, their accident rate is actually lower than that for workers with normal vision (Shephard, 1974).

Nevertheless, employment prospects for the average disabled person remain relatively poor. Kofsky and Shephard (1985) found that of those who had left school, roughly equal numbers of paraplegics were employed and unemployed. Moreover, the proportion of habitually physically inactive subjects was much higher in the unemployed than in those who were employed. Overall, about 50% of the paraplegic group were living at or below the poverty line for Ontario (an income of $16,000 per year at the time of their survey, 1978-1984). Further, the proportion earning more than $25,000 per year was only about half of that anticipated in the general population, and the proportion earning $5,000 or less was about 5 times greater than the Canadian national average.

Among the blind, 60% are over the age of 65 years, so in many instances the issue of gainful employment does not arise. However, only 12 to 15% of blind students are regarded as employable; particular difficulty is encountered in placing older people with multiple handicaps (Shephard, 1974).

Habitual Activity

Price (1987) found that following spinal trauma, the leisure satisfaction of the injured individual in general decreased. This finding was uninfluenced by the life stage at which disability had begun or the period that had elapsed subsequent to onset of the handicap. Participation in sports, games, outdoor pursuits, and other forms of physically active self-actualization was likely to decrease relative to the individual's pretrauma situation, whereas the time allocated to more passive pursuits was likely to increase.

The Canada Fitness Survey (1986) reported data for that 13.7% of their sample who described themselves as functionally disabled and were willing to be tested. From both the incidence of disability relative to other statistics (see chapter 2) and other information presented in the Canada Fitness Survey, it appears that the type of disability discussed, although chronic, was in many instances not very severe. Some 50% of the disabled group regarded themselves as physically active, their most popular reported activities being walking, gardening, cycling, swimming, and home exercises rather than pursuits that required community facilities. Most of the inactive half of the disabled population indicated that nothing would increase their level of physical activity.

The Canada Fitness Survey made enquiry about health behaviors. Some 50% of the active disabled but only 23% of the inactive regarded exercise as an important health behavior. The active disabled were more likely than the inactive to be nonsmokers, to have a good breakfast regularly, and to take 7 or 8 hours of sleep per night.

Among the various clinical types of disability studied by Kofsky and Shephard (1985), the least active group were those affected by multiple sclerosis. This probably reflects in part the fact that whereas specific sports organizations have been formed for the spinally injured, amputees, the blind, the deaf, the cerebral palsied, and the mentally retarded, little has been done to promote an increase of physical activity among those with multiple sclerosis (the NWAA nevertheless does accept competitors with multiple sclerosis).

Smoking Habits

Kofsky and Shephard (1985) found that the proportion of smokers among their wheelchair disabled (49% of men, 45% of women) substantially exceeded provincial norms; these disturbing figures were apparently uninfluenced by either the level of the lesion or the pattern of habitual activity. However, the heavy smokers (> 25 cigarettes/day) were predominantly those with a Type B personality on the Rosenmann scale;[1] as in studies of the able bodied, they tended to have an external locus of control. They were also trusting, shy, and of below average intelligence; in general, they claimed to be unaware of the health hazards associated with smoking and regarded physical activity as a challenge that they probably could not meet.

---

[1]This scale distinguishes the time-conscious Type A personality from the more relaxed ("laid back") Type B personality.

Alcohol Consumption

It is notoriously difficult to obtain accurate information on alcohol consumption from self-reports. Kofsky and Shephard (1985) found that 68% of their sample of paraplegics described themselves as no more than occasional social drinkers, and only 12% admitted taking more than six alcoholic drinks per week. Those who reported heavy drinking were the more intelligent members of the group, with a bold and undisciplined type of personality on the Cattell scale.

Personality of the Disabled

Inevitably, the social problems discussed previously tend to have an adverse influence not only on lifestyle but also on the manifest personality of the disabled person; although some disabled athletes have as high a level of self-actualization as the able-bodied (Sherrill, 1986c; Sherrill & Rainbolt, 1987), many disabled people show evidence of maladjustment, retarded emotional development, and social alienation, with feelings of self-pity, rejection, depression, excessive submissiveness, and sometimes attempts at compensation including egocentricity and passive hostility (Adedoja, 1987; Bruininks, 1978; Bryan, 1976; Cohen, 1977; Cratty, 1980; Harper & Richman, 1980). Such changes in turn affect attitudes toward physical activity (Flynn & Salomone, 1977; Glick, 1953; Harper, 1978; Harper & Richman, 1978; Katz et al., 1978, Lazar, Demos, Gaines, Rogers, & Stirnkorb, 1978).

Immediately following spinal injury, ego strength is low and depression scores are very high (D.J. Dunn, 1969). In subsequent months, disabled individuals have considerable problems adjusting to their handicaps (Glick, 1953; E. Miller, 1958). Physical activity may be of considerable therapeutic and psychological benefit during the early phase of rehabilitation, helping the patient develop a sense of self-efficacy (Bandura, 1977; Lewko, 1981) and an awareness that it is not necessary to accept a life of total inactivity and dependency (Owens, 1968).

Subsequent participation in athletic competition is also important to many disabled people, not only because of the gains in physical condition that result from precontest preparation, but also because of the social respect, approval, and prestige that is gained (N. Croucher, 1976; Dendy, 1978; Goode, 1978; Gouldner, 1965). Involvement in sport holds the prospect of deinstitutionalization and reintegration into able-bodied society (Ross, 1983).

Tucker (1968) found that the Cattell 16 PF score (Institute for Personality and Ability Testing, 1972) of physically handicapped persons reflected greater intelligence, more introversion, and a less practical attitude than able-bodied subjects, whereas Harper (1978), using the Minnesota Multiphasic Personality Inventory (MMPI), noted that the disabled were particularly prone to problems of social adjustment. Goldberg and Shephard (1982) further examined this issue, applying a number of standard psychological tests including Cattell's 16 PF test, McPherson's body image scale, and the locus of control test of Nowicki and Strickland (1973) to nine wheelchair athletes and eight moderately active spinally injured paraplegics. Kofsky and Shephard (1985) subsequently extended this investigation to encompass 163 male and 97 female lower-limb disabled adults. Mastro and French (1986) recently examined the status of the blind athlete, with particular reference to anxiety levels and mood states.

Before interpreting details of these various results, certain general limitations of the data must be stressed. As with any paper-and-pencil test of attitudes or personality, the results depend on the truthfulness of the subjects; only one of the several instruments to be discussed incorporated any "lie scale" (the Cattell test) and even this is of doubtful validity (Braun & LaForo, 1968). Although the subjects appeared cooperative and well motivated, some may (consciously or unconsciously) have provided answers that they thought the investigators wanted to hear or were appropriate to popular stereotypes of their disability. Moreover, all of the available, normative scores were designed for use with able-bodied populations, taking no account of the peculiar problems faced by disabled people in their attempts to integrate with society.

In the study of Goldberg and Shephard (1982), the more active half of those tested were wheelchair athletes, and any differences between them and the general disabled population might reflect the social status accruing to individuals with publicized achievements in athletic competition, rather than a more specific response to vigorous training. Because most of the available studies of the disabled are cross-sectional in type, there is no proof as to whether an increase of physical activity is responsible for the favorable psychological characteristics of groups such as wheelchair athletes or whether initially favorable psychological characteristics have allowed such subgroups to undertake more vigorous activity subsequent to the onset of their disability.

Cattell Test Scores

The Cattell test is a well-accepted psychological questionnaire that yields information on 16 orthogonal[2] personality traits; the score for each trait is presented in normalized fashion using a Standard Ten (STEN) score (normal value 5.5 ± 1.0) relative to a pair of contrasting characteristics (e.g., cautious/venturesome). In an initial survey of a small sample of spinally injured paraplegics, Goldberg and Shephard (1982) found no significant differences of test scores relative to the general population. However, wheelchair athletes were distinguished from more sedentary paraplegics by high scores on Factors B (intelligence), H (venturesomeness), and I (tough mindedness). Moreover the wheelchair athletes differed significantly from the general wheelchair population with respect to Factor H.

This could imply that much of the achievement that marks the disabled athlete is due not to some peculiarity of physiological endowment but rather to a strength of personality and an achievement orientation that has assured a willingness to undertake vigorous training (Szyman, 1980). Alternatively, a favorable response to training and an ability to undertake unexpected feats may have strengthened a feeling of toughness and venturesomeness among the more active segment of the disabled population.

In a larger sample of paraplegics, Kofsky and Shephard (1985) confirmed an association of activity with intelligence and venturesomeness in male subjects.

---

[2]Showing no significant correlation with other test factors.

Other authors have had similar findings both in the disabled (Shatin, 1970) and in healthy women athletes (Mushier, 1972). Moreover, in the sample as a whole, Kofsky and Shephard (1985) found that 12 of the 16 personality factors differed from the published normal standards. In most instances, the deviations were in a direction that would be regarded as disadvantageous to the paraplegics (see Table 8.3). Relative to an able-bodied individual, the paraplegic demonstrated traits described as reserved, intelligent, neurotic, pessimistic, expedient, shy, tough minded, practical, shrewd, conservative, temperamental, and maladjusted. However, it is possible to argue, particularly with traumatic paraplegia, that these personality characteristics contributed to the accident rather than resulted from it. The female paraplegics also differed from the males, being more conscientious, timid, troubled, and tense than their male counterparts (see Table 8.3). Such differences seem in essence an exaggeration of normal, culturally determined sex differences.

Goldberg and Shephard (1982) reported that individuals with severe high-level lesions (ISMGF Classes I-III) had high scores on Factor O (placid vs. apprehensive), but those with low-level lesions (Classes IV-VI) showed relatively normal scores for apprehension. Kofsky and Shephard (1985) further found that men with high-level lesions were more detached, humble, and serious but also more resourceful than those with less severe disabilities.

Body Image

Tests of body image provide a numerical expression of how the self is perceived, both physically and socially (Mueller, 1962). If the image is poor, a substantial gap develops between the ideal and the perceived body image. Early research suggested devaluation of self in various types of disability (Geis, 1972; Shontz, 1978; Simon, 1971; Vargo, 1978; Wylie, 1961). Harper (1978) found that paraplegics often had problems of self-perception and a poor body image, although he found no difference of scores between those with congenital and those with traumatic lesions. Likewise, Brinkmann and Hoskins (1979) noted a poor self-concept in hemiplegic patients; after a period of training, the researchers reported significant gains on several subscales of the Tennessee self-concept scale, including identity, physical self, personal self, and social self. Patrick (1986) applied acceptance-of-disability scale and the Tennessee self-concept scale; 5 months after their first competition, novice wheelchair athletes showed a significant improvement on both of these scales. In contrast, Lazar et al. (1978) found no perceptible differences of social adjustment or attitudes between paraplegics and able-bodied university students; however, they commented that the disabled were more oriented toward cognitive goals, possibly reflecting years of hard work in proving that they were superior to their able-bodied peers.

The Kenyon/McPherson instrument is one measure of body image. It develops scores for items such as ''My body is as I would like it to be'' and ''The real me'' from a series of Likert scales, spanning contrasting adjectives such as beautiful and ugly. Goldberg and Shephard (1982) found that the gap between the perceived and the desired body image, as measured by this test, was larger in moderately active spinally injured than in those who had achieved the status of

Table 8.3 Cattell's 16 Personality Factors: Standard Ten Scores (Mean ± SD) for Male and Female Paraplegic Subjects

Personality factor	Males (n = 87)	Females (n = 46)
Factor A (Reserved vs. outgoing)*	5.0 ± 2.2	5.7 ± 2.0
Factor B (Less vs. more intelligence)*	6.2 ± 2.1	5.9 ± 2.0
Factor C (Emotional vs. unemotional)*	4.8 ± 2.0	4.3 ± 1.8
Factor E (Humble vs. assertive)	5.7 ± 2.0	5.3 ± 1.7
Factor F (Sober vs. enthusiastic)*	5.4 ± 2.1	4.9 ± 2.0
Factor G (Expedient vs. conscientious)*	5.4 ± 1.4**	6.3 ± 1.7
Factor H (Shy vs. venturesome)*	5.8 ± 2.4**	4.8 ± 1.9
Factor I (Tough minded vs. sensitive)	5.1 ± 1.9	5.3 ± 1.9
Factor L (Trusting vs. suspicious)	5.3 ± 1.9	5.4 ± 2.1
Factor M (Practical vs. imaginative)*	5.1 ± 2.1	4.9 ± 1.8
Factor N (Forthright vs. shrewd)*	5.9 ± 1.9	6.2 ± 2.0
Factor O (Placid vs. apprehensive)	5.7 ± 2.0**	6.5 ± 2.1
Factor Q1 (Conservative vs. experimenting)*	5.4 ± 2.1	4.7 ± 1.9
Factor Q2 (Dependent vs. self-sufficient)*	6.2 ± 1.8	6.2 ± 2.1
Factor Q3 (Undisciplined vs. controlled)*	4.7 ± 1.6	4.9 ± 2.0
Factor Q4 (Relaxed vs. tense)	5.5 ± 2.1**	6.8 ± 2.1

Note. Based on data from "Factors Influencing Fitness and Life Adjustment of Disabled Individuals" by P.R. Kofsky and R.J. Shephard, 1985, *Final Report to Grant 6605-1915-46.* Ottawa: Health & Welfare Canada.

*Significant difference from normal. **Significant sex difference.

wheelchair athletes (see Table 8.4). In the former group the difference from the able-bodied approached statistical significance (Goldberg & Shephard, 1982). However, no consistent difference of body image was seen between those with high- and low-level spinal lesions.

Kofsky and Shephard (1985) confirmed both the advantage of active over inactive paraplegic individuals and the lack of influence of lesion level upon body image. Not surprisingly, they also noted a poorer self-image in women than in men, and in both sexes the gap between ideal and perceived image was much larger for lesions that were due to disease than those that were due to trauma.

Nevertheless, Siller and Peizer (1957) and Siller (1960) commented that feelings of inferiority and shame were also an important part of the reactions in children after limb amputations for trauma. Current society places such a heavy emphasis upon health and beauty that the negative self-image of the disabled person is hardly surprising (Simon, 1971). Any handicapped patient is in turn adversely influenced by the negative perceptions of outsiders (Katz et al., 1978; Shontz, 1978; Simon, 1971; Vargo, 1978). A full adjustment to disability requires not only a personal acceptance of the handicap but also a willingness to learn, understand, and tolerate the misconceptions of a relatively unsympathetic society (Vargo, 1978; B.A. Wright, 1983). In particular, the majority of the able-bodied react more favorably to war heroes than to patients who are injured at work, with a corresponding negative impact upon the self-concept of the latter group (Katz et al., 1978).

Fortunately, the younger generation seems to be adopting a more positive attitude toward the disabled, irrespective of the cause of the lesion (Lazar et al., 1978). The process of accepting the handicapped can probably be helped further by specific instruction of physical educators and schoolchildren (S.C. Anderson,

Table 8.4 Body Image: Discrepancy From Desired Value on Kenyon/McPherson Scale

Normals			Paraplegics			
Middle-aged men	Old men	Old women	Athletic men	Moderately active men	Active women	Inactive women
23.8	21.8	26.6	30.2 ± 15.1	34.6 ± 16.0	—	—
			27.9 ± 18.8	42.0 ± 19.4	45.0 ± 23.9	47.9 ± 19.4

Note. Based on data from "Personality Profiles of Disabled Individuals in Relation to Physical Activity Patterns" by G. Goldberg and R.J. Shephard, 1982, *Journal of Sports Medicine and Physical Fitness*, **22**, pp. 477-484 and from Kofsky and Shephard, 1985 (see note to Table 8.3). Mean $\pm$ *SD*. A high score indicates a large discrepancy from desired body image.

1980; Aufsesser, 1982; Jansma & Schultz, 1982), by a mainstreaming of disabled pupils into classes for the able-bodied (Auxter, 1981; Beuter, 1983; Dibner & Dibner, 1973; see chapter 9), and by a correction of physical barriers to sports and leisure participation (Hutchison, 1980; see chapter 6).

Locus of Control

The locus of control scale examines the extent to which an individual perceives an ability to control her or his environment. External control is assumed when a person perceives events as unpredictable or the result of luck, chance, or fate, whereas internal control is deduced if events are seen as contingent upon personal behavior (Nowicki & Strickland, 1973; Rotter, 1975).

In the studies of Goldberg and Shephard (1982), the locus of control for the wheelchair-disabled individuals was usually external, the average score being almost twice that described for young able-bodied people (Nowicki & Strickland, 1973). However, patients with high-level spinal lesions (ISMGF Classes I-III) had the same scores as those with low-level lesions.

Kofsky and Shephard (1985) obtained much lower scores (implying a more internal locus of control), perhaps because many of their group had the initiative to attend laboratory exercise training sessions (see Table 8.5). Nevertheless, they confirmed that the locus of control of the spinally injured person was uninfluenced by the level of the lesion or by habitual physical activity. In their study, the women had a stronger belief in an external locus of control than did the men.

Self-Actualization

Formal measurements of self-actualization in elite ISOD competitors, made using the personal orientation inventory of Shostrom (Sherrill, 1986c; Sherrill & Rainbolt, 1987), demonstrated fairly high levels of self-actualization. Relative to non-elite competitors, the subjects scored higher on the two scales most closely related to self-actualization (time competence and inner directedness), although they showed less time competence than able-bodied adults. They also had higher

Table 8.5   Locus of Control

Normals		Paraplegics			
Men	Women	Men	Women	Highly active men	Moderately active men
9.2	9.5	10.7*	12.7*	21.9	22.9
±4.1	±3.9	±4.7	±4.3	±2.3	±2.6

Note. Based on data from Goldberg and Shephard, 1982 and Kofsky and Shephard, 1985 (see note to Table 8.4). A low score denotes an internal locus of control.

*Many members of this sample were willing to attend exercise training sessions in the laboratory. Mean ± *SD.*

scores than the non-elite competitors for self-actualizing values, feeling reactivity, and capacity for intimate contact.

In terms of functioning, the researchers suggested that the elite subjects were less worried about pleasing others and less likely to resort to manipulative behavior; they had liberated themselves from a rigid adherence to social pressures and social expectations and tended to autonomous, independent functioning. Relative to the non-elite, they were less burdened by guilt, regrets, and resentments from the past and tended to live in the present.

Anxiety

Many disabled groups such as the blind become acutely anxious following the onset of disability, fearing that they will be unable to support themselves and any dependents (Klemz, 1977). Several reports suggest that the blind competitor is particularly prone to state anxiety during competition because of the lack of normal visual cues (Hardy & Cull, 1972; Peake & Leonard, 1971; Wycherly & Nicklin, 1970). The main evidence that anxiety had developed was a high heart rate during exertion, although plainly this could have arisen in part from poor posture or a low mechanical efficiency rather than from any psychological disturbance. Mastro and French (1986) applied the state/trait anxiety inventory of Spielberger, Gorsuch, and Lushene (1970), finding that in general scores did not differ between elite blind athletes and normal individuals, either between or before their participation in international competitions. However, the authors admitted that because of practical difficulties, they were unable to collect responses very close to the time of actual competitive events. Mastro, French, Henschen, and Horvat (1986) nevertheless confirmed a high state and trait anxiety in the blind, their subjects being golfers.

Henschen, Horvat, and French (1984) applied the same instrument to wheelchair athletes, finding an average level of state anxiety and a low level of trait anxiety, much as in able-bodied athletes. However, Levine and Langness (1983) suggested that mentally retarded basketball players were more anxious than normal adults.

Monnazzi (1982) applied a clinical instrument (the Middlesex Hospital questionnaire) to 22 paraplegic athletes and 19 nonathletes. A cross-sectional comparison of test scores for these two groups suggested to Monnazzi that sport participation may have attenuated anxiety, phobia, and translation of physical problems into psychoses (somatization), and depression.

Profile of Mood States (POMS)

The POMS test is a simple, one-page questionnaire examining immediate mood state. It is widely used in sports psychology. Henschen et al. (1984) obtained POMS scores from 33 male wheelchair athletes, and Canabal, Sherrill, and Rainbolt (1987) studied 39 cerebral palsied athletes attending the 1984 ISOD Games. Both groups observed the "iceberg" profile typical of an able-bodied competitor (a high score for vigor and low scores for tension, depression, fatigue, and confusion). The one difference from healthy competitors was that the disabled group manifested high scores on the anger scale, particularly if they had difficulty in ambulation, anger being negatively correlated with sports classification (Canabal, Sherrill, & Rainbolt, 1987). Mastro, Sherrill, Gench, and French (1987) also observed a typical iceberg profile in elite, visually impaired athletes, with even higher vigor scores that able-bodied competitors. In contrast, Mastro et al. (1986) found blind golfers to have a POMS profile similar to that of the general population.

Minnesota Multiphasic Personality Inventory (MMPI)

The MMPI is a well-respected, extended paper-and-pencil assessment of basic personality traits. Application of this procedure revealed little difference of scores between those with congenital and those with traumatic lesions (Harper, 1978). However, relative to those with a cleft palate, orthopedic disabilities led to an isolative and passive orientation. When compared with normal subjects, significantly lower scores were seen on Scales Hs (hypochondriasis), D (depression), Mf (masculinity/femininity), Sc (schizophrenia), and Ma (megalomania).

Overall Impact

G.M. Davis et al. (1980, 1984a) found that current self-reported personality attributes discriminated relatively effectively (86% correct classifications) between spinally injured individuals with three different lesion levels (C6-C8; T1-T10; T10-S2; Figure 8.1). Factors contributing to the discriminant function included Cattell's 16 PF test (five items), the locus of control test, and five attitudes toward physical activity as assessed on the Kenyon scale. The implication was that a more severe lesion led to a greater psychological disturbance.

Effects of Training

It seems logical that a favorable personality profile would increase the ability to undertake training (Flynn & Salomone, 1977), whereas an increased ability to perform daily activities and live an independent life would have a positive influence on the body image and psychological profile of the disabled person (Roberts, 1974). Some studies indicate that this expectation has been realized. In children with mental retardation, participation in appropriately adjusted types of competition has had a very beneficial impact upon self-image and social interactions (Bell, Kozer, & Martin, cited by J. Wright & Cowden, 1986; Fisher, 1980; Kinney, 1979; Rarick, 1971; J. Wright & Cowden, 1986). Barnes (cited in J. Wright & Cowden, 1986) found that for mentally retarded adults, also, Special Olympics participation offers a valuable alternative to the usual sedentary lifestyle.

Nevertheless, for the physically disabled much depends on the establishment of a training program with realistic goals and expectations. Trainers must take account of inherent shifts in mood state and avoid making excessive physical or emotional demands that could further damage an already fragile self-image. Roberts (1974), himself a paraplegic with a T9 spinal injury, suggested that the primary cause of disillusionment during rehabilitation was fatigue. In the long term, exercise should help to counter this handicap, but in the early stages of

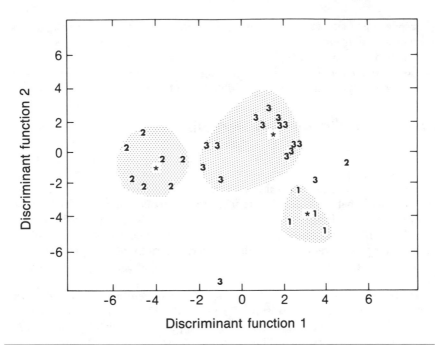

Figure 8.1. Discrimination of anatomical disability grading, based on two discriminant functions developed from various self-reported psychological attributes. Subjects were 28 male wheelchair users, aged 19 to 59 years, with (1) cervical (C6-C8), (2) thoracic (T1-T10), or (3) low-level (T10-S2) lesions. Based on data from G.M. Davis, Jackson, & Shephard, 1984.

rehabilitation patients need a slow introduction to relatively undemanding sports, set in the context of others who face similar problems through a matched level of disability.

Ankenbrand (1972) conducted one of the few longitudinal studies of self-image. He found that an 8-week bowling program led to significant gains of skill, self-concept, and self-acceptance in disabled subjects, all of these gains being much larger than the responses observed in able-bodied controls during a comparable period of physical activity.

Dalton (1980) noted a significant decrease in depression scores for disabled men and women following 8 weeks of endurance training. However, interpretation of these results is complicated by the fact that vitamin B_{12} supplements were provided during the training period.

The cross-sectional results of Goldberg and Shephard (1982) offer some further support to the hypothesis of Roberts (1974). A high level of physical activity was associated with a bold and sociable personality, a willingness to try new things, and an ability to face grueling emotional situations. In contrast, those individuals who undertook only moderate activity tended to be withdrawn, cautious, and impeded in self-expression and to have feelings of inferiority.

Despite much suggestive evidence that sports participation can enhance the psychosocial adjustment of the disabled, conclusive proof is as yet lacking. In particular, if we can demonstrate benefit, we must still weigh carefully the relative merits of sports, fitness, and recreation programs and compare the effectiveness of specially adapted versus integrated programs.

Exercise Motivation and Compliance

Both initial recruitment to an activity class and subsequent compliance with a prescribed exercise regimen are major problems even among able-bodied subjects. Well-designed programs attract no more than 20 to 30% of eligible adults, and as many as half of those who are recruited drop out of the organized activity within 6 months (Dishman, Sallis, & Orenstein, 1985; Shephard, 1985a, 1985b). Variables influencing this discouraging situation include attitudes toward physical activity, behavioral intentions (determined in turn by personal attitudes, beliefs, and social norms), and environmental factors that encourage socialization into sport.

Plainly, the factors discouraging exercise recruitment and continued sports participation are even more formidable in the disabled than in an able-bodied person. G.M. Davis (1985) examined the compliance of spinally injured paraplegics with a laboratory training program that required attendance at three sessions of arm ergometer exercise per week. After 8 weeks, adherence was 92%, but it dropped to 63% after 16 weeks and 54% after 24 weeks. The most frequently cited reasons for lack of compliance were much as in the general population (lack of interest, 28%; lack of time or distance from the training site, 36%; health or medical problems, 36%).

However, the medical problems encountered in his series were more serious than for the able-bodied, including pressure sores, respiratory and renal infections, and back injury. Disposable income is also smaller than for the able-bodied, free time may be more limited, and even a short journey to an exercise facility can pose major problems of accessibility. Moreover, the exercise itself is more demanding and less pleasant for the participant, attendance may be interrupted by intercurrent infections, and loss of sensation predisposes to the onset of medical complications such as pressure sores. Relative to the able-bodied, a disabled person must generally spend a much longer time before physical activity becomes an intrinsically rewarding pursuit, and in the interim, a greater reliance must be placed upon external reward systems (Danielson & Danielson, 1979), particularly the strong encouragement provided by a sympathetic class leader.

Recent research with disabled subjects has examined such issues as attitudes toward physical activity (Cooper et al., 1986; Goldberg & Shephard, 1982; Kennedy, 1980), behavioral theories of exercise participation (Colantonio, Davis, Shephard, Simard, & Godin, 1986; Shontz, 1978), specific motivational techniques for the disabled (McLeish, 1983; Sandler & McLain, 1987), and reasons for competing (M. Cooper et al., 1986).

Attitudes Toward Physical Activity

The Kenyon instrument examines the instrumental value to the individual of a global concept of exercise in seven specific domains (six domains in earlier versions of the test). A series of contrasting adjectives (e.g., good/bad) rate the corresponding concepts (e.g., exercise as a means to fitness and health).

Delforge (1973) applied the Kenyon instrument to students at the University of Arizona, finding no differences between handicapped and nonhandicapped individuals. Goldberg and Shephard (1982) likewise found that paraplegics perceived five of the seven Kenyon domains much as did able-bodied individuals (see Table 8.6). However, the wheelchair athletes showed more interest than the general population in exercise as "the pursuit of vertigo" (swift accelerations being a characteristic feature of wheelchair sport) and exercise as an ascetic experience (probably a marked feature of endurance training from a wheelchair). The moderately active but nonathletic paraplegics showed parallel differences on these two scales.

Kennedy (1980) applied the Kenyon instrument to 84 paraplegic and amputee athletes; some of their scores differed substantially from all-Canadian samples, but relative to the able-bodied athlete, the disabled group showed more interest in activity as the pursuit of vertigo, as an ascetic challenge, as a means of catharsis, and as a means of fitness; furthermore, the disabled subjects' scores were higher on each of the six scales if the disability had been incurred after the individual had reached an age of 17 years (see Table 8.6).

Kofsky and Shephard (1985) further observed significant differences of attitudes between male and female paraplegics (see Table 8.6); the males valued activity as the pursuit of vertigo and as an ascetic experience, and the females valued the aesthetic aspects of exercise. M. Cooper et al. (1986) reported data for 170 participants in a national competition for the cerebral palsied. This group scored highly on each of Kenyon's attitudinal scales, in some instances even exceeding the results reported by Goldberg and Shephard (1982).

When scores for the various domains of attitude were classed in terms of the extent of disability, Goldberg and Shephard (1982) found that the more severely restricted individuals (ISMGF Classes I-III) differed significantly from those with low-level lesions, the former group placing more value on exercise as an aesthetic experience. However, subsequent studies (M. Cooper et al., 1986; Kennedy, 1980; Kofsky & Shephard, 1985) found no difference of attitudes between those with high- and low-level lesions. Unfortunately, Kenyon's inventory does not clearly distinguish personal physical activity from a more general appreciation of spectator sport, and it is unclear whether the severely disabled subjects in the study of Goldberg and Shephard (1982) still valued light but aesthetically pleasing movements from a personal viewpoint or whether they merely enjoyed the spectacle of such activity.

Formal studies in other types of disability seem relatively few. M. Cooper, Sherrill, and Marshall (1986) examined 464 adult participants in the U.S. National Cerebral Palsy Games, noting that although attitudes toward physical activity were

Table 8.6 Attitudes Toward Physical Activity in Normal Adults, Able-Bodied Athletes, Spinal Cord–Injured Amputees and Cerebral Palsied Athletes

Attitude	Normal adult men	Athletic men (able-bodied)	Athletic men	Moderately active men	Paraplegic		Paraplegia + amputation	Cerebral palsy
					Male	Female		
Aesthetic	47.7	43.2	45.3	50.5	48.7	45.2*	39.3	47.0
Social	45.9	40.2	47.0	49.4	43.9	45.9	40.2	47.6
Fitness	45.7	39.2	47.0	50.0	44.5	45.0	41.5	46.9
Catharsis	46.5	36.1	44.2	45.1	45.9	43.8	39.2	46.4
Vertigo	33.7	35.1	39.9**	43.9**	38.7	30.6*	35.9	41.5
Ascetic	32.2	29.4	40.6**	42.4**	32.0	37.1*	36.3	41.4
Games of chance	30.4	—	34.9	32.3	32.6	32.2	—	—

Note. Based on data from ''Social and Psychological Dimensions'' edited by C. Sherrill, 1986b, *Sport and Disabled Athletes*. Champaign, IL: Human Kinetics and from Goldberg and Shephard, 1982 and Kofsky and Shephard, 1985 (see note to Table 8.4).

*Significant difference from men. **Significant difference from normal adults.

generally positive, subjects showed less interest in sport as a thrill and as long, hard training than as a social experience and a way to achieve health, fitness, beauty, and tension release. Dummer, Ewing, Habeck, and Overton (1987) also studied athletes with cerebral palsy, noting that they emphasized "winning" less than did the general population. Moreover, irrespective of the outcome (winning or losing), the subjects had a greater than normal tendency to attribute the result to external factors such as luck. Dummer et al. (1987) suggested that this might be due in part to the substantial intraindividual variations of disability in cerebral palsy.

Specific Motivational Techniques

The importance of external motivation by a sympathetic class leader or coach in the early stages of training has already been stressed. Vigorous and repeated stimulation is particularly important in increasing the motivation of the mentally retarded (McLeish, 1983). In children with multiple handicaps, Sandler and McLain (1987) found that response-contingent vestibular stimulation is much more effective than traditional reinforcing devices such as food or praise.

Perceived Reasons for Participation

M. Cooper (1986) used a paired comparison test to rank the main perceived reasons why the disabled individual participated in sport. The first seven reasons were, in order, challenge of competition, fun and enjoyment, love of sport, fitness and health, knowledge and skills relating to sport, contribution to sport, and the team sport atmosphere. These seven items were all ranked significantly higher than items such as liking for other team members, travel, liking for the coach, and status.

Sherrill, Rainbolt, and Ervin (1984) had athletes list the six main areas in which sport had contributed to their lives. The items cited by 201 cerebral palsied athletes were fitness, socialization/friendships, self-concept/mental health, interesting/exciting use of leisure time, release of tension/relaxation, and development of motor skills. The ranking was similar for 100 blind athletes, except for interchanges of rank between socialization and self-concept and between use of leisure time and tension release. Participation was more important than winning for 79% of the cerebral palsied and 82% of the blind competitors. Likewise, in mental retardation, Levine and Langness (1983) suggested that self-esteem and a "normalizing experience" were more important motives than winning when playing a game of basketball, and J. Wright and Cowden (1986) found positive effects of an "Olympic" swim-training program upon self-concept.

Behavioral Modeling

The able-bodied individual's immediate intention to exercise can be explained largely in terms of Fishbein's theory of reasoned action (Godin & Shephard, 1986; Riddle, 1980). This assumes that the intention to undertake a particular action is shaped by a weighted combination of attitudes and social norms. The attitudes reflect beliefs about a given behavior and the personal appraisal of such beliefs, whereas the social norms reflect the perceived attitudes of significant others and the motivation to comply with such norms (see Figure 8.2).

The factors influencing the disabled person's exercise behavior seem somewhat different than in the able-bodied (Colantonio et al., 1986; Godin, Colantonio, Davis, Shephard, & Simard, 1986). It is possible to explain 35% of the observed variance in the habitual activity of a spinally injured paraplegic group from behavioral data using instruments of the type suggested by Fishbein and Ajzen (1975). The strongest predictor of active behavior was behavioral intention. However, in contrast to the researchers' studies on the able-bodied, none of the standard Fishbein model variables (attitudes or social norms) helped in describing actual exercise behavior. Exercise habits accounted for about 7% of the total variance in current exercise behavior. Investigators thus hypothesized that relative to able-bodied subjects, factors extraneous to the standard model (such as the cause of disability and the prior strength of the exercise habit) played a more significant role as determinants of active behavior in this type of individual.

Socialization Into and Via Sport

Many authors have noted that minority groups show a lack of social integration and that this influences their involvement in recreation and sport. It is thus important to recognize that most types of disability confer the undesirable status of membership in a visible minority (Hill, 1974). In consequence, disabled individuals generally show poor social relationships and a limited integration into their immediate society (Martinek & Karper, 1981). Potential expressions of maladjustment include shyness, timidity, fearful behavior and other forms of withdrawal, concealment, refusal to recognize reality, and actual delusions (Barker, Wright, & Gonick, 1983).

Involvement in sport can sometimes help the process of integration (Marr, 1987; Sherrill, Pope, & Arnhold, 1986; Sherrill & Rainbolt, 1986), but whether it is effective (particularly in the long term; Anderson, Grossman, & Finch, 1983) depends not only on the attitude of the disabled individual but also on the reactions of physical education majors and society as a whole (Rowe & Stutts, 1987). Too often, teachers begin work with negative, stereotyped attitudes toward the disabled (Gargiulo & Yonker, 1983), or they develop such attitudes due to frustrations encountered in instructing the disabled (Chasey, Swartz, Chasey, Brogman, & Sandler, 1975; Rizzo, 1984). Programs that sensitize teachers (Aufsesser, 1982), teachers in training (Conine, 1969; Jansma & Schultz, 1982; Naor & Milgram, 1980; Patrick, 1987), students (G. Clark, French, & Henderson, 1985), and the general public (Anderson, 1980) to the potential of the disabled can thus be of considerable practical value in increasing the social integration of special populations. Close personal contact with the disabled seems much more effective in this regard than the mere provision of information (Hamilton & Anderson, 1983; Kisabeth & Richardson, 1985).

Loy and Ingham (1973) and Hopper (1986) noted that people can be both socialized into sport and socialized by sport. A study of socialization into sport examines

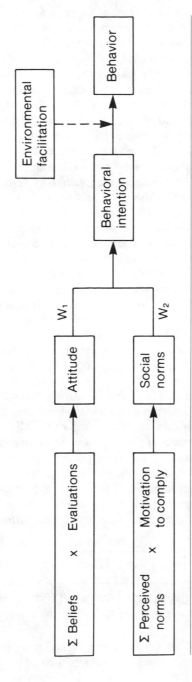

Figure 8.2. Fishbein's model of reasoned behavior.

factors that cause the individual to become active, whereas socialization via sport considers the impact of physical activity upon aspirations (athletic, educational, and occupational) and associated changes of self-esteem.

Kennedy (1980) concluded from a cross-sectional study that the age of onset and the severity of disability were not significant determinants of socialization into sport. This view was supported by Sherrill et al. (1986b), who questioned blind and cerebral palsied athletes regarding the specific factors that had influenced their involvement in sport. Whereas it is common to find that the parents of able-bodied competitors were also once highly athletic, in the blind and the CP samples the attitudes of the parents and siblings toward physical activity were generally neutral; indeed the majority of relatives had never shown any great personal interest in sport. Among the blind, a physical education teacher had usually done most both to attract the subject to sport and to provide specific instruction; attitudes toward school-based experiences are much more favorable than those centered on community or family (Sherrill et al., 1984). For wheelchair-bound CP athletes the influence of peers and friends was dominant, but for ambulatory patients the family had exerted the most important influence; the mean age of first competition (18.5 years) was much older in the cerebral palsied than in the able-bodied (Sherrill & Rainbolt, 1986).

Ruckert (cited in Sherrill, 1986b) had somewhat similar findings in a survey of disabled athletes, mainly paraplegics and amputees; the primary perceived stimuli to sports involvement in this group were the initiative of the individual participant (29%) and the encouragement of disabled friends (27%), able-bodied friends (27%), or family (9%). As in other situations where the effectiveness of the physician in promoting active behavior has been formally tested, only 8% of the sample considered that their family doctor had been the primary stimulus to enhanced personal activity.

Hopper (1986) found that 31% of the socializing variance of sport in wheelchair athletes was directed toward educational aspirations, 24% to athletic aspirations, and 12.5% to self-esteem. The younger the individual, the greater the educational and athletic impact of participation. Somewhat surprisingly, Hopper found an inverse relationship between self-esteem and commitment to sport. Hopper (1986) suggested that other factors such as career and domestic happiness may have had a larger impact upon self-esteem than did success in wheelchair competition. In support of this view, he noted that as the athletes became preoccupied with sport, their educational aspirations suffered.

Key Ideas

1. Stigmatization and stereotyping on the part of both the able-bodied and those with less severe forms of disability add to the physical handicaps of the disabled.

2. Many of the disabled are better motivated and more productive than able-bodied workers, yet because of prejudice, their employment prospects remain poor.

3. A poor lifestyle, a low level of habitual activity, and other bad habits such as cigarette smoking and alcoholism can compound disability.

4. Difficulty in adjusting to the various problems encountered in daily life has a negative effect on personality, with many disabled subjects showing a low ego strength, a poor body image, and a reactive depression. Disabled subjects' scores on many of Cattell's 16 personality factors differ from scores of the able-bodied. The disabled commonly perceive an external locus of control and may have high anxiety levels. Involvement in an exercise program, particularly if this involves adapted competition, can alleviate many of these psychological problems.

5. Compliance with exercise programs is difficult to sustain in the disabled. In addition to the usual problems of time management reported by the able-bodied, the disabled have limitations of disposable income, limited mobility, and medical problems attributable to the disability.

6. Those involved in wheelchair sport have a particular appreciation of the vertiginous aspects of activity.

7. The disabled can be socialized into sport by significant others, and such involvement makes a substantial contribution to their integration with society.

Practical Applications

1. Why would one class of disabled individuals stigmatize or stereotype another class of the disabled?

2. What practical measures could improve the employment prospects of the disabled?

3. Why do many of the disabled adopt a negative lifestyle?

4. Are all of the personality characteristics of the disabled secondary to physical disability?

5. What practical measures could be suggested to improve recruitment to and compliance with an exercise program?

Chapter 9

Effective Program Design

From the previous discussion, it appears that regular physical activity would benefit most categories of disabled individuals. However, prior to training, both their physical endurance and their self-concept are often inadequate, limiting both recreation and productive employment. There are formidable obstacles to the goal of making wheelchair exercise a "respectable" and accepted pursuit. One recent survey of people with physical, emotional, or mental handicaps attending a vocational rehabilitation program (Day, 1984) found that only 3% of such subjects rated sports as their first choice of leisure activity, although a further 8% opted for walking. This chapter offers some practical suggestions regarding program objectives, appropriate methods of satisfying these objectives, and methods of encouraging both recruitment to and continued participation in exercise programs.

Objectives of Exercise and Sport Programming

Exercise and sport programs may be advocated because of anticipated gains in self-concept, mood state and socialization, improvements of metabolic control, muscle building, increase of flexibility, development of aerobic power, habituation to physically demanding situations, learning of exercise techniques, and medical benefits. We will review the various objectives with particular emphasis upon the type of exercise prescription needed to yield the suggested benefit.

Psychological Gains

Particularly for younger individuals, an important objective of any program of increased physical activity is to counter the negative impact of disability upon self-image and mood state (see chapter 8.). The type of program most likely to satisfy this objective varies with the initial physical and psychological state of the individual. Someone who is in poor physical condition may become embarrassed or discouraged if the exercise prescription seems demanding relative to ability. On the other hand, a person who is already physically active may judge a low-level exercise class as a waste of time or even as stigmatization as a "cripple." Such problems are best resolved by grading exercise classes in terms of initial ability and where possible by personalizing the exercise prescription.

An extrovert with an external locus of control will tend to respond best to opportunities for exercise in a group setting, whereas an introvert with an internal locus of control may respond more favorably to an individual program (Massie & Shephard, 1971); a "thinking" type of individual will want a program that accords with his or her personal beliefs regarding exercise and health (Fishbein & Ajzen, 1985), certainly with feedback of data and information, possibly with an associated health education program (Becker & Maiman, 1975). On the other hand, a person who is guided by feelings will be influenced more by the general ambience of the exercise sessions, attitudes toward the instructor or other class members, and the sensations experienced while exercising (e.g., an appreciation of the beauty of movement, the thrill of a contest, or the vertigo induced by rapid turns in a wheelchair; Kenyon, 1968a, b).

Many disabled people will benefit from exercising as a group, not only because of the physical activity undertaken in this setting but also because of the support offered by the class leader and other members of the organization (Franklin, 1988). Participants can discuss practical problems of daily living, share solutions, obtain advice regarding improvements of lifestyle, and obtain treatment for any intercurrent medical conditions.

Any form of physical activity should have an arousing effect (Martens, 1974), due both to a stimulation of the limbic system of the brain by an increased proprioceptive input and the mere fact of exposure to an environment outside of the home. The extent of proprioceptive stimulation depends on such factors as spindle receptor density (greater in the muscles of the arms than in those of the legs) and the vigor of the movement that is undertaken. However, a change of environment can be realized with only a modest expenditure of energy. The goal of an elevation of mood may thus be satisfied if a person with a spinal cord injury operates a wheelchair gently through pleasant parkland or a blind person takes a nature walk along a trail where the texture of bark and the appearance of beautifully scented flowers are discussed by a sighted guide or an electronic aid.

An alternative short-term basis for an exercise-induced elevation of mood would be an increased secretion of beta-endorphins (Harber & Sutton, 1984). This requires a prolonged and intensive bout of activity and is thus an unlikely explanation of mood changes in the average disabled person. However, it could conceivably be a factor in groups such as wheelchair marathoners (who are vigorously active for 2 or more hours).

In the more long term, exercise could improve mood state through an enhancement of body image (Dishman, 1985; Morgan, 1982); this is likely to occur if the individual senses gains in both physical performance and the ability to cope with the demands of daily living as a result of participation in the exercise classes. The instructor should thus interpret current physical performance with this emphasis; attention should be drawn to a longer distance covered without fatigue or the accomplishment of a task previously regarded as impossible. In this regard, it is important that the expectations of the instructor are realistic. Many disabled people are initially greatly discouraged by their handicap, and some may require quite strong external motivation in order to improve their condition. However, the instructor must strike a careful balance between encouragement and excessive pressure; unrealistic expectations can have a strongly negative effect upon motivation. Much discussion has centered around the relative merits of adapted and integrated programs (Sherrill, 1986c) and their respective impacts on perceived competence and self-concept.

In the case of schoolchildren, the current consensus is that although the body image of the child may develop more favorably through participation in normal classes than through restriction to adapted classes, much depends on the level of disability; ideally there should be a need-based continuum of opportunities from segregated to fully integrated instruction (Winnick, 1987). A further source of argument has been the merits of competition (see chapter 2). Some authors maintain that suitably adapted types of competition provide the disabled person with a new source of excitement, greatly enhancing the mood of the winners. Others have pessimistically questioned whether the poor image of a disabled individual can handle the trauma of losing a contest against others who are disabled.

Metabolic Control

A second argument in favor of increased activity is that it will improve metabolic regulation. Studies in the able-bodied have shown that increased activity can help control blood sugar (reducing the risk of diabetes; Holm & Krotkiewski, 1985), improve the blood lipid profile by a decrease of LDL and total cholesterol (Wood, Haskell, & Blair, 1983), and diminish body fat as a better balance is struck between the intake and the usage of food energy (Brownell & Smoller, 1985).

The essential element in achieving these metabolic benefits is to prescribe a regimen that assures a slightly negative energy balance. A reduction of body fat and a decrease of total cholesterol could be achieved merely by rigorous dieting, but the disabled individual hardly needs the added depression of mood associated with adherence to such a plan (Shephard, 1982b). Alternatively, the daily level of physical activity could be increased and the daily intake of food energy held constant. As each gram of body fat is equivalent to some 29 kJ of energy, an obese person must carry out a substantial amount of physical work in order to consume excess adipose tissue. Prolonged steady exercise is preferable to bursts of high intensity activity that are difficult to sustain; the consumption of fat relative to carbohydrate is greater with moderate exercise, and there is less danger of overloading a heart that probably suffers from some degree of coronary atherosclerosis.

Quite moderate intensities of activity seem effective in improving the blood lipid profile. Thus in able-bodied postal carriers, both Arnold, Shephard, and Kakis (1985) and Cook et al. (1986) found that a daily round of some 8 km (walked at 4-5 km/hr) was sufficient to increase HDL2 cholesterol levels. Wood et al. (1983) proposed that the threshold distance for this type of benefit is a weekly walking or jogging distance of 18 to 20 km (i.e., about 4 hours of walking per week). Likewise, in the wheelchair disabled, benefit has been seen in comparisons of athletes and inactive individuals. Because the energy cost of ambulation is at least as great as when walking at a comfortable speed, the threshold for augmentation of HDL cholesterol should be no more than 4 hours of wheeling per week.

Muscle Building

Therapeutic exercise to maximize residual muscle function is helpful in many forms of disability (Kraus, 1963). In the wheelchair disabled, the development of the arm and shoulder muscles is desirable, both to permit the strong isometric contractions needed to propel a chair up a curb or a steep gradient, and to counter the cardiac afterloading problem that arises when attempts are made to sustain the perfusion of weak skeletal muscles that are contracting at a large fraction of their total force. In many forms of disability, muscle training has the further advantage of maximizing function in accessory muscles not affected by the primary disorder.

As with cardiorespiratory fitness, gains in muscle strength and endurance reflect the frequency, intensity, and duration of training relative to the initial condition of the muscles (Hettinger, 1961). A typical muscle-building regimen might thus call for three sets of 10 isotonic contractions by a given muscle group, each made against a load representing a substantial fraction of maximum force; some degree of muscle overload seems essential if training is to occur. Given an appropriate choice of strength-training regimen, the subject may anticipate hypertrophy of the exercised muscles with an increase of fiber size and local increases in the concentration of enzyme markers of anaerobic metabolism (see chapter 6).

Flexibility

One of the hazards presented by many forms of disability is that the loss of muscle function is not distributed equally between flexor and extensor muscles. Given also some associated muscle spasm, it is easy for a limb to be held for long periods in an abnormal and awkward position and eventually for a contracture to develop, with an increase of disability (Sherrill, 1986b).

An important objective of flexibility training is thus to preserve the full range of movement at a given articulation. In general, this is best accomplished by taking the joint gently through its full range of motion on a regular basis. Gentle stretching at the ends of the range of motion is also acceptable, but bouncing or unduly forcible attempts to extend the range of motion merely lead to spasm, with a further limitation of movement.

Aerobic Power

In general, an endurance-training program is expected to increase the individual's maximum oxygen intake, or aerobic power. Much of the strain imposed upon the body by a bout of physical activity depends upon the intensity of the required effort, expressed as a percentage of the individual's maximum aerobic power (Shephard, 1969b). Thus, if the individual's aerobic power is increased, the strain of performing a given external task is proportionately reduced. One may anticipate a parallel reduction in the perception of effort (Borg, 1971) and the sensation of fatigue, with positive implications for heart rate, cardiac work rate, myocardial ischemia, and the risk of a cardiac catastrophe while exercising (Shephard, 1981).

When a person performs exercise with the legs (e.g., treadmill or cycle ergometer training), a training response develops progressively over several months or even years. There may be some contribution from such factors as an increase of aerobic enzymes in the working muscles, a redistribution of blood flow from the skin or viscera to the working tissues, and an increase of hemoglobin level (allowing a larger maximum arterio-venous oxygen difference), but the main benefit accrues from an increase of stroke volume and thus maximal cardiac output (Shephard, 1982b). In some instances, the well-trained individual may also show an increase of oxygen transport during brief bouts of activity, and endurance is enhanced over 30- to 60-minute periods of exercise, particularly when work must be performed in a hot climate. When the training program involves only the relatively small muscle mass of the arms and shoulder girdle, an increase of peak cardiac output and oxygen transport seems likely if the aerobic power is tested during arm work, but it is less clearly established that the training response is generalizable to exercise involving other parts of the body (Clausen, 1973, 1977).

The type of training needed to induce a gain of aerobic power depends somewhat on the initial fitness of an individual (Shephard, 1969b, 1977). In general, it is necessary to engage 60 to 70% of the heart rate reserve (the difference between the resting and the maximum heart rate for a given mode of exercise) in order to increase the absolute maximum oxygen intake (L/min). However, if body mass decreases over the course of training (e.g., due to a reduction in the percentage of body fat), this will in itself increase the relative aerobic power (expressed in oxygen transport units of ml/kg • min). Because wheelchair operation is normally weight supported, the training responses of the paraplegic are best considered in absolute units (oxygen transport units of L/min rather than ml/kg • min).

Habituation and Learning

When a subject is first evaluated in the laboratory, a given exercise load often induces a substantial tachycardia due to anxiety. As the task is repeated, the subject finds the process less threatening. Anxiety diminishes, and by a process of negative conditioning the excessive heart rate is overcome with a resultant reduction in cardiac work rate (Shephard, 1969a). Although to date the process has only been examined in the able-bodied, it seems likely that a first encounter with laboratory equipment is even more threatening to the disabled. An exaggeration of the normal habituation responses might thus be anticipated in a disabled subject.

A similar type of habituation can occur in response to repeated bouts of vigorous exercise in the gymnasium or on the field. Particularly among disabled individuals, there is again an initial anxiety that the prescribed activity is dangerous, unrealistic, or impossible (see chapter 8). However, with repetition of the prescription, such fears are overcome; the excessive response of the sympathetic nervous system progressively disappears, the exercise heart rate becomes slower, and the outpouring of catecholamines is greatly reduced. These changes in turn have implications for the safety of a given type and intensity of exercise. Moreover, if an emergency arises in which the subject must combine an acceptance of psychological stress with vigorous physical effort, the output of catecholamines is likely to be much smaller than in naive subjects, and the likelihood that ventricular fibrillation or cardiac arrest will develop during the burst of activity is correspondingly reduced (Shephard, 1981).

The ability of a subject to make good use of the available muscle force and aerobic power depends greatly upon his or her learning an appropriate biomechanical technique (see chapter 7). Whereas efficient movements are important to an able-bodied individual, they are even more vital for the person with acquired disability. The latter is required to relearn a wide range of movement patterns and must carry out many tasks with less than a normal complement of functioning muscles. The learning of technique can thus be an important aspect of training. It can be identified, for example, by an increase of steady-state maximum power output without any change of maximum aerobic power. If this type of training response is sought, the most effective approach is a frequent repetition of the required skill under the watchful eye of a well-trained physiotherapist or coach.

When teaching more efficient movement patterns to subjects with various types of brain damage, the trainer must note that initially even simple, gross motor skills may be absent. Thus, rather than attempting to introduce complex motor behaviors for which there is little foundation, the trainer should break down instruction into its simplest elements (Croce, 1987).

Medical Benefits

A final important benefit of training is a reduced likelihood of developing the various medical problems that are associated with the adoption of an inactive lifestyle. Many medical consultations are sought because the individual has a poor perception of personal health, in the absence of any specific organic pathology (Herzlich, 1973). The incidence of perceptually based complaints is linked to mood state and is thus greatly reduced by physical activity that elevates mood and improves body image. Bar-Or (1983) and Shephard (1985c) discussed other potential health benefits of regular exercise with reference to children and adults, respectively. In a long-term perspective, the inactive lifestyle of the disabled undoubtedly predisposes them to such conditions as myocardial infarction and osteoporosis. To reduce the likelihood of ischemic heart disease, trainers should recommend prolonged bouts of moderately intense aerobic effort. Weight or load bearing must be added to such activity in order to avoid problems of calcium loss from disabled limbs.

Content of Fitness Programming

General considerations regarding the content of an appropriate fitness program are much as for an able-bodied individual and indeed have been largely considered in preceding chapters (see particularly chapter 5). Sherrill (1983) has discussed specific approaches to those with severe disabilities, such as the nonambulatory, the nonverbal, and the quadriplegic. For such individuals, she has recommended the Van Dijk coactive teaching model. This comprises six elements—resonance behavior (building of body schema, anticipatory behavior, and self-help skills), coactive movements (moving with the teacher but with a progressive increase in the intervening distance), nonrepresentational reference (learning body parts and pointing behavior), deferred motor imitation (imitation of the teacher with an increasing time lapse), natural gesturing (e.g., representing a ball by a throwing action), and language development.

It is important to offer as wide a range of options as possible so that the disabled person can discover and select those activities relevant to personal needs (Topsfield, 1974). The trainer must also give due thought to the needs of those who are severely disabled. Among possible modes of exercise are vigorous daily activity, laboratory training sessions, fitness classes, and participation in suitably adapted individual and group sports. Whatever the mode chosen, it is important that the subject move from skill to skill in an ordered manner. Past experience, motivation, an understanding of the activities, and self-confidence all influence the level of attainment at any given point in the course of rehabilitation.

In addition to effectiveness, considerations of cost, convenience, free time, aptitudes, interest, and personality may influence the choice between these various program options. In the United States, disabled children have specific rights under item PL 94-142—the Education of all Handicapped Children Act, 1975, of the Federal Individualized Education Program (Appenzeller, 1983; Sherrill, 1986c; Werder & Kalakian, 1985). The program administrator (ideally a suitably trained physical educator, but often a special educator or educational diagnostician) must document (a) the student's current educational performance, (b) annual goals and short-term objectives, (c) specific educational and related services to be provided, (d) the child's capability to participate in normal school classes, (e) a timetable for initiation and continuation of services, and (f) objective procedures for evaluating progress.

Vigorous Daily Activity

Many disabled people still live unnecessarily sheltered lives. The blind may make only rare outdoor excursions with a cane, a guide dog, or an experienced companion, or those with motor dysfunction may only venture out of their homes using a specially adapted car or power-operated wheelchair. However, with appropriate counseling, these people can find valuable training for a wide range of muscle groups in vigorous performance of the ordinary activities of daily living.

The main advantages of encouraging an increase of daily activity are as follows: (a) The individual does not need to invest money in specialized sports equipment and club membership fees, (b) only a limited amount of time must be invested in the exercise program, and (c) regular participation is stimulated by the normal schedule (e.g., the daily walk of a blind person to the subway station). The main disadvantages of relying upon normal, everyday activities as a source of training are as follows: (a) The intensity of the activity chosen may be too light to induce a conditioning response (see chapter 6), and (b) if participation is of appropriate vigor, the exerciser may be embarrassed by an accumulation of sweat and may lack suitably adapted shower facilities at the place of work.

Camping (Trowbridge, 1974) can be considered an extension of normal daily activity. It seems a particularly effective approach for disabled children, providing fun, a holiday, and a chance to learn new activities and meet new people; in many cases it also offers a welcome break to the parents. Some authors have recommended more vigorous outdoor programs to adolescents and adults, particularly the emotionally disturbed.

Laboratory Exercise Training

With this type of approach, the disabled individual might make three or more 30-minute visits to the laboratory each week in order to perform standard ergometer exercise (typically controlled at 60-70% of maximum oxygen intake). The main advantage of laboratory exercise training is that the intensity, frequency, and duration of effort can all be closely monitored. This is particularly valuable at the beginning of the rehabilitation process, when little is known about the subject's condition or the potential reactions of a weakened heart to vigorous training. The subject can be taught the sensations associated with an appropriate intensity of effort, for example, the onset of moderate breathlessness, some sweating, and a perception of moderate effort on the Borg (1971) scale. The trainer can also watch for anginal pain and ventricular premature systoles and can warn the subject to exert moderate effort or to return to the laboratory for reevaluation if such symptoms are detected. The addition of simple, self-administered tests of physical fitness can greatly enhance motivation, contributing to the further development of fitness and the enhancement of health learning (Shephard, 1980).

One important limitation to laboratory-based training is its cost. Provision of a battery of ergometers and trained supervisory staff is unacceptably expensive, except for experimental programs involving a relatively small number of subjects. A second obstacle to regular laboratory training, particularly in a large city, is its "opportunity cost" (Shephard, 1986a). It may be necessary to invest as much as 2 to 3 hours of travel time in order to achieve a half hour of exercise. The travel problem is particularly acute for many of the disabled. Some 4% of the population are "transportation handicapped" (Canadian Transportation Development Centre, personal communication). These people often lack or cannot operate cars, the service provided by municipal adapted transportation is at best unpredictable, and the menial nature of their jobs restricts the possibility of either renting an adapted taxi or taking prolonged periods away from work.

A laboratory-based program is thus unlikely to be acceptable to most disabled individuals, except during the early stages of training. Subsequently, a cooperative program might be developed between a university laboratory and an organization for the disabled, or the subject could be asked to continue an equivalent exercise at home; in the latter instance, compliance with the prescribed regimen should be monitored by the completion of suitable diary sheets (Kavanagh, 1980) and periodic return of the subject to the supervising laboratory.

Group Exercise Sessions

Suitably graded gymnasium-type classes can be arranged for the disabled (see Table 9.1). The disabled need to train for balance, postural orientation, contacts

Table 9.1   Possible Items for Inclusion in a School Program for Disabled Students

---

Small equipment gymnasium-type activities—ropes, jump ropes, balls, hoops, logs, inner tubes, chairs, barrels, parachutes, ladders, boxes, and beanbags.

Large equipment gymnasium-type activities—horizontal ladders, jungle gyms, climbing ropes, turning bars, cargo nets, obstacle courses, mazes, pipes, and concrete blocks.

Sedentary or remedial programs—for problems of posture or locomotion, weakness, instability, or inadequate range of movement at individual joints.

Partner activities—calisthenics, combative games, and dual stunts.

Aquatic activities—swimming and aquabics.

Circuit training

Informal recreation—walking, hiking, and cycling.

Self-assessment—for both learning and motivation.

Note. Information in this table is based largely on suggestions from AAHPER, 1975.

with exterior objects, and receipt and propulsion of an object during the period of rehabilitation. A specific program may thus include mobility training, all types of balance activities, progressive development of basic motor functions, movement exploration, rhythmic activities to improve motor ability, and recreational and sports activities (Crowe et al., 1981; Sherrill, 1986c; see Appendix A).

To avoid medicolegal liability, exercise leaders should provide substantial supervision, particularly in the early phases of rehabilitation (e.g., one paramedical professional for 5-10 participants). When players are limited by muscular weakness, leaders can reduce the amount of activity by using a smaller playing area. Larger balls may help to slow the tempo of some games, and in other group activities a lighter ball or striking instrument may be useful.

The primary difficulty for the deaf individual is communication with both the instructor and teammates. Amplification of auditory signals helps those with partial hearing loss, and special signs and symbols have been devised to facilitate instruction of the totally deaf (Eichstaedt & Seiler, 1978; Schmidt & Dunn, 1980). Stewart (1986) stressed that the widely used American Sign Language differs from any spoken language in both its lexicon and syntax, so that the totally deaf tend to live in a unique culture.

If lighting is good and participants are close to the instructor, some deaf individuals can use lipreading in sports, but only about 4% of the deaf population are skilled in this method of communication. Inability to hear or interpret instructions or regulating whistles can frustrate attempts to integrate a deaf child into a group activity. Modern dance, synchronized swimming, and free gymnastics are useful forms of group exercise for some deaf students, but others have difficulty with pursuits that demand rhythm or balance. Many deaf individuals want to swim with their heads out of water, but special underwater lighting can be arranged to replace the feedback a synchronized swimmer would normally obtain from hearing.

The blind have particular difficulties with games that use moving objects or that require visual assessments of rapidly changing conditions. A high intensity of illumination and the bright painting of balls and markers will help the partially sighted, whereas the totally blind require balls fitted with beepers, buzzers, or bells and other auditory or tactile cues.

Irrespective of the type of disability, group exercise classes have the attraction of camaraderie and mutual support, but participants who are working adults must face problems of cost and travel time. The level of disability varies widely from one person to another; carefully graded programs, preferably with an individualized prescription, are thus needed. Talented students must be allowed to learn at an accelerated pace, and the pace of learning must be decelerated for those who are less talented.

With good organization, educators can organize the appropriate grading of activities in the mainstream of a normal classroom or community exercise facility. When arranging such grading, the teacher must note that disability is rarely uniform for all types of exercise. A child may thus be at Grade 6 for tumbling but Grade 11 for archery. A circuit arrangement of the gymnasium allows the individual to be suitably challenged on each of a variety of activities. Group pool exercises such as "aquabics" (Lawrence, 1981) are also helpful, particularly to those individuals who are limited by severe muscle spasm.

If an individual exercises in a gymnasium or play area containing specialized equipment (e.g., guide wires, handrails around the track, or sighted guides for the blind), there is a danger that he or she may come to think that exercise is possible only when such equipment is provided. Thus in one study, blind students showed a substantial loss of physical condition over a summer vacation period (DiNatale et al., 1985); many of the individuals concerned complained that exercise had been restricted during the summer months because they lacked sighted guides. No training or rehabilitation program can be really effective unless the techniques taught are generalizable from the supervised training situation to the community environment (Auxter, 1983).

One way of providing greater supervision is by the use of paired teaching techniques. A child with a specific disability may be paired with a neighbor of similar age for one-to-one teaching; those students with one type of disability can also serve as squad leaders, assistants, or peer teachers to those with another type of disability. Indeed, such responsibility is an important motivating force, increasing the interest of the peer teacher in physical activity. In some instances, parents can also serve as a valuable resource to augment and reinforce professional programs of adapted physical education (J.M. Dunn, 1983; Folsom-Meek, 1984; Horvat, 1982; Lynch & Stein, 1982).

Group and Team Sports

With some imagination, leaders can adapt the rules of most sports to allow the participation of the disabled (see Table 9.2). The journal *Palaestra* provides much current information on modifications of rules and equipment to accommodate specific types of disability. Jones (1984) prepared an extensive sports manual for the cerebral palsied, and other valuable resources include the texts of Guttmann

Table 9.2   Modifications of Sport, Play, and Teaching for Various Classes of Handicap

Type of disability	Modifications of sport and teaching
Blindness	*Archery*—pegs to mark appropriate stance *Running and swimming*—guide ropes *Softball*—sand paths with raised bases *Class management*—ordered environment, with clear reference points on field or floor, auditory cues to obstacles *Teaching*—clear auditory signals, braille instruction manuals, manual guidance, addressing player by name *Safety*—protect eyes and/or eyeglasses, soft ball and striking object, hazard-free play area, avoidance of high-speed passing of other players
Mentally retarded and learning disabled	*Class management*—pictures or stick symbols, distraction-free environment, footprints and handprints to guide direction of body parts *Teaching*—simple and concise instructions with simultaneous verbal modeling
Physically handicapped	Handrails, nonslip pool bottom, safety belts, and soft mats in gymnasium
Deafness	Protect hearing aid

Note. Based in part on data from *Principles and Methods of Adapted Physical Education and Recreation* by W.C. Crowe, D. Auxter, and J. Pyfer, 1981. St. Louis: Mosby.

(1976a), Adams et al. (1982), and Sherrill (1986c), together with a series of 20 paperback Special Olympics Instructional Manuals. For example, additional players can be added to a team, the number of points or the permitted duration of play can be shortened, and rules for substitution of players can be eased (Crowe et al., 1981).

The Australian Council for Rehabilitation of the Disabled (1974) provided some specific examples of how cricket and table tennis can be adapted to the needs of the blind. Balls or baskets can be equipped with beepers, buzzers, or bells, and both bats and balls can be made of materials such as sponge, foam, plastic, vinyl, or leather to minimize the risk of injury (Ward, 1985). However, blind individuals usually gain maximum satisfaction from a sport when there has been only minimal alteration of rules or equipment (C. Buell, 1983; Morisbak, 1980).

Guide rails were once used when blind athletes competed in track events. However, experience has shown that the coach's voice provides sufficient direction for a 100-m run or swim. Over longer distances, a guide is tethered to the athlete by a short rope. Electronic head sets are sometimes used to provide assistance to both blind and deaf athletes, but unless such equipment is available to all competitors, it confers an unfair advantage.

Group sports offer the important advantages of mutual encouragement and motivation by competition (A. Brown, 1982). However, as with participation in laboratory and group exercise sessions, cost and travel time are disadvantages. Moreover, the general organizational pattern of disabled sports has tended to promote the segregation of performers, officials, and spectators, rather than their integration into the able-bodied world (Thorpe-Tracy, 1976). Finally, poorly motivated individuals may find excuses for their current nonparticipation in the lack of a suitably matched team, or may be discouraged from future involvement by their poor current performances relative to those judged as having similar types of disability.

Individual Exercise Participation

The individual participant commonly follows an exercise prescription (e.g., walking or jogging) as offered by the supervising physician. A typical recommendation specifies the distance to be covered (km), the pace (min/km), the number of repetitions per week, and any warning symptoms that may be anticipated. Compliance can be monitored by the completion of weekly diary sheets (Kavanagh, 1980).

Individual exercise participation is best suited to the introvert with a strong internal motivation (Shephard, 1985a, b). Cost and travel time can be matched to personal inclination, but if the subject is not conscientious, failure to participate regularly can pass undetected by the program supervisor. Moreover, if the types of activity prescribed carry a risk of physical injury, then the dangers posed by an accident are increased unless the activity is pursued by groups of two or more individuals.

One major obstacle to individual exercise participation is that most municipal recreation departments have done little to make either community programs or local facilities accessible to special populations (Andreas, 1970; Hayes & Smith, 1973; P.F. Wilkinson, 1984; P.A. Witt, 1977). This is unfortunate, as minor changes to facilities, programming, and attitudes would open up such resources to many of the disabled.

Music and Rehabilitation

Bright (1974), Bitcon (1976), and Sherrill (1983) discussed the role of music in education and rehabilitation. Music seems particularly valuable when treating the mentally retarded. Individuality is encouraged as the subject chooses a favorite tune. Even within the oppressive setting of an institution, personal likes and dislikes can be expressed through the musical selection, and the choice also presents an opportunity for social interaction. The rhythm further encourages physical effort to be both initiated and maintained, and finally the music itself can provide a new source of interest and mental stimulation.

Adventure Programs

Adventure recreation programs are particularly helpful in building self-esteem, group cooperation, and trust among adolescents with psychological disturbances (Langsner & Anderson, 1987; Witman, 1987). Outdoor programs also seem more effective for blind students than traditional gymnasium activities, particularly in terms of developing balance and spatial veering (Black, 1983).

Feasibility of Physical Activity

The program of physical activity recommended to a disabled person must often steer a careful balance between too low an intensity (with lack of an effective training stimulus) and too high an intensity (leading to a dangerous overdose of exercise). In some cases, the setting of an appropriate prescription that is both effective and safe poses a severe problem. This is particularly true if the subject (and possibly friends or relatives) have a limited intelligence or lack basic skills (e.g., individuals with a congenital defect of sight or hearing; Ward, 1985).

The main barriers to physical activity perceived by the disabled (see Tables 9.3 and 9.4) were explored by Quintner (1974) and by the Canadian Fitness Survey (1986; Shephard, 1986b). Quintner (1974) found that among Australians, the physical disability itself was the limiting factor in 42% of subjects; other frequent citations were cost (15%), lack of facilities (14%), and problems of transportation (10%). In the Canadian sample, items cited were generally similar to those observed in the general population; in addition to the primary problem of general health, participation was limited by intercurrent problems such as bladder infections, along with secondary difficulties such as pressure sores in those with neurological deficiencies.

Difficulties of access (both barriers inherent in the physical design of facilities and problems of transportation) may preclude the translation of an intention to exercise into exercise behavior (see chapter 8). Stairs or steps may exclude those with walking aids or wheelchairs. Limited function of a hand or arm may deny access to a building equipped with taps, handles, manual switches, and control buttons (M.J. Fox, 1974). Special thought is needed in the design of toilets, lifts, telephone booths, showers, doors, and passageways. Particularly if blind participants are anticipated (Buell, 1987), all aspects of a facility require a high level of maintenance. Holes must be filled and approach paths must be smooth, easy to comprehend, and free of obstacles. If living accommodation is provided for competitors, exits must be well marked with both auditory and visual warning systems; preferably, severely disabled members of a team (including the deaf and blind) should be accommodated on the ground floor. Blind athletes also need provision for the feeding and housing of guide dogs (Ward, 1985). Possible tactics to increase accessibility (M.J. Fox, 1974) include publicity to promote public awareness, legislation assuring a right to access, municipal legislation establishing disabled transport and ensuring parking concessions, city guides detailing facilities open to the handicapped, and architectural awards to facilities that cater to special populations.

The disabled may find a lack of time to be as great or even a greater barrier than do the able-bodied (Hill, 1974). Problems of the cost of participation are compounded by low and uncertain incomes. Finally, certain important facilitating factors can increase the exercise participation of the disabled, such as the existence of suitable adapted programs and the support of significant others (see

Table 9.3   Barriers to Exercise Perceived by the Disabled

	Percentage who would be encouraged to exercise by correction of barrier	
Perceived need	Currently active (%)	Currently sedentary (%)
Leisure time	32	16
Closer or better facilities	23	22
People with whom to participate	23	16
Interest of family	15	13
Less expense	20	15
Interest of friends	15	15
Fitness classes	12	10
Fitness test and program	11	9
"Nothing would increase activity"	38	95

Note. Based on data from *Physical Activity Among Activity-Limited and Disabled Adults in Canada*, Canada Fitness Survey, 1986. Ottawa: Canada Fitness and Lifestyle Research Institute.

Table 9.4   Possible Factors That Would Encourage Greater Physical Activity

Factor	Percent citing	Factor	Percent citing
More leisure time	29	Common interest of family	19
Better or closer facilities	22	Common interest of friends	15
Less expensive facilities	18	Information on benefits	7
People with whom to participate	22	Employer/union-sponsored activities	6
Organized fitness classes	11		
A fitness test and program	11		

Note. See note to Table 9.3. Based on data for disabled adults over the age of 20 years.

Table 9.4). In this regard, friends and community agencies seem more important than immediate family to both the cerebral palsied and the blind (Sherrill, Rainbolt, Montelione, & Pope, 1986).

Although less severely disabled individuals react well when integrated into normal school or community programs, those with gross disabilities or multiple handicaps appreciate the advantages of small classes, good equipment, and close contact with teachers who can use special methods of communication such as braille and sign language (Ward, 1985). In the case of the mentally retarded, the development of "lead-in" skills is also an important first step to participation in many activities (Luyben, Funk, Morgan, Clark, & Delulio, 1986).

Motivation

The central principles of exercise motivation in the disabled can be gleaned from the foregoing discussion, including our analysis of personality, behavior, and social adjustments (see chapter 8). The principles are much like those for sport (Silva & Weinberg, 1984) and exercise programs (Dishman, 1988) in the able-bodied, although we must make due allowance for the frustrations and slower rate of progression inherent to most forms of disability.

In general, the educator's objective is to provide the sport or exercise participant with immediate external motivation until the internal rewards of participation become apparent (Danielson & Danielson, 1979). The period of external motivation is likely to be longer for a person with an external locus of control than for someone who is internally motivated; many of the disabled fall into the former category (Goldberg & Shephard, 1982).

Reasoned Behavior

In accordance with Fishbein's model of reasoned behavior (Ajzen & Fishbein, 1980), educators can strengthen exercise intentions through a development of beliefs in the value of exercise and a favorable personal evaluation of such beliefs, together with an enhancement of behavioral norms. The data from the Canada Fitness Survey (1986) suggest that the provision of more "fitness" information would be relatively ineffective in shaping exercise behavior (see Table 9.4), but this may be because to date such information has been presented in a fashion that fails to shape personal evaluations of the suggested actions. On the other hand, perhaps because the disabled are a relatively dependent group of individuals, the influence of significant others (i.e., family and friends) upon exercise participation appears to be quite strong. In the Fishbein model, accessibility factors limit the translation of a behavioral intention into an overt behavior. The larger the number of steps that intervene between intention and behavior, the less the likelihood that the behavior will be realized. One major gap in the basic Fishbein model is that too little attention is directed to previous experience of physical activity (Godin & Shephard, 1986).

Many of those disabled by trauma or disease have had positive or negative experiences with exercise before the onset of their disability, and indeed in some instances the disability itself has been caused by an athletic injury. Prior experience with physical activity is thus very likely to influence the translation of intention into an overt behavior. A second weakness in the standard Fishbein model is that insufficient attention is directed to feelings. Briggs-Myers (1986) proposed a classification of personality into 16 types, based upon introversion versus extroversion, sensing versus intuitive, feeling versus thinking, and perceptive versus judging. These various characteristics all undoubtedly influence reactions to both personal beliefs and subjective norms. For example, a "judging" type of person may react positively to the theoretical benefits of exercise, whereas the type of person who is influenced mainly by personal feelings will need to experience activity (and to make a positive evaluation of the resultant feelings) before being encouraged to further participation.

External Motivation

The nature of external motivation can be very varied. In Skinnerian terms (Danielson & Danielson, 1979; J.M. Dunn, 1983), behavioral modification can be achieved if the subject is either rewarded for participation or punished for failure to participate. Rewards may be symbolic (badges, pins, T-shirts, awards, or membership of an elite club), material (money, prizes, release time, assistance with club dues, or demonstration of physiological gains), or psychological (encouragement from the instructor, recognition of achievement, or attention and friendship). In many special populations, adaptation of reinforcement is needed. For example, displaying on a bulletin board photographs of students engaged in physical activity substantially increases the activity patterns of mentally retarded children (Katz & Singh, 1986). In mentally retarded adults (Cauette & Reid, 1985), auditory reinforcement (the playing of music while a specified intensity of ergometer pedaling is maintained) seems more effective than visual reinforcement (a display of colored lights also linked to the ergometer).

Punishments can be classified in similar fashion to positive reinforcement, although some are deliberate, and others are an unavoidable consequence of the early stages of training: symbolic (exclusion from the group), material (fines for noncompliance, costs of tuition, clothing and equipment, time loss, or physical effort and fatigue), or psychological (discouragement or ridicule from the instructor, family, or friends; failure to achieve the anticipated goals; family complaints about program involvement or absence from home; or psychological fatigue due to the program). In general, a successful experience (positive reinforcement) makes a more useful contribution to learning than failure (negative reinforcement); in many people, negative reinforcement merely increases the likelihood of defection from an exercise program.

As with industrial performance (Shephard, 1974), the most effective external motivation is a variable schedule with a variable size of reward. However, the continual devising of new rewards is exhausting for an exercise instructor; thus the class leader should encourage when possible an appreciation of the internal rewards of exercise. The student's attention can be drawn to improved self-image, mood, and performance capability and (in peer-learning arrangements) to the satisfaction of helping others improve personal fitness. Devices that encourage self-motivation depend upon the age and intelligence of the subjects and can include the construction of a decisional balance sheet, contracting, and (if intelligence is limited) repeated explanation of cause-and-effect relationships between vigorous activity and improved functional capacity.

Key Ideas

1. Fitness programming may induce gains of psychological state, metabolic control, muscle development, flexibility, aerobic power, habituation, mechanical efficiency, or health status. Differing intensities and durations of activity are needed to satisfy these differing objectives.

2. Possible program options include an enhancement of normal daily activity, laboratory exercise sessions, gymnasium classes, involvement in sport, and individual activity programs. Considerations of cost, convenience, free time, aptitudes, interests, and personality influence the individual's preference among these options.

3. Perceived barriers to an increase of physical activity among the disabled are commonly as reported for the general population. Medical problems may have a factual basis, but other perceived barriers do not withstand critical examination.

4. The disabled commonly need external motivation to increase physical activity in the early stages of an exercise program. Instructors can provide material, symbolic, and psychological rewards in accordance with Skinnerian principles. The development of internal motivation can be encouraged by such tactics as drawing up a decisional balance sheet and contracting. For school students, the contract might usefully specify participation in vigorous activities outside of normal class times; in this way, the disabled person develops confidence in his or her ability to assume responsibility for the development and maintenance of physical condition.

Practical Applications

1. Which of the possible objectives of fitness programming do you think are the most important for a disabled individual?

2. If you were affected by a major physical disability, which of the possible program options would be most appealing to you? Why?

3. Why do both able-bodied and disabled subjects develop perceived barriers to exercise participation? If such barriers appear to have little material substance, what can be done to remove them?

4. What novel rewards can you suggest to sustain the exercise motivation of the disabled? Would you ever use punishment to increase compliance? If not, why not?

5. A decisional balance sheet is said to help exercise motivation. Try drawing up such sheets for a T-6 paraplegic and for a person who has been blind from birth.

Chapter 10

A World View

In this final chapter, we look briefly at key international organizations and consider comparative aspects of legislation, programs, and treatment, noting the increasing trend to uniformity of opportunities for the disabled in developed countries. Possible factors contributing to the matching of programs and services between nations include (a) governmental contacts (such as the International Conference of Ministers and Senior Officials responsible for Physical Education and Sport for Youth in the context of lifelong education, convened by the United Nations Educational, Scientific, and Cultural Organization, UNESCO, in 1976), (b) surveys initiated and literature distributed by agencies such as UNESCO during the International Year of the Disabled, and (c) more informal contacts established through international athletic competition. Presently, differences within a given country tend to be larger than differences between nations (J.U. Stein, 1986). Nevertheless, even in superficially similar cultures (for example, Canada vs. the United States), differences remain that are related to political structures and the importance accorded to personal versus collective interests (Ziegler, 1976).

International Organizations

The first International Congress on Physical Education was held in Paris in 1889. At that time, much rivalry existed between the Swedish system of remedial exercises, the German emphasis on gymnasium work, and the British interest in sport (Bennett, 1978). By 1910, tension between the various groups reached the point that a separate International Congress of Pedagogical, Military, and Aesthetic Gymnastics was organized by supporters of the Swedish system. A second meeting of the Swedish group at Odense, Denmark, in 1911 led to formation of the International Institute of Physical Education, which in 1930 became the International Federation of Ling Gymnastics, and in 1953, the Féderation International d'Education Physique (FIEP). Another initiative of this period was the foundation of the International Federation of Sports Medicine (FIMS) at the Olympic Games in Amsterdam (1928).

We have already commented on the emergence of international organizations governing sport for disabled athletes—ISMGF for the spinally paralyzed, CP-ISRA for the cerebral palsied, ISOD for amputees and les autres, IBSA for the blind,

Special Olympics Inc. for the mentally retarded, CISS for the deaf, and the overall coordination of ICC, which represents disabled athletes at the level of the International Olympic Committee (IOC).

Although the average person may sometimes be stimulated and challenged by the achievements of the international competitor, this is not always the case. UNESCO, working through its International Committee on Sport and Physical Education (ICSPE, founded in 1959), has been concerned with promoting "Sport for All" on an international basis (McIntosh, 1980). The primary roles of the committee are education, exchange of ideas, and moral persuasion, although it also attempts to gather funds from more wealthy nations to allow the development of matching opportunities in poorer countries. In cooperation with the relevant national agencies, UNESCO has received various regional reports, such as an assessment of needs of physical education and sport in the African nations (Lillis, 1977), a parallel earlier report to the Council of Europe (1970), and a study of physical culture and sport in socialist societies (Pavlov, 1980).

In April 1976, a conference for Ministers of Sport was held at UNESCO House in Paris, with 101 of the 150 member states represented, and three key recommendations of this conference were endorsed by the general conference of UNESCO, which met in Nairobi later that year: (i) establishment of a permanent intergovernmental committee on physical education and sport, (ii) creation of an international fund for the development of physical education and sport, and (iii) development of an international charter for physical education and sport.

The International Charter was adopted by UNESCO in November 1978, and Article 1 stipulates, "The practice of physical education and sport is a fundamental right for all." It notes specifically (in Item 1.3), "Special opportunities must be made available . . . for the handicapped to develop their personalities to the full through physical education and sport programmes suited to their requirements" (McIntosh, 1980).

In 1982, UNESCO joined forces with the WHO to develop a plan of action for implementing the global strategy of "Health for All by the Year 2000." National agencies cooperating in this task include the U.S. President's Council on Physical Fitness, Fitness Canada, Recreation Canada, ParticipACTION (Canada), Trim (Denmark, Japan, the Netherlands, Norway, and Sweden), Trimm (West Germany, BRD), Sport for All (U.K. and Columbia), Deportes Para Todos (Spain and Brazil), Kuntourheilu (Finland), the Spartakiads of Eastern Europe, Life Be In It (Australia) and Come Alive (New Zealand). Initiatives have been more limited in Third World countries, although Sport for All programs have emerged in Egypt, Tunisia, and the United Republic of the Cameroons.

The United Nations declared 1981 The International Year of the Disabled with the Declaration on the Rights of Disabled Persons. This stated that it has become the responsibility of all to ensure that the education of the disabled becomes an integral part of cultural development, with full social integration, and equality of access to leisure facilities. Expression of this commitment was seen in 1985, when many national and international plans for the UNESCO-sponsored International Youth Year gave clear recognition to the potential and achievements of handicapped youth.

The interests of UNESCO and the Geneva-based WHO have overlapped substantially, with many initiatives being sponsored jointly. WHO also relies heavily upon persuasion and education, with frequent regional and international meetings of small expert groups to consider specific health issues. In our present context, WHO has initiated research and sponsored program reviews in health education (World Health Organization 1969, 1974), examined the medical and social problems of the disabled (Kallio, 1982), considered issues of human rights and health ethics, joined UNESCO in establishing a committee on teacher preparation for health education, cooperated with the Pan-American Health Organization in organizing interregional conferences on the postgraduate education of health workers, and sponsored study tours allowing an examination of different systems of health education. WHO publishes statistics on health and morbidity quarterly and annually, and it maintains international digests of health legislation, health economics, and health expenditures.

A third agency of international cooperation is the professionally oriented International Council for Health, Physical Education and Recreation (ICHPER), which has national counterparts such as AAHPERD and CAHPER. ICHPER was founded in 1959. A section of this organization has specific interest in the disabled. Cooperative endeavors with UNESCO include international surveys on the place of sport in education, teacher training for physical education and the development of physical education and sport for the physically and mentally handicapped (J.U. Stein & Gepford, 1982), the hosting of an international symposium on the same topic at College Park, Maryland in November 1982 (UNESCO, 1982), and the publication of the quadrilingual *International Journal of Physical Education*.

International research on physical activity for the disabled has been coordinated through the International Federation for Adapted Physical Activity (see chapter 2). This was founded in Québec City in March 1977, and in addition to sponsoring biennial symposia, the organization's international board of directors promotes an ongoing exchange of information on research, programs, and personal preparation.

Legislation

Specific legislation directed to the needs of the disabled has evolved progressively over the past decade, in part as a response to the UNESCO and WHO initiatives discussed previously. Among other issues, such legislation now covers the establishment of government agencies that provide for the fitness needs of the disabled, requirements for physical education of the disabled in state schools, requirements for employment of the disabled by private companies, and regulations requiring access to private sports clubs.

The majority of the communist nations of Eastern Europe have included statements on physical culture and sports in their constitutions (Bennett, Howell, & Simri, 1983). Pooley (1978) argued that Western nations saw sport as a means to benefit the individual and humankind, whereas communist nations saw the benefits of sports in terms of increased production and improved defense. Nevertheless, in constitutional democracies and military dictatorships alike, a nonpartisan observer would accept that many of the earliest governmental initiatives in both East and West have apparently had motives of wartime patriotism or peacetime defense.

North America

The dominant concern of national defense is well exemplified by Canada. Thus the Canadian parliament gave its assent to a National Fitness Act in 1943, under pressure to find fit recruits to fight in World War II. This act was subsequently repealed in 1956. More recently, interest has reflected a desire to win a larger share of medals at the Olympic Games and to reduce spiraling health care costs. Thus, in 1961, Canada passed Bill C-131, "An Act to Promote Fitness and Amateur Sport." As central bureaucracy and overall government involvement has grown, other political objectives have emerged, particularly the promotion of national unity in the face of regional separatism (MacIntosh, Franks, & Bedecki, 1986; Ziegler, 1976). Elements of the program have included Fitness Canada, Sport Canada, Recreation Canada, ParticipACTION (a promotional agency), a central office block for all sports agencies, and a scientific information and documentation center (see Shephard, 1977, for details). The government has directed efforts largely to the able-bodied, but occasional initiatives have considered problems of providing equal opportunities for all (Howell, 1978), including the disabled. For example, a comprehensive computer search of literature on sport in the disabled has recently been published, and two specific conferences on fitness for the disabled were hosted in 1979 and 1981.

The U.S. President's Council on Physical Fitness was established during the relative peace of 1956; nevertheless, President Kennedy wrote in one of the council's early brochures "If we are to retain this freedom . . . we must be willing to work for those physical goals on which the courage and skill of the person so largely depend. Only in this way . . . can the spirit and strength of America be constantly renewed" (U.S. President's Council on Physical Fitness, 1963). President Nixon's administration set more modest goals applicable to the disabled, recognizing that not every citizen could become a top athlete. The President's Council unfortunately has no funds for distribution but works through education, persuasion, and award programs. A further component in United States policy is the U.S. Olympic Committee; this committee now operates an Olympic Center in Colorado Springs, which tests and trains top athletes. The Amateur Sport Act of 1978 recommended the promotion of sports for the handicapped (Howell, 1978) and thus opened the way for a Committee on Sports for the Disabled within the U.S. Olympic Committee. This group has established a computerized literature search on sports for the disabled and also has a research committee on sports for the disabled (Sherrill, 1986c).

Europe

In Britain, the British Sports Council was established by Royal Charter in 1972; the Council has coordinated recent efforts to promote both health-related fitness and athletic success (G.B. Wright, 1986). The chairperson and members are appointed by a Minister of State within the Department of the Environment, and government funding is provided, but this may be spent (within broad limits) as the council sees fit.

A second key agency is the Central Council for Physical Recreation (CCPR), which coordinates the activities of 240 governing bodies for sport and recreational activities. First established under royal patronage in 1935, CCPR cooperated with the British Medical Association in pressuring the government to pass the Physical Education and Recreation Act in 1937. Subsequent to World War II, CCPR has played a major role in the establishment of a series of discipline-specific National Sport Centres. The CCPR also established the Wolfenden Committee in 1957, and when the report of this committee was received by the CCPR in 1960, a major recommendation was the establishment of the Sports Council, an independent body of 6 to 10 experts reporting directly to the Lord President of the Council. Subsequently, the Sports Council has assumed a "cabinet" executive function, with the CCPR continuing as the "parliament" of the sports associations.

A further important influence in Britain and other European countries has been the Council of Europe, with its Sport for All program (J.U. Stein, 1986). Expressions of the Council of Europe's concern for the disabled include a technical study entitled *Sports for the Handicapped* (the Third Conference of European Ministers Responsible for Sport, in 1981) and the Seminar on Sport for the Mentally Handicapped, hosted in Brussels in 1980. Other specific target groups (McIntosh, 1980) have included vacationers (Sweden: "Trim during the holidays" campaign), the family (Spain), people over 50 (Belgium), and workers in factories and offices (USSR).

The European model of sport promotion may be illustrated by the government-sponsored Swedish Sports Federation, which encompasses 13,467 sports clubs covering all of the various athletic disciplines (Brattnas, 1974); although elite, medal-seeking competition is one goal of the Federation, it also requires clubs to include a fitness program or sport for all campaign. Likewise, in Norway, existing sports clubs have been asked to welcome "Trimmers" (people participating in the national Trim program) who lack affiliation with existing sports organizations.

In Central Europe, sport is regarded as closely linked to "Kultur" (Lüschen, 1970). Eastern Bloc countries also provide constitutional guarantees of fitness. Thus, the Soviet constitution of 1977 requires the government to promote both physical culture and sport (in Article 24), and specifies the right of each citizen to harmonious development with protection of health through participation in such activities (in Article 41). The Committee for Physical Culture and Sport, which comes under the USSR Council of Ministers assumes governmental responsibility for this requirement. The All Union Council of Trade Unions, which organizes voluntary sport societies in each of the 15 Soviet republics supplements these efforts. The creation of national unity in a vast federation is a major internal objective, whereas the international promotion of communism through sporting achievements is a central external objective (Jefferies, 1986b).

Sports policy in most other Eastern Bloc nations is modeled on the Soviet pattern. Article 35 of the 1974 constitution of East Germany (DDR), for example, states that "physical culture, sport and tourism as elements of socialist culture serve the all-round physical and mental development of the citizens." A significant feature of the DDR statement is its insistence that athletic activities be viewed as elements of socialist culture; practical expression is given to this emphasis in the training of instructors, one third of their courses being devoted to a study of Marxist-Leninist principles. Sport and pedagogy have thus become firmly intertwined (Morton, 1963). In the Soviet system, responsibility for fitness promotion lies with the unions and an elaborate network of volunteer coaches, although a Committee for Physical Culture and Sport coordinates their activities (McIntosh, 1980).

Other Countries

Australia faced many of the same pressures as Canada during World War II, and its first National Fitness Act was passed in 1941 (Baka, 1986), with limited funding for community centers, coaching, and physical education programs. More recently, interest has shifted to producing (through capital grants for facilities and support of sports associations) medal winners in specific sports such as swimming and to promoting the health of the sedentary population (through an awareness campaign known as Fitness Australia). An attitudinal survey was conducted in the State of Victoria, and it was decided to meet the second objective by emphasizing moderate-level activities in places where people congregated, with government-sponsored opportunities for people to begin learning specific skills. The program was adopted nationwide by the Australian Recreation Ministers' Council in 1977. A well-equipped, national sports center opened in Canberra in 1982. In 1983, the newly returned Labour Party greatly increased federal spending on sport, one specific consequence being the establishment of a National Sports Commission, an advisory and monitoring body for all sport issues.

The New Zealand Council for Recreation and Sport advises government on appropriate methods of administering and financing recreation and sport but has little budget within its control. In the Chinese People's Republic, the four aims of the state sport program have been "to improve the physical constitution of the population, to develop bonds of friendship among the Chinese, to permit increases of production, and to contribute towards the country's defence in the event of an attack" (McIntosh, 1980). The emphasis has been upon traditional forms of Chinese exercise such as t'ai chi and wu-shu, with instructors from Institutes of Physical Culture leading groups of 500 or more citizens in early morning activity sessions in city parks.

In Indonesia, physical education is perceived by the government as a means "to build a better future generation, able to fulfil and maintain the independence of the country" (McIntosh, 1980). Singapore has established an active Sports Council with a National Aerobic Fitness Award and mass surveys of aerobic fitness, these activities being sponsored jointly by the Post Office Savings Bank and the Singapore National Heart Association.

School Programs

UNESCO (1964) recommended that 1/3 to 1/6 of the school timetable be devoted to physical education. Required school programs of physical education were introduced in Scandinavia in the early 19th century (e.g., Denmark in 1814, and Sweden in 1820; see Shephard, 1977, for details). Interest in childhood physical education spread gradually to other European countries, and many nations now have either included a physical education section in the general legislation covering education or have introduced a comprehensive law covering various aspects of sport and physical education for the growing child.

North America

In Canada, the requirement to organize physical education classes, including details of their scope, frequency, and age range remains largely a matter of judgment for individual boards of education. There are thus widely discrepant programs and facilities from one part of the country to another (Bailey, 1974). At the primary school level classes are generally required, but teachers are often poorly prepared, whereas in the later years of high school programs are commonly optional and sometimes not even available to students (see Table 10.1). In Ontario, passage of Bill 82 in the Provincial Parliament now requires integration of disabled students into mainstream physical education programs, where possible.

Sports participation in Canada is in part through schools and in part through various national and provincial sports associations. At the national level, 59% of funding comes from the federal government, with additional support from private sponsors (17%), fund-raising efforts (11%), and registration fees (6%). An important recent development has been the introduction of a national certification program, with five levels of instruction in theory, technique, and practice. To date, about 150,000 coaches have shared in this program, although it has yet to be extended to the disabled.

In the United States, Public Law 749 of 1966 provided universities with funding for programs to train physical educators for the disabled. A subsequent law (PL-170, 1967) extended funding to the training of physical education and recreational personnel who would work with disabled children (Clumpner, 1986).

Section 504 of the Rehabilitation Act of 1973 (Public Law 93-112) directed specific attention to the handicapped student. This legislation prohibited discrimination against an individual in the areas of education and sports on the basis of a physical or mental handicap. It advocated specific measures to increase accessibility for the disabled (Winnick et al., 1980). Physical education is the sole item of the school curriculum specifically mentioned in Public Law 94-142 (the Education for All Handicapped Children Act), signed by President Gerald Ford in 1975 (U.S. Office of Education, 1977). This law requires that all disabled students be provided with physical education instruction in the least restricted environment possible (Appenzeller, 1983; Rizzo, 1984; Sherrill, 1986b; Winnick, 1984).

The majority of handicapped students in the United States are expected to attend normal physical education classes, and instructors are required to carry out

Table 10.1 Hours Devoted to School Physical Education in Selected Schools

Location	Grade	Frequency (per wk) & duration (min)	Specialist teacher	Required course
Saskatoon, Canada	1-8	2 × 30	No	Yes
	9-10	2 × 45	Yes	Yes
	11-12	2 × 45	Yes	No
United Kingdom*	1-6	2 × 45	No	Yes
	7-12	3 × 45	Yes	Yes
Denmark	1-4	2 × 50	No	Yes
	5-9	3 × 50	No	Yes
	10-12	3 × 50	Yes	Yes
West Germany	1-9	3 × 45	No	Yes
	10-13	3 × 45	Yes	Yes
East Germany	1-6	4 × 45	No	Yes
	7-12	4 × 45	Yes	Yes
Japan	1-6	3 × 45	No	Yes
	7-9	3 × 50	No	Yes
	10	4 × 50	Yes	Yes
	11	3 × 50	Yes	Yes
	12	2 × 50	Yes	Yes
Brazil	1-4	2 × 45	No	Yes
	5-12	3 × 45	Yes	Yes

Note. Based in part on data from "Exercise, Fitness and Physical Education for the Growing Child" by D.A. Bailey, 1974, in W.A.R. Orban (Ed.), *Proceedings of the National Conference on Fitness and Health* (pp. 13-22). Ottawa: Health & Welfare Canada.
*Much higher figures at some private schools.

periodic assessments to ensure that such classes are effective in assuring the physical maturation of the disabled student. The Education for All Handicapped Children Act also specifies that equal opportunity be allowed in extracurricular activities such as athletics. The immediate practical consequence has been an extensive upgrading of qualifications by those teaching in ordinary state schools. By 1983, Cowden and Tymcson (cited by Winnick, 1984) noted that eight states had introduced teacher certification in adapted or special education, and a further 11 states were developing such a program.

Europe

In England, schools are governed by the Education Act of 1944, which prescribes the minimum level of facilities that must be provided for physical education classes. State schools do not provide specialist teachers at the primary school level (S.C. Campbell, 1986), and despite the dedication of well-trained professionals, facilities may also be rather rudimentary at some secondary modern schools for older, industrial-stream students. In contrast, many of the more prestigious private schools have beautiful sports facilities, and the students of such schools spend most afternoons on the playing fields. The decline of interest in sports after leaving school remains a major concern of the British Sports Council, and in recent years the Council has attempted to sustain this interest through the development of community sports centers (see Shephard, 1986a, for details). Passage of the Warnock Committee's Report addressed the specific needs of the disabled. This report has similar provisions to Ontario Bill 82 and U.S. Public Law 94-142.

In the Soviet Union (Morton, 1963) and other Eastern Bloc countries, a clear distinction is drawn between elite sport programs for athletically gifted students (typically conducted at residential schools) and the average school programs of sport and physical education. An estimated 39% of the 46 million children in the general school system are involved in some type of sport program (Kirillyuk, 1981). Other opportunities for vigorous physical activity arise through pioneer camps (attended by about 26% of students); the Komsomol youth organization that coordinates such competitions as soccer, swimming, ice hockey, and cross-country skiing (Jefferies, 1986a); and extracurricular sports "collectives." A strong emphasis on the productive use of free time encourages adolescents to attend the various available sports programs (Jefferies, 1986b). Nevertheless, the student who does not attend an elite sports school faces many handicaps, including limited access to facilities and severe shortages of athletic equipment and clothing.

Other Countries

In Australia, the primary emphasis of both school and community programs has been upon competitive sport. This approach seems quite successful with preadolescent students, as 75% of boys and 67% of girls become involved in at least one sport (Robertson, 1986). However, the subsequent dropout rate is high even among the able-bodied, with the stress of programming and the behavior of adults frequently cited as reasons for abandoning sport. Formal tests of attitudes (Kenyon, 1970) show that students are somewhat less enthusiastic about physical activity than they are in Canada and the United States.

Brazil provides an example of a developing country with enormous contrasts between rich and poor families. Brazil's Ministry of Education has decreed that physical education be provided to all students 2 times per week in Grades 1 through 4 and 3 times per week thereafter (Rocha-Ferreira, 1986). The wealthy private schools have readily met this requirement, but public schools have had problems of implementation due to lack of both physical facilities and money to pay special physical education teachers. Fiscal support for upgrading programs is sought not only through the National Fund for Education Development, but also through the National Fund for Social Development (Sport Lottery), property taxes, endowments, and other sources of private support. Private sports clubs play an important role in the development of elite athletes, but because visibility and financial support depend on competitive success, the less gifted children are rapidly eliminated. Despite the size of the national population (around 100 million), serious research is hampered because few journals or modern textbooks are translated into Portuguese. There is also a pressing need to develop activities that appeal to girls, indigenous children, and the underprivileged children of the urban ghettos. In other developing countries, the same problems exist on an even greater scale; much of South America, for example, is still in the process of ensuring basic reading ability for all except a small and wealthy elite.

Employment

The original approach to employment in several countries was to develop sheltered workshops, partially supported by charity, where the disabled could work under less pressure than in the commercial world. However, as with other forms of segregation, this led to stigmatization and a loss of self-esteem.

North America

In the United States, protection has recently been afforded to the disabled through the Rehabilitation Act of 1977, with the Office of Civil Rights Equal Employment Opportunities Commission (EEOC) as the main enforcer. Civil rights legislation of this type is designed to counter obvious prejudice and stereotyping, but it leaves the disabled person who wishes employment the responsibility of demonstrating a level of performance matching that of the able-bodied. Indeed, in certain forms of employment where public safety is an issue, people having specific categories of disability may be automatically excluded from employment by this same legislation. In Canada, current human rights legislation follows a similar pattern to that adopted by the EEOC in the United States. Specific instances of alleged discrimination are heard by a Human Rights commissioner in a quasilegal process.

Europe

Britain has also maintained for many years a special register of 650,000 persons who are substantially handicapped in holding employment on account of injury, disease, or congenital deformity. All substantial employers (operations with 20 or more personnel) are required to accept a standard percentage of employees from the disabled register, and in certain occupations well suited to the employment of people with a particular form of handicap, an increased percentage is required.

In France, legislation was originally designed to secure the employment of war pensioners (Law of 26 August, 1924). Currently, under Book 3, Chapter 3 of the Code du Travail, commercial and industrial establishments and offices must accept a total of 10% of designated employees, at least 3% being handicapped. However, this percentage varies somewhat with the degree of disability; Category A (mild disability) counts as only half a placement, whereas Category C (severe disability) counts as two placements (Desoille, Scherrer, & Truhaut, 1984).

Sports Organizations

In the past, many sports organizations have tended to be a law unto themselves, but this view is increasingly challenged by legislation such as PL-94-142 in the

United States. Likewise, the British High Court ruled in 1978 that a sports ground was a public place (Bennett et al., 1983). This ruling has obvious implications for assuring accessibility and countering discrimination against the disabled.

Physical Education and Sport Programs

UNESCO conducted an international survey on the development of physical education and sport for the physically and mentally handicapped (J.U. Stein & Gepford, 1982). UNESCO collected information on program development and administration, facilities and equipment, instructional methods and techniques, personnel preparation, documentation, research, and international cooperation and coordination. Although the report found considerable agreement on optimal programs, the report also demonstrated a substantial variation of actual practice within most of the countries surveyed.

In a number of nations, the initiation of activity programs for disabled adults has relied largely upon the initiatives of national sports organizations for the disabled. A further force has been ICHPER, which has stimulated adapted program development with the strong moral support of UNESCO and WHO.

North America

The earlier pattern of tightly segregated physical activity for the disabled is changing rapidly in Canada and the United States. The current emphasis is upon the return of disabled schoolchildren (including preschoolers) to the normal classroom (at first termed *mainstreaming* but more recently described as *integration*); likewise, disabled adults are being moved from institutions into the community (Benson & Williams, 1979; Field, Roseman, DeStefano, & Koewler, 1982; Ispa, 1981; Pomeroy, 1983). Although normal classroom teachers have little initial knowledge of disabling conditions (Bird & Gansneder, 1979; Rizzo, 1984), it has been argued that they have the fundamental skills needed to handle disabled students (Forest, 1984) with the specific exception of multiple-disability blind and deaf students.

Teacher confidence thus grows as teachers are exposed to the disabled (Salend & John, 1983). Moreover, segregation is undesirable, as it limits social experiences and interactions for all students—able-bodied and handicapped alike. The teachers (Karper & Martinek, 1985) and the able-bodied members of a class (C.C. Stewart, 1988) need to learn tolerance and constructive attitudes toward the disabled (G. Clark et al., 1985; Kilburn, 1984). Likewise, those who are handicapped need able-bodied peer models who will challenge them to develop both physical potential and community-related skills rather than the attitudes and values typical of many handicapped groups.

Certainly there is no harm in integrating older mentally retarded students (Rarick & Beuter, 1985). However, some authors have gone much further, assuming uncritically that social benefits stem from a fully integrated program, irrespective of the age of the child or the type and severity of disability. Watkinson and Titus (1985) tempered this optimism, suggesting that a minimum level of physical competence is necessary for successful integration. Integrated programs may therefore fail to achieve increases of either habitual activity or social interaction (Titus

& Watkinson, 1987). Winnick (1987) suggested the need for a continuum of programs reflecting the nature and severity of the handicap and the ability to perform as related to a specific sport. The goal becomes a positive interaction between able-bodied and disabled, rather than total integration, with free movement of the individual along the continuum from integration to segregation as circumstances dictate (French & Jansma, 1982).

Whether full integration or a continuum of programs is adopted, in-service training is desirable to ensure that teachers develop a capacity for individualized instruction adapted to the needs of special students (Knowles, 1983). Current certification programs help in this regard.

Residential institutions are currently reserved for people with exceptional needs, and even such institutions have the same requirement for physical education as a normal school or community. One important obstacle to effective integration of the disabled into active North American society remains the continued emphasis of many able-bodied school programs on competitive sports.

Another recent trend has been the development of outdoor recreation and adventure programs for disabled students (see chapter 9). Godfrey (1980) described courses for the blind and the hearing impaired at the Outward Bound School in Minnesota; lakeside camping for the blind is also popular in Ontario. Such programs seem particularly effective for individuals with associated emotional disturbances.

Europe

In Europe, mountain resorts (called Kurhausen) have a long tradition of catering to the disabled. At such centers, outdoor physical activities are combined with specific therapies such as massage, hydrotherapy, natural mineral baths, special diets, and relaxation training in a delightful rural setting (Badal, 1966; Beckmann, 1966; Kirchhoff, 1966; Venediktov, 1966). A West German law of 1957 allowed trade unions to establish such institutions for their members, costs of attendance being met by the union membership fees (Blohmke, 1966). In West Germany, the Bavarian Sports Association for the Handicapped sponsors similar camps that offer a variety of indoor and outdoor sports, including international camps that attract guests from as many as 10 different countries at any one time.

Union-operated Kur-Resorts have been seen as fulfillment of Articles 119 and 120 of the Soviet constitution—"the provision of a wide network of health resorts for the use of the working people" (Venediktov, 1966, p. 378). One current responsibility of Soviet trade unions is to share with governmental health authorities the task of developing special training programs for the disabled.

As was once the case in North America, the traditional European approach to the education of children with more severe forms of physical or mental disability was to sequester the affected students in some dismal institution, with limited facilities for any type of education and particularly little chance to develop physical skills. In West Germany, there are still 10 different types of school, catering to the blind, the partially sighted, the deaf, the hearing impaired, the physically disabled, the mentally retarded, the socially deviant, and those with speech disorders, learning disabilities, and other medical conditions (Doll-Tepper, 1983).

This reflects a continuing interest in special forms of movement education for the mentally retarded and for those with other types of disability (Irmischer, 1980; Kiphard, 1983; Kiphard, 1979; Kiphard & Leger, 1975).

Nevertheless, there is a trend to educate the disabled in the normal classroom in countries such as England, Norway, Israel, and Holland (Bennett et al., 1983). Likewise, in the Soviet Union (Shneidman, 1978), students diagnosed by their physician as having temporary or permanent medical disabilities attend the normal physical education classes with their peers, although if they are not able to participate in the general program special remedial classes are arranged. The main problem of full integration is that if students need special help and individual assistance, an effective personal program demands a low student-teacher ratio.

A. Brown (1982) described a program for the teaching of team sports to children with severe spastic paralysis who attend an English special school. He argued that although the disorder may be so severe as to prevent active play, the learning of rules and tactics is helpful in enabling the affected individuals to become intelligent spectators and (if they so wish) to join a supporters' club.

In Scandinavia (Brattnas, 1974), the emphasis of normal school physical education programs is upon training and recreation (as opposed to the sports emphasis of many U.S., Canadian, and Australian schools). This may be one reason why higher figures have been reported for the physical working capacity of the disabled in Sweden than in the U.S., Canada, and Australia (Snaith, 1974).

Other Countries

Many of the developing countries lack the basic knowledge to undertake integrated programs, and countries such as the United States and Canada thus have a responsibility to share not only financial resources but also technical information. ICHPER has played a valuable role in facilitating such sharing, stimulating formation of the Caribbean and Central American Commission on Physical Education for the Handicapped, with the support of the Organization of American States. This group has not only hosted major conferences but has also provided followup workshops and in-service activities in Central America, identifying resource personnel and developing exemplary demonstration programs.

There is undoubtedly further scope for such action. Lillis (1977) writes with respect to Africa: "The lack of finance is the biggest single hindrance. . . . The present overall position is very haphazard . . . optimum efficiency is not obtained from present investments. The multiplicity of interests, often the lack of harmony amongst donors means that money and energy are being dissipated. One area that ICSPE/UNESCO might very usefully research is the origin of finance for physical education and sports projects and its effective direction for future planning and development."

Therapy

Both the nature of disability and patterns of treatment show considerable cultural differences. In the less developed parts of the world, substantial concentrations of those disabled by infections (e.g., conditions such as poliomyelitis, leprosy, and conjunctival infections) remain, whereas the toll of spinal injuries from road accidents is quite small. In some primitive cultures, the incidence of persistent congenital disabilities was also quite low until recently, largely because physically imperfect babies were killed (Friedmann, 1972; Menon, 1970). On the other hand, both Hindu scripture (the Rigveda) and the Bible describe appliances to help the ambulation of the lower-extremity disabled (Ghosh, 1980), and ancient Buddhist (Jayasuriya, 1974), Greek, and Roman civilizations made liberal use of massage and various types of hydrotherapy. Patterns of exercise therapy for the disabled have undergone a substantial degree of standardization from one part of the world to another over the past 10 years, although techniques remain influenced by local resources, interests, and traditions.

North America

In the United States, the typical pattern of treatment has supplemented sports and recreation by physical and occupational therapy. The physical therapist has used a variety of tools to improve muscle and joint function, such as deep heat (both diathermy and ultrasound), superficial heat (infrared radiation and hydromassage), cold therapy, massage, passive stretching, specific muscle exercises (see Table 10.2), and electrical muscle stimulation. Considerable excitement has attended the work of Petrofsky (1986), who showed that normal exercise rehabilitation could be assisted by high-technology, computer-assisted stimulation of paralyzed muscles. Those using this approach claim an appreciable restoration of lean tissue, and some paraplegics have been enabled to operate a wheeled vehicle with their legs or even walk short distances with partial support from a frame. Occupational therapy has sought to complement recreational and physical therapy, providing the individual with interesting tasks to develop strength endurance and dexterity in specific muscle groups, particularly the hands.

Other Countries

In less developed countries, many of the forms of therapy considered routine in North America are not practicable. Even if funds can be found to purchase a wheelchair, rutted dirt roads and primitive housing make this form of ambulation excessively tiring. For some populations, even a second-hand crutch can be a most welcome donation from North America. Likewise, a braille-signed gymnasium and electronic beeper balls may be totally unrealistic in a society where few able-bodied people can read and no ready source of electricity is available. Among such populations, therapists must focus upon the most basic forms of clinical treatment and the simplest forms of physical therapy.

The Chinese have shown interest in the ability of T'ai Chi (Zhuo, 1985) and yoga (Singh & Chhina, 1974) to increase joint flexibility, reduce muscle spasm, and prevent a progressive restriction of movement. The exerciser combines the gentle, slow movements of T'ai Chi with relaxation of the wrists, arms, shoulders, chest, abdomen, and back; such movements are directed by thought rather than strength, the exerciser concentrating attention upon each movement. In the early stages of paralytic lesions, Chinese rehabilitation teams also apply massage–

Table 10.2 Specific Therapeutic Activities Used by the Physiotherapist in the Treatment of Patients With Neurological Disorders

---

Muscle stretching—to relieve contractures, prevent deformities, and increase range of movement

Gravity exercises—to lift the body part against gravity

Muscle awareness exercises—to control specific muscles

Neuromuscular re-education—to stimulate proprioception

Reciprocal exercises—to strengthen protagonists

Tonic exercises—to prevent atrophy

Relaxation training—to relieve contractures, rigidity, and spasms

Postural alignment and gait training

Body mechanics—to maximize use of large muscles

Proprioceptive facilitation—to maximize excitation of motor units

Ramp climbing—to improve balance and ambulation

Note. Based in part on data from *Principles and Methods of Adapted Physical Education and Recreation* by W.C. Crowe, D. Auxter, and J. Pyfer, 1981. St. Louis: Mosby.

deep kneading or stroking for flaccid muscles and surface stroking for spastic muscles. Finally, therapists recommend acupuncture in the first 6 months after most types of injury.

Yoga (Singh & Chhina, 1974) involves various cleansing rituals, followed by eight physical, moral, and physiological practices—yama (abstention), niyama (observance), asana (physical postures), pranayama (breath control), pratyahara (control of sensory perception), dhyana (fixed attention), dháraná (contemplation), and samadhi (absolute concentration). Not all of these practices have specific value for the disabled. However, the postural exercises can help relaxation and improve coordination. During the breathing exercises, considerable degrees of hypoxia and hypercarbia can arise; again the practice has profound effects on muscle tone and oxygen consumption, and such changes may be quite helpful to a person with severe muscle spasm.

Key Ideas

---

1. Services available to disabled populations have become more uniform through both intergovernmental contacts and informal exchange of ideas at athletic competitions.

2. Legislation is progressively assuring the disabled of appropriate fitness programming, including access to physical education in state schools and participation in private sports clubs. Special registers of the disabled and equal rights legislation also increase access to employment.

3. Programs for disabled adults have developed largely at the initiative of national sports organizations for the disabled, although in some regions initiatives of UNESCO, WHO, and ICHPER have also made a valuable contribution.

4. Traditionally, schoolchildren have been sent to disability-specific residential schools. Although this pattern of organization still persists in some parts of Europe, in North America there is rapid progress toward the integration of all except severely handicapped students into the normal school system. This presents an urgent need for the development of appropriate skills by normal classroom teachers.

5. Patterns of disability-causing diseases still vary substantially from one part of the world to another. Cultural factors strongly influence local attitudes toward the disabled and toward acceptable patterns of therapy.

6. Assuming that the current trend toward high-technology medicine persists, in the future we may see increasing use of approaches such as programmed electrical stimulation in the restoration of function in the quadriplegic.

Practical Applications

1. Good practical ideas for the disabled sometimes take substantial time to move from one region to another. How could this process be accelerated?

2. Could any additional legislation help the disabled in your country, province or state, or municipality? Is legislation the best method of obtaining equality of opportunity for the disabled? What are its disadvantages?

3. What initiatives do you think your government should introduce to help the disabled?

4. Do you think integration is a desirable method of education for the disabled child? What practical difficulties may be encountered in implementing such a strategy?

5. In what ways could the voluntary organizations in your city offer more effective help to the disabled?

6. Do you agree that the current trend toward ''high-tech'' medicine holds great promise for the disabled? Do you see any disadvantages in such an emphasis?

7. Is there a role for traditional medicine in the treatment of disabled individuals in developing countries and in the native societies of North America?

Other Reference Texts in Adapted Physical Education

General Textbooks Used in Adapted Physical Education Courses

Arnheim, D.D., & Sinclair, W.A. (1975). *The clumsy child* (2nd ed.). St. Louis: C.V. Mosby.

Arnheim, D.D., & Sinclair, W.A. (1985). *Physical education for special populations: A developmental, adapted, and remedial approach*. Englewood Cliffs, NJ: Prentice-Hall.

Auxter, D., & Pyfer, J. (1985). *Principles and methods of adapted physical education and recreation* (5th ed.). St. Louis: C.V. Mosby. Fourth edition (1981) was by Crowe, Auxter, and Pyfer. Senior author on other editions was Arnheim.

Clarke, H.H., & Clarke, D.H. (1978). *Developmental and adapted physical education* (2nd ed.). Englewood Cliffs, NJ: Prentice-Hall.

Cratty, B.J. (1975). *Remedial motor activity for children*. Philadelphia: Lea & Febiger.

Cratty, B.J. (1980). *Adapted physical education for children and youth*. Denver: Love.

Danicls, A.S., & Davies, E.A. (1975). *Adapted physical education* (3rd ed.). New York: Harper and Row.

Eichstaedt, C.B., & Kalakian, L.H. (1987). *Developmental/adapted physical education: Making ability count* (2nd ed.). Minneapolis, MN: Burgess.

Fait, H.F., & Dunn, J.M. (1982). *Special physical education: Adapted, corrective, developmental* (5th ed.). Philadelphia: W.B. Saunders.

Folio, M.R. (1985). *Physical education programming for exceptional learners*. Rockville, MD: Aspen Systems Corporation.

French, R.W., & Jansma, P. (1982). *Special physical education*. Columbus, OH: Charles E. Merrill.

Geddes, D. (1978). *Physical activities for individuals with handicapping conditions* (2nd ed.). St. Louis: C.V. Mosby.

Geddes, D. (1981). *Psychomotor individualized education programs for intellectual, learning, and behavioral disabilities*. Boston: Allyn and Bacon.

Groves, L. (Ed.). (1979). *Physical education for special needs*. Cambridge, England: Cambridge University Press.

Appendix A was previously published in *Leadership Training in Adapted Physical Education* (pp. 467-470) edited by Claudine Sherrill, 1988, Champaign, IL, Human Kinetics and is reprinted here with the permission of the editor.

Gubbay, S. (1975). *The clumsy child*. Philadelphia: W.B. Saunders.

Masters, L.F., Mori, A.A., & Lange, E.K. (1983). *Adapted physical education: A practitioner's guide*. Gaithersburg, MD: Aspen Systems Corporation.

Miller, A.G., & Sullivan, J.V. (1982). *Teaching physical activities to impaired youth*. New York: John Wiley & Sons.

Seaman, J., & DePauw, K. (1982). *The new adapted physical education: A developmental approach*. Palo Alto, CA: Mayfield.

Sherrill, C. (1986). *Adapted physical education and recreation: A multidisciplinary approach* (3rd ed.). Dubuque, IA: Wm. C. Brown.

Vannier, M. (1977). *Physical activities for the handicapped*. Englewood Cliffs, NJ: Prentice-Hall.

Vodola, T. (1976). *Project ACTIVE Maxi-Mini Kit*. Oakhurst, NJ: Township of Ocean School District. Includes nine adapted physical education manuals. Based on Vodola, T. (1973). *Individualized physical education program for the handicapped child*. Englewood Cliffs, NJ: Prentice-Hall.

Wessel, J. (1977). *Planning individualized education programs in special education: With examples from I CAN physical education*. Northbrook, IL: Hubbard.

Wessel, J., & Kelly, L. (1986). *Achievement-based curriculum development in physical education*. Philadelphia: Lea & Febiger.

Wheeler, R.H., & Hooley, A.M. (1976). *Physical education for the handicapped* (2nd ed.). Philadelphia: Lea & Febiger.

Winnick, J.P. (1979). *Early movement experiences and development: Habilitation and remediation*. Philadelphia: W.B. Saunders.

Wiseman, D.C. (1982). *A practical approach to adapted physical education*. Reading, MA: Addison-Wesley.

Specialized Textbooks Used in Specific Adapted Physical Education Courses

Assessment

American Alliance for Health, Physical Education, and Recreation. (no date, circa 1976). *Testing for impaired, disabled, and handicapped individuals*. Washington, DC: Author.

McClenaghan, B., & Gallahue, D. (1978). *Fundamental movement: A developmental and remedial approach*. Philadelphia: W.B. Saunders.

Werder, J., & Kalakian, L. (1985). *Assessment in adapted physical education*. Minneapolis, MN: Burgess.

Winnick, J., & Short, F. (1985). *Physical fitness testing of the disabled: Project UNIQUE*. Champaign, IL: Human Kinetics.

Curriculum and Instruction

Morris, G.S.D. (1980). *Elementary physical education: Toward inclusion*. Salt Lake City: Brighton.

Morris, G.S.D. (1980). *How to change the games children play* (2nd ed.). Minneapolis, MN: Burgess.

Mosston, M. (1981). *Teaching physical education* (2nd ed.). Columbus, OH: Charles E. Merrill. (1st ed., 1966)

Wessel, J., & Kelly, L. (1986). *Achievement-based curriculum development in physical education*. Philadelphia: Lea & Febiger.

Physical Education for Severely Handicapped Students

Dunn, J., Morehouse, J., & Fredericks, H.D.B. (1985). *Physical education for the severely handicapped: A systematic approach to a data based gymnasium* (2nd ed.). Austin: Pro-Ed. (1st ed. Dunn, J., et al. 1980) *A data based gymnasium*. Monmouth, OR: Instructional Development Corporation.

Jansma, P. (Ed.). (1984). *The psychomotor domain and the seriously handicapped* (2nd ed.). Lanham, MD: University Press of America.

Wessel, J. (1981). *I CAN adaptation manual: Teaching physical education to severely handicapped students*. East Lansing, MI: Michigan State University.

Legal, Historical, and Philosophical Foundations, Teacher Training Methodology, and Administration

Appenzeller, H. (1983). *The right to participate: The law and individuals with handicapping conditions in physical education and sports*. Charlottesville, VA: Michie.

Sherrill, C. (Ed.). (1987). *Leadership training in adapted physical education*. Champaign, IL: Human Kinetics.

Research Collections and Readings in Adapted Physical Education and Sport

Berridge, M., & Ward, G. (Eds.). (1986). *International perspectives on adapted physical activity*. Champaign, IL: Human Kinetics.

Eason, R., Smith, T., & Caron, F. (Eds.). (1983). *Adapted physical activity: Proceedings of the Third Symposium of the International Federation of Adapted Physical Activity*. Champaign, IL: Human Kinetics.

McLeish, E. (Ed.). (1985). *Adapted physical activities: Proceedings of the Fourth Symposium of the International Federation of Adapted Physical Activity*. London: Author.

Sherrill, C. (Ed.). (1986). *Sport and disabled athletes*. Champaign, IL: Human Kinetics.

Sports for Disabled Individuals

Adams, R.C., Daniel, A.N., McCubbin, J.A., & Rullman, L. (1982). *Games, sports, and exercises for the physically handicapped* (3rd ed.). Philadelphia: Lea & Febiger.

Guttmann, L. (1976). *Textbook of sport for the disabled*. Aylesbury, England: HM & M.

Sherrill, C. (Ed.). (1986). *Sport and disabled athletes: Proceedings of the International Scientific Congress*. Champaign, IL: Human Kinetics.

Special Olympics, Inc. (1981 on). *Sports skills instructional manuals*. Washington, DC: Author.

Van Hal, L., Rarick, G.L., & Vermeer, A. (1984). *Sport for mentally handicapped: Mentally handicapped sport symposium of The Netherlands—USA Bicentennial*. Haarlem, The Netherlands: Vitgeverij de Vrieseborch. (U.S. distributor is Human Kinetics)

Early Childhood Adapted Physical Education

American Alliance for Health, Physical Education, and Recreation. (1976). *Early intervention for handicapped children through programs of physical education and recreation*. Washington, DC: Author.

Evans, J. (1980). *They have to be carefully taught*. Reston, VA: American Alliance for Health, Physical Education, Recreation, and Dance.

McClenaghan, B., & Gallahue, D. (1978). *Fundamental movement: A developmental and remedial approach*. Philadelphia: W.B. Saunders.

Adapted Physical Education Focusing on One Disability

Adams, R.C., Daniel, A.N., McCubbin, J.A., & Rullman, L. (1982). *Games, sports, and physical exercises for the physically disabled* (3rd ed.). Philadelphia: Lea & Febiger.

Buell, C.E. (1983). *Physical education for blind children* (2nd ed.). Springfield, IL: Charles C Thomas.

Colvin, N.R., & Finholt, J.M. (1981). *Guidelines for physical educators of mentally handicapped youth: Curriculum, assessment, IEPs*. Springfield, IL: Charles C Thomas.

Hackett, L. (1975). *Movement exploration and games for the mentally retarded* (5th printing). Palo Alto, CA: Peek.

Moran, J.M., & Kalakian, I.H. (1977). *Movement experiences for the retarded or emotionally disturbed child* (2nd ed.). Minneapolis, MN: Burgess.

Rarick, G.L., Dobbins, D.A., & Broadhead, G.D. (1976). *The motor domain and its correlates in educationally handicapped children*. Englewood Cliffs, NJ: Prentice-Hall.

Norms for Fitness Tests

Test results are substantially affected by the environment—both internal and external—in which they are conducted. Researchers should thus take environmental conditions into account and note them for further reference; ideally all tests should be conducted under the same conditions whenever reassessment is needed. All of the following variables are important:

- time of day
- temperature (dry bulb, wet bulb, globe)
- wind and ground conditions (for field tests)
- fatigue level (tests preferably preceded by 24 hr of rest)
- time since last meal (tests best carried out 2-3 hr after a light carbohydrate meal)
- freedom of subject from acute injury or infection
- level of anxiety—this should be minimized by allowing preliminary practice of all required tests (habituation)
- motivational level—this can be made more consistent if the same observer is used throughout

Body Composition

Ideal Body Mass

Body mass is evaluated relative to standing height. Values listed in Table B.1 are "ideal" from the actuarial viewpoint. An excess mass normally reflects an accumulation of body fat. However, mass/height relationships are distorted by unusual height (stunted growth or spinal deformity), muscle wasting, loss of bone density, amputation, or limb deformity.

Skinfold Readings

Skinfold readings can be used to predict body fat. Widely accepted equations for the general population are based upon the sum of biceps, triceps, subscapular, and suprailiac folds, ΣS (Durnin & Womersley, 1974):

$$
\begin{aligned}
\text{Body density (boys)} &= 1.1533 - 0.0643 \log_{10} \Sigma S \\
\text{(girls)} &= 1.1369 - 0.0598 \log_{10} \Sigma S \\
\text{(men)} &= 1.1631 - 0.0632 \log_{10} \Sigma S \\
\text{(women)} &= 1.1599 - 0.0717 \log_{10} \Sigma S
\end{aligned}
$$

$$\text{Body fat } (\%) = (4.570/D - 4.142)\ 100 \qquad \text{(Behnke, 1961)}$$

A recent paper (Bulbulian et al., 1987) argued that it is preferable to use a somewhat different formula when making the calculation in subjects whose arms have undergone extensive hypertrophy from wheelchair ambulation:

$$\text{Body density} = 1.09092 + 0.00296S_1 - 0.00072S_2 - 0.00182C_1 + 0.00124C_2$$

where S_1 is the thickness of the chest skinfold, S_2 the thickness of the subscapular skinfold, C_1 the waist circumference, and C_2 the calf circumference. Body fat is then calculated from density D, using the formula of Siri (1956): Body fat (%) = ([4.95/D] − 4.50) 100.

The optimum percentage of body fat thus calculated is 14% or less in a young man and 18% or less in a young woman, but many disabled subjects have much higher values. A simpler alternative is to interpret the skinfold readings in their own right. An appropriate basis for comparison is provided by the thickness of the folds observed in young adults approximating the ideal body mass (see Table B.2). The central type of fat distribution, typical of the male and associated with an increased risk of ischemic heart disease, can be assessed from the ratio of chest to suprailiac readings.

Muscle Strength

Anaerobic Power and Capacity

Anaerobic power and capacity can be tested by all-out effort on a cycle ergometer (Table B.3). Anaerobic power can also be assessed by a staircase sprint or by a 50-yard (45.7 m) sprint (Table B.4).

Isometric Muscle Force

Normative data is available for handgrip force (Table B.5), the lifting force of the back (Table B.6), and for upper body strength (Table B.7).

In field situations, performance is expressed as the number of times the body mass can be displaced against gravity, either timed or untimed (e.g., bent-knee sit-ups, see Table B.8, or push-ups, see Table B.9). Scores in this type of test depend on the ability of the subject to understand the required procedure, motivation to do well, and the body mass to be displaced, as well as any local development of the arm and shoulder muscles.

Isokinetic Muscle Force and Endurance

An isokinetic dynamometer such as the Cybex II can record the forces developed during fixed-speed rotation of the major joints. In all measurements, it is vital to align the axis of rotation for the machine and the joint. Some authors report the peak force, expressed in newtons, but this depends somewhat on the damping of the force record (see Table B.10). Others report the average force sustained over the entire contraction. The speed of rotation can vary from 30 to 300° per second; the slow contractions reflect predominantly the action of the slow twitch muscle fibers, whereas the fast contractions reflect largely the action of the fast twitch fibers.

Isokinetic endurance is commonly expressed as the decrease in force observed over 50 contractions, measured for instance at a rotation speed of 180°/s.

Aerobic Power

The aerobic power reflects the ability to sustain activity by aerobic metabolism. It can be expressed in terms of the performance of physical work at a specified heart rate (e.g., the PWC at a heart rate of 170 beats/min; see Table B.11) or the equivalent steady-state transport of oxygen (traditionally expressed in ml/kg • min [see Table B.12] but more recently reported also as μmol O_2/kg • min, ml/kg • min $- 44.6 \ \mu$mol/kg/min). The aerobic power is assumed to be a measure of cardiorespiratory function and is thus reported for a large muscle exercise (uphill treadmill running, bench stepping, or cycle ergometry). In the able-bodied, the aerobic power seen during arm exercise is only about 70% of that for leg exercise, but in disabled individuals with hypertrophy of the arm and shoulder girdles, the upper-limb figure (measured on an arm ergometer or wheelchair ergometer) may approach much more closely to lower-limb norms (see Table B.13).

In field surveys of the able-bodied, the maximum oxygen intake can be predicted with a coefficient of variation of about 10%, using such devices as the Åstrand monogram (Åstrand, 1960). This calculates a formula of the type:

$$\text{For young men,} \quad \dot{V}O_2\text{max} = \frac{(193 - 128) \ 2}{(P - 63)} \ \dot{V}O_2$$

$$\text{For young women,} \quad \dot{V}O_2\text{max} = \frac{(203 - 138) \ 2}{(P - 73)} \ \dot{V}O_2$$

where P is the observed heart rate between 50 and 100% of maximum aerobic power and $\dot{V}O_2$ is the corresponding oxygen consumption. In older adults, this figure must be adjusted downward to allow for a decrease of maximum heart rate, using constants of the type shown in Table B.14. Tests with amputees (Kavanagh & Shephard, 1973) and the wheelchair disabled (Kofsky et al., 1983b) suggest that the standard Åstrand nomogram can be applied with moderate success to such populations.

In those with use of the legs, we can measure the distance covered in 12 or 15 minutes (see Table B.15), and the same type of test can be carried out in a wheelchair (see Table 4.6), although norms for the latter are by no means clearly established. Scores for timed performance depend on an understanding of the test, motivation, coordination, and an appropriate choice of pace; other key variables are body mass, ground conditions, and (for the wheelchair user) the design of wheelchair.

Flexibility

Flexibility is highly joint specific even in the able-bodied, and independent testing must thus be undertaken at each of the major articulations. The passive range of motion can be ascertained by aligning a goniometer with the principal axis of rotation of each of the major joints in turn (see Table B.16). A simple overall measure of active flexibility for the hips and lower back is provided by having the subject perform a sit-and-reach test (see Table B.17).

Table B.1   Ideal Body Mass in Relation to Standing Height

Height (cm) (no shoes)	Ideal body mass (kg) (indoor clothing)	
	Male	Female
147.3	—	48.5
149.9	—	49.9
152.4	—	51.2
155.0	—	52.6
157.5	57.6	54.2
160.0	58.9	55.8
162.6	60.3	57.8
165.1	61.9	60.0
167.6	63.7	61.7
170.2	65.7	63.5
172.7	67.6	65.3
175.3	69.4	66.8
177.8	71.4	68.5
180.3	73.5	—
182.9	75.5	—
185.4	77.5	—
188.0	79.8	—
190.5	82.1	—
193.0	84.3	—

Note. (1) A subject can have substantially less than the ideal mass and yet be in good health; many primitive peoples weigh 10-15 kg below the ideal. (2) A well-muscled subject may exceed the ideal mass; "excess weight" must thus be interpreted in conjunction with observations on body fat and skeletal dimensions. (3) A reduction of body mass may reflect loss of lean tissue rather than fat. Based on data from *Build and Blood Pressure Study*, Society of Actuaries, 1959. Chicago: Author.

Table B.2   Thickness of Selected Skinfolds in Young Adults Approximating the Ideal Body Mass

Skinfold	Male (mm)	Female (mm)
Chin	5.8 ± 8.7	7.1 ± 2.8
Triceps	7.8 ± 4.1	15.6 ± 6.2
Chest	12.0 ± 7.9	8.6 ± 3.7
Subscapular	11.9 ± 5.1	11.3 ± 4.2
Suprailiac	12.7 ± 7.0	14.6 ± 8.0
Waist	14.3 ± 8.2	15.3 ± 7.5
Suprapubic	11.0 ± 6.4	20.5 ± 8.2
Knee (medial aspect)	8.6 ± 4.1	11.8 ± 4.2
Average (all folds)	10.4 ± 4.9	13.9 ± 5.1

Note. Based on data from *Endurance Fitness* (2nd ed.), by R.J. Shephard, 1977. Toronto: University of Toronto Press.

Table B.3   Anaerobic Capacity and Power

	Males	Females
Anaerobic power		
Staircase sprint (W/kg)	11-18	9-11
5-s cycle ergometer test (W/kg)*	8-11	8-10
5-s arm ergometer test (W/kg)**	1.7-2.3	—
Anaerobic capacity		
30-s cycle ergometer test (J/kg)*	105-135	83-113
30-s arm ergometer test (J/kg)**	50-66	—

Note. Based on data from *Pediatric Sports Medicine for the Practitioner* by O. Bar-Or, 1983. New York: Springer-Verlag; from "A Comparison of 'Anaerobic' Components of O$_2$ Debt and the Wingate Test" by B. Goslin and T.E. Graham, 1985, *Canadian Journal of Applied Science*, **10**, pp. 134-140; and from "An Outline for Setting Significant Tests of Muscular Performance" by R. Margaria, 1966, in H. Yoshimura and J.S. Weiner (Eds.), *Human Adaptability and Its Methodology*. Tokyo: Society for the Promotion of Sciences for the able-bodied; and from "Aerobic and Anaerobic Power of Canadian Wheelchair Athletes" by K. Coutts and J.L. Stogryn, 1987, *Medicine and Science in Sports and Exercise*, **19**, pp. 62-65 for the wheelchair disabled.

*Able-bodied. **Wheelchair disabled.

Table B.4   Time Required to Cover a Distance of 50 Yards

Age (years)	Boys 50th	Boys 25th	Girls 50th	Girls 25th
	percentile		percentile	
10	8.3	9.0	8.7	9.2
11	8.0	8.7	8.4	9.0
12	7.8	8.3	8.1	8.8
13	7.4	8.0	7.9	8.5
14	7.1	7.6	7.9	8.4
15	6.9	7.2	7.8	8.3
16	6.7	7.0	7.9	8.4
17	6.6	7.0	8.0	8.5

Note. Based on data from *National School Population Fitness Survey*, 1985, Washington, DC: President's Council on Physical Fitness and Sports and from *AAHPER Youth Fitness Test Manual*, 1976. Washington, DC: AAHPER. Scores depend greatly on running surface and prior experience of the test.

Table B.5   Peak Handgrip Force for the Dominant Hand (kN)

Age (years)	Males (kN)	Males (kN/kg)	Females (kN)	Females (kN/kg)
8	154	5.5	138	4.9
11	226	5.8	201	5.1
14	337	6.5	280	5.4
17	488	7.3	308	5.4
20-29	545	7.4	312	5.4
30-39	541	7.1	320	5.2
40-49	525	6.7	314	4.9
50-59	490	6.3	286	4.4
60 +	443	5.7	266	4.1

Note. Based on data from Canada Fitness Survey, 1983 (see note to Table 9.3). Results are up to 10% lower for the nondominant arm; the standard deviation of data in the able-bodied population is about ± 15% of the mean score. Results for the upper body strength of the wheelchair disabled are shown in Table B.7.

Table B.6   Peak Back Lifting Force as Measured by Dynamometer

Fitness level	Males	Females
Excellent (> 90th percentile)	550-580	375-405
Very good (75-85th percentile)	505-535	332-361
Good (60-70th percentile)	460-490	287-317
Average (45-55th percentile)	415-445	242-272
Fair (30-40th percentile)	370-400	198-227
Poor (15-25th percentile)	325-355	153-183
Very poor (< 10th percentile)	280-310	108-138

Table B.7   Upper Body Strength of the Wheelchair Disabled

Fitness level (SD)	Males (N/kg)	Females (N/kg)
Excellent (+1.8 to +3.0)	> 23.6	19.0
Above average (+0.6 to +1.8)	18.2-23.6	13.4-19.0
Average (−0.6 to +0.6)	12.7-18.1	7.6-13.3
Below average (−1.8 to −0.6)	7.1-12.6	1.9-7.5
Poor (−3.0 to −1.8)	< 7.1	< 1.9

Note. Based on data from Kofsky et al., 1986 (see note to Table 6.3). Upper body strength represents the sum of peak isometric force for elbow flexion, elbow extension, and shoulder extension.

Table B.8   Bent-Knee Sit-Ups Performed Over an Interval of 1 Minute

Age (years)	Males	Females
8	28.0	28.1
11	34.9	32.6
14	38.5	33.7
17	38.2	31.6
20-29	33.7	26.1
30-39	27.1	19.5
40-49	22.2	14.5
50-59	19.9	12.3
60 +	12.6	7.2

Note. Based on data from Canada Fitness Survey, 1983 (see note to Table 9.3) for able-bodied subjects, ankles held by assistant, knees bent to 90°, hands clasped behind head. At the 25th percentile, the number of sit-ups is about 75% of that at the 50th percentile. Scores are influenced by both muscular endurance and the mass of the upper half of the body.

Table B.9   Push-Ups Performed Over an Interval of 1 Minute

Age (years)	Males	Females
8	10.6	15.0
11	13.1	20.0
14	17.0	21.3
17	25.6	20.8
20-29	24.7	17.4
30-39	18.9	15.5
40-49	14.4	13.3
50-59	11.4	10.8
60 +	9.7	9.1

See note to Table 9.3 (data for able-bodied, using the toes as the pivotal joint in males; the knees as pivotal joint in females). Scores are influenced by both muscular endurance and body mass.

Table B.10   Peak Isokinetic Muscle Force at Knee Joint (Torque, Newton-Meters, at Specified Speeds of Rotation) for Well-Trained Late Adolescent and Young Adult Able-Bodied Soccer Players

Speed of rotation (degrees/s)	Males		Females	
	Extension	Flexion	Extension	Flexion
30	183	108	—	—
60	161	96	105	59
180	111	79	62	49
240	100	70	—	—
300	81	55	44	41

Note. Based on data from "Specific Muscular Development in Under-18 Soccer Players" by P. Leatt, R.J. Shephard, and M. Plyley, 1987, *Journal of Sport Sciences,* **5**, 165-175. The decrease of performance of 50 repetitions at 180°/s is approximately 50%.

Table B.11   Physical Work Capacity at a Heart Rate of 170 B/Min Leg Ergometer Exercise, Expressed in Watts/Kg

Age (years)	Males	Females
7	2.0	1.6
8	2.1	1.8
9	2.1	1.7
10	2.1	1.7
11	2.2	1.7
12	2.2	1.7
13	2.3	1.5
14	2.3	1.4
15	2.1	1.4
16	2.2	1.4
17	2.2	1.4

Note. Based on data from *The Physical Work Capacity of Canadian Children 7-17 Years* by M.L. Howell and R.J. MacNab, 1968. Ottawa: CAHPER. A more recent survey has shown values some 10% higher in boys and up to 20% higher in older girls (Gauthier, Massicotte, Hermiston, & MacNab, 1983). Values at the 25th percentile are some 20% lower than those at the 50th percentile.

Table B.12   Maximum Oxygen Intake of Able-Bodied Subjects

Age (years)	Males (ml/kg • min)	Females (ml/kg • min)
8	49.9	42.7
11	50.4	42.8
14	50.7	42.5
17	49.3	40.9
20-29	46.4	38.4
30-39	44.4	37.3
40-49	39.5	34.7
50-59	32.6	29.1
60 +	27.5	24.2

Note. Based on data from Canada Fitness Survey, 1983 and *Fitness of a Nation: Lessons from the Canada Fitness Survey* by R.J. Shephard, 1986. Basel: Karger. Calculations are based on attained rate of stepping. Coefficient of variation for data ($\pm$ 1 *SD*) of approximately 20% at any given age. In the able-bodied, values for arm work are approximately 70% of those recorded on the treadmill, step test, or cycle ergometer. Data for the wheelchair disabled are shown in Table B.13.

Table B.13   Peak Oxygen Intake of the Wheelchair Disabled During Arm Ergometry

Fitness level (*SD*)	Males (ml/kg • min)	Females (ml/kg • min)
Excellent (+1.8 to 3.0)	> 44.9	> 38.0
Above average (+0.6 to 1.8)	33.5-44.9	27.2-38.0
Average (−0.6 to +0.6)	22.0-33.4	16.3-27.1
Below average (−1.8 to −0.6)	10.5-21.9	5.4-16.2
Poor (−3.0 to −1.8)	< 10.5	< 5.4

Note. Based on data from Kofsky et al., 1986 (see note to Table 6.3).

Table B.14   Constants Used to Correct the Åstrand Prediction of Maximum Oxygen Intake for the Decrease of Maximum Heart Rate With Age

Age (years)	Correction factor
10	1.10
25	1.00
35	0.87
45	0.78
55	0.71
65	0.65

Note. Based on data from "Aerobic Work Capacity in Men and Women with Special Reference to Age" by I. Åstrand, 1960, *Acta Physiologica Scandinavica*, **49** (Suppl. 169), pp. 1-91.

Table B.15   Relationship Between the Distance Covered in 12 Minutes and the Corresponding Maximum Oxygen Intake (ml/kg • min)

Distance covered (km)	Corresponding estimate of maximum oxygen intake (ml/kg • min)
1.6	28.0
2.0	34.0
2.4	42.0
2.8	52.0
> 2.8	> 52.0

Note. Based on data for able-bodied young adults from "A Means of Assessing Oxygen Intake" by K.H. Cooper, 1968, *Journal of the American Medical Association*, **203**, pp. 201-204. The normal score of a young adult male is about 46 ± 8, dropping to about 28 ± 6 ml/kg • min at the age of 65 years. Corresponding figures for women are 38 ± 7, dropping to 24 ± 6 ml/kg • min.

Table B.16   Normal Range of Passive Motion at Major Joints

Joint movement	Moller et al. (1985) (degrees)	Oberg et al. (1984) (degrees)
Hip abduction	40	33
Flexion	79	81
Extension	81	81
Knee flexion	145	139
Ankle dorsiflexion	21	22

Note. Based on data from "Stretching Exercise and Soccer: Effect of Stretching on Range of Motion in the Lower Extremity in Connection With Soccer Training" by M.H.L. Moller, B.E. Oberg, and J. Gillquist, 1985, *International Journal of Sports Medicine*, **6**, pp. 50-52 and from "Muscle Strength and Flexibility in Different Positions of Soccer Players" by B.E. Oberg, M.H.L. Moller, J. Ekstrand, and J. Gillquist, 1984, *International Journal of Sports Medicine*, **5**, pp. 213-216. Data for able-bodied males (results for women are commonly 20% larger).

Table B.17   Normal Scores for Sit-and-Reach Test

Age (years)	Males	Females
8	27.9	31.8
11	26.5	30.9
14	26.2	32.8
17	29.8	34.1
20-29	30.3	32.7
30-39	28.8	31.8
40-49	24.9	29.9
50-59	24.6	29.5
60 +	22.1	27.6

Note. Based on data from Canada Fitness Survey, 1983 (see note to Table 9.3). Scale is positioned so that a reading of 25 cm coincides with the ability to touch the floor with the tips of the fingers.

Placement on the Integration Continuum

In the United States, Federal Public Law 94-142 regulates plans for special education. This law requires each state to develop a regional implementation plan in order to assure federal funding of adapted physical education. Each handicapped child must have the opportunity to participate in the normal physical education program, unless the child is enrolled full-time in a separate facility or needs specially designed physical education as a part of an individualized educational program (IEP).

In order to receive the specially designed physical education program, the student must be declared handicapped according to a clearly defined process (Sherrill, 1986c). The child may be identified by the teacher or the parent; with the parent's consent, eligibility data are collected (usually by the physical education teacher). A pre-IEP meeting determines the need for further testing, and a written report is prepared at this stage. A multidisciplinary team, including an adapted physical education specialist, then undertakes a comprehensive individual assessment (with parental notification of rights and consent). The formal IEP meeting includes the child's teacher, one or both parents, the child (when appropriate), a representative of the public agency qualified to provide or supervise special education, and other individuals at the discretion of the parent or agency. As a result of the IEP meeting, the program is then implemented, with provisions for annual program review and transfer to full-time regular education if the child's condition permits.

The least restrictive environment is determined from a physical, mental, and social viewpoint. For many activities, this will be the normal classroom, but for some it may be a special education setting. The detailed report for each child specifies special equipment and facility needs, any required changes of teaching methods or means of communication, and required changes in class or grading requirements.

Performance scores on tests of the type described in chapter 4 and Appendix B have been proposed in a number of states to provide objective evidence of the need for special education. The cut-off level has been set in various jurisdictions at the 15th to the 30th percentile of age-specific scores, or a developmental delay of 1 to 2 years. However, educators are increasingly recognizing that simple field tests can provide no more than a very general indication of where a person should be placed on the continuum linking fully integrated with fully segregated sport and physical education.

First, the error inherent in any test of physical performance must be acknowledged. For instance, a direct measurement of maximum oxygen intake has an error of 4 to 5%, even if it is performed by an able-bodied person under ideal conditions in a well-equipped laboratory. The coefficient of variation for a routine assessment may deteriorate to 8 to 10%, particularly when testing a disabled person. Submaximal predictions of aerobic power have a coefficient of variation of 10 to 12% relative to directly measured values (although a part of this discrepancy is due to the error of the direct measurement). In the disabled, abnormalities of maximum heart rate (due to loss of sympathetic innervation, reliance on arm work, and impaired mechanical efficiency) may further boost the error to 20% or more. Given that the difference between a fit and an unfit person is often only 20%, the limited information content of the fitness test must be acknowledged.

Problems inherent in test design are compounded by intraindividual variation. Even in the able-bodied, a temporary relaxation of training due to a severe cold or a bout of influenza may reduce aerobic power by 20%, with a corresponding deterioration in many performance measures. Such variations in condition from one test to another are an even greater problem in the disabled person, particularly when performance is limited by a variable amount of muscle spasm.

A further source of difficulty is lack of construct validity for the school, work, or sports field. Thus poor motivation, a lack of understanding of required procedures, or a poor choice of technique may limit laboratory measurement of aerobic power. However, these limitations may have little relevance when the subject attempts a simple and familiar task that she or he wishes to complete.

Last, loss of function is not uniform from one test to another. If an individual has a very low aerobic power and yet a good muscular endurance, that person may be able to accomplish a desired task by working very slowly and patiently. The ability to compensate in this manner depends greatly upon personality, intelligence, and motivation. With much persistence, an investigator might be able to set minimum levels of aerobic power compatible with various levels of program integration. When a given deficit of aerobic power is combined with other handicaps such as mental retardation, restriction of vision, poor balance, and muscular spasm, the investigator may be able to use laboratory or field tests to make an arbitrary and very crude classification of ability to undertake a specific sport, but making useful categorization with respect to the multifaceted demands of school or employment becomes virtually impossible.

Glossary

actualization—Realization of personal potential; a concept developed by Abraham Maslow

aerobic—Dependent upon oxygen; aerobic fitness implies an enhanced ability to delivery oxygen to the working tissues

afterload—The impedance to ventricular ejection

angina—An intense pain, felt in the midline of the chest and spreading down the inner side of the left arm, associated with transient myocardial ischemia; rapidly relieved by removal of the precipitating cause (e.g., halting exercise)

anisomelia—Developmental disorder with an asymmetry of the limbs of more than 7 cm (10 cm in swimmers)

ankylosing spondylitis—Chronic, progressive disease of rheumatoid origin involving the joints between the articular processes of the vertebrae, costo-vertebral joints, and sacroiliac joints and leading to ankylosis with a loss of back flexibility

ankylosis—Stiffness or fixation of a joint

arthrodesis—Operative fusion of a joint

arthrogryposis—Permanent flexion or ankylosis of a joint

arthrosis—Disturbance of joint function due to degeneration of articular surface

atherosclerosis—Infiltration of the arterial wall by lipids, with secondary degenerative changes, resulting in a localized narrowing of the vessel with a relative ischemia of distal tissues; in the coronary vessels, artherosclerosis may cause angina or myocardial infarction, whereas in the brain it may cause a "stroke" or a progressive deterioration of cerebral function

athetosis—Alternating bouts of excessive and inadequate muscle tone

atrophy—Reduction in size of an organ due to disuse or degeneration

autism—Self-centered mental state associated with normal intelligence but also marked by disturbances of speech and repetitious, purposeless movements.

beta blocker—Drug-blocking beta-adrenergic activity

body image—Perception of self

bradycardia—Slow heart rate

Buerger's disease—Vascular degeneration that usually affects the arterial supply to the leg muscles; the affected individual becomes increasingly liable to ischemic pain in the calf when attempting to walk

calculi—"Stones"; the risk of formation of urinary calculi is enhanced by lack of mobility and demineralization of bone

callus—An area of thickened and hardened skin

carpal tunnel syndrome—Syndrome characterized by a compression of the median nerve as it passes through the carpal tunnel

catecholamines—Norepinephrine and epinephrine

catharsis—Relief of a feeling such as anger or tension

chondromalacia patella—Painful condition in which cartilage is lost from the back side of the patella

clonus—Series of movements characterized by alternating contractions and relaxations

contractility—Ability to develop a force by contraction, typically used to describe the status of the ventricle

contracture—Permanent shortening of a muscle due to spasm, paralysis, or fibrotic change in the surrounding tissues

decibel—Logarithmic unit of pressure used for expressing the difference in energy level between various sound signals

diplegia—Paralysis of similar parts on the two sides of the body

Down's syndrome—A form of mental retardation associated with a mongoloid appearance and an abnormal chromosome count

Duchenne's dystrophy—A form of locomotor ataxia with an associated muscular weakness and pseudohypertrophy of the muscles

dwarfism—Physical growth departing from the norm by an arbitrary amount (e.g., three standard deviations below the normal age standard)

dyskinesia—Impairment of the power of voluntary motion

dysmelia—Developmental disorder characterized by the absence of the arms or legs

efficiency—Ratio of work performed to energy cost; net efficiency subtracts the cost of resting or basal metabolism, whereas delta efficiency involves the slope of the relationship of work performed to energy cost

ego strength—Self-confidence

Ehlers Danlos syndrome—Hyperextensibility of the joints, with an unusual tendency toward articular dislocation

electromyography—The recording and study of electrical impulses that arise during contraction of muscles

ergometer—Mechanical device allowing a subject to perform external work at a measured rate

ergonomics—Study of work, generally concerned with improvement of the match between humans and items of equipment in the home or in industry

esotropia—Inwardly crossed eyes

etiology—Study of the cause of disease

Frank/Starling mechanism—Increase of ventricular stroke volume induced by an increased end-diastolic filling of the ventricle

Friedrich's ataxia—A rare inherited condition involving incoordination of voluntary movements

gangrene—Death of a part such as a foot due to failure of the local blood supply

genu recurvatum—Backward curvature of the knee joint

glaucoma—Condition of the eye marked by an increased intraocular pressure that eventually causes blindness

glycolytic—Prone to breakdown of glycogen by anaerobic pathways

glycosaminoglycans—Polysaccharides that attach to specific proteins to form the ground substance of connective tissues, including bone

Guillain Barré syndrome—Disorder of the peripheral nerves—characterized by an ascending muscular weakness, impairment of reflexes, and sensory disorders—often following a febrile illness; essentially an infectious polyneuritis

habituation—Form of negative conditioning in which the anxiety of the subject is diminished by repetition of the required test procedure

hemianopsia—Blindness in a half of the visual field

hemiplegia—Paralysis on one side of the body

hemophilia—Inherited disease with a great prolongation of the time required for coagulation of the blood

hyperkinesia—Tendency to excessive habitual movement

hyperplasia—Formation of additional muscle fibers (e.g., in response to training)

hypertension—Pathological increase of resting blood pressure, commonly a systolic reading of more than 160 mm Hg or a diastolic reading of more than 90 to 95 mm Hg

hypertrophy—Increase in size (e.g., of individual muscle fibers)

impedance—Combination of forces opposing an action (e.g., muscular-vascular impedance—the forces opposing flow of blood into the working muscles)

incidence—Proportion of individuals from a population who present for treatment of a given clinical condition over a specified period, usually 1 year

intelligence quotient (IQ)—Performance of the individual on a standard test of intelligence, relative to a normal population of the same age

ischemic heart disease—Disease associated with a reduced oxygen supply to the heart muscle, including such clinical manifestations as angina, myocardial infarction, and sudden death

joule—SI unit of energy, equal to 4.186 calories

kinesthesis—Appreciation of the position of body parts

Kurhaus—German form of health spa, generally located in mountainous area with access to mineral springs

law of Laplace—Physical law used to relate the tension in the ventricular wall to the intraventricular pressure and the average radius of the ventricular cavity

les autres—Heterogenous category of disabled sports competitors other than paraplegics, amputees, blind, deaf, and cerebral palsied

locus of control—Psychological concept that distinguishes those who are directed by external events from those with an inner sense of direction (internal locus of control)

mainstreaming—Return of disabled children to normal classroom programs

multiple sclerosis—Patchy focal degeneration of the central nervous system that leads to progressive muscular weakness

muscular dystrophy—Progressive wasting disease of muscles, apparently due to peripheral rather than central nervous degeneration

orthosis—Straightening of a deformity; also a device used for correction of a deformity, support of the body, or control of involuntary movements

osteogenesis imperfecta—Condition in which the bones are unusually brittle and vulnerable to trauma

osteomyelitis—Infection of the bone marrow

osteoporosis—Progressive decrease in the mineral content of the bone, seen as a consequence of lack of weight-bearing activity, which predisposes the affected body part to fractures

paraplegia—Paralysis of the lower limbs (a diagnosis based on the anatomical level rather than the cause of the lesion)

paresis—Partial paralysis

Parkinsonian degeneration—Degeneration of that portion of the midbrain that normally inhibits the gamma reflex loop at the spinal level; results in general increase of muscular tone, spasticity, and a tremor most apparent during voluntary movement

phobia—Irrational fear

phocomelia—Absence of the middle segment of a limb due to a disorder of development

poliomyelitis—More properly, anterior poliomyelitis; a viral infection that localizes in the anterior horn cells of the spinal cord and causes paralysis of the affected motor units

polyarthritis—Inflammation of many joints

polyneuritis—Inflammation of more than one nerve (usually many, as in the Guillain Barré syndrome)

preloading—Diastolic filling pressure applying a load to ventricular muscle as contraction begins

prevalence—Proportion of individuals affected by a given condition in a specific population, as ascertained by a careful survey

proprioception—Appreciation of body or limb position

prosthesis—Artificial body part, in the present context an artificial limb

pulk—Special type of toboggan used by paraplegic athletes who wish to participate in winter sports

quadriplegia—Paralysis of all four limbs

rate-pressure product—The multiple of heart rate and systolic blood pressure, used as a simple approximation of the relative work rate of the left ventricle

scoliosis—Permanent lateral curvature of the spine

self-efficacy—Belief that one is in control of one's life and can meet requirements (such as participation in a training program)

serotonin—5-hydroxytryptamine; a chemical important to the transmission of nerve impulses in the brain

somatization—Translation of physical problems into psychotic symptoms

spina bifida—A congenital defect with incomplete closure of the spinal canal; cerebral spinal fluid and sometimes nerve tissue protrude through the defect in a hernial sac

state—Psychological characteristic of a person at a given time

syringomyelia—Chronic disease that leads to the formation of cavities in the spinal cord and loss of the senses of pain and heat; occasionally involves spread of lesions to the lateral and anterior horns of the gray matter, with muscle weakness in the affected motor units

tachycardia—Rapid heart rate

tetraplegia—Paralysis of all four limbs

torque—Turning moment; the product of force and lever length

trait—A relatively permanent characteristic of a person's psychological makeup

ventilatory equivalent—Ratio of ventilation to oxygen consumption

vertigo—Sensation induced by swift accelerations

References

AAHPER. (1975). Testing for impaired, disabled, and handicapped individuals. Washington, DC: Author.

AAHPER. (1976). *AAHPER youth fitness test manual* (rev. ed.). Washington, DC: Author.

Abbasi, A. (1981). *Echocardiographic interpretation*. Springfield, IL: Charles C Thomas.

Abernathy, E.M. (1936). Relationships between mental and physical growth. *Monographs of the Society for Research in Child Development*, 1(7).

Adams, R.C., Daniel, A.N., McCubbin, J., & Rullman, L. (1982). *Games, sports and exercises for the physically disabled* (3rd ed.). Philadelphia: Lea & Febiger.

Adams, T.D., Yanowitz, F.G., Fischer, A.C., Ridges, J.D., Lovell, K., & Pryor, T.A. (1981). Non-invasive evaluation of exercise training in college aged men. *Circulation*, **64**, 958-965.

Adedoja, T.A. (1987). Psychological and social problems of physical disability: State of the art and relevance to physical education. In M. Berridge & G. Ward (Eds.), *International perspectives on adapted physical ability* (pp. 25-31). Champaign, IL: Human Kinetics.

Adelson, E., & Fraiberg, S. (1974). Gross motor development in infants blind from birth. *Child Development*, **45**, 114-126.

Ajzen, I., & Fishbein, M. (1980). *Understanding attitudes and predicting social behavior*. Englewood Cliffs, NJ: Prentice-Hall.

Alderton, H.R. (1966). A review of schizophrenia in childhood. *Canadian Psychiatric Journal*, **11**, 276-285.

American College of Sports Medicine. (1978). The recommended quantity and quality of exercise for developing and maintaining fitness in healthy adults. *Medicine and Science in Sports and Exercise*, **10**, vii-x.

Ammons, D.K. (1986). World games for the deaf. In C. Sherrill (Ed.), *Sport and disabled athletes* (pp. 65-72). Champaign, IL: Human Kinetics.

Anderson, S.C. (1980). Effectiveness of an introduction to therapeutic recreation courses on students' attitudes toward the disabled. *Leisurability*, **7**, 13-16.

Anderson, S.C., Grossman, L., & Finch, H. (1983). Effects of a recreation program on the social interaction of mentally retarded adults. *Journal of Leisure Research*, **15**, 100-107.

Andreas, C. (1970). The status of municipal recreation for the mentally retarded. *Therapeutic Recreation Journal, 4*(1), 1-3.

Andrew, G.M., Reid, J.G., Beck, S., & McDonald, W. (1979). Training of the developmentally handicapped young adults. *Canadian Journal of Applied Sport Sciences, 4*, 289-293.

Ankenbrand, R.J. (1972). An investigation of the relationship between achievement and self-concept of high risk community college freshmen. *Dissertation Abstracts International, 13*(8A), 4338.

Anthony, W.A. (1979). *The principles of psychiatric rehabilitation.* Boston: Human Resources Development Press.

Appenzeller, H. (1983). *The right to participate: The law and individuals with handicapping conditions in physical education and sports.* Charlottesville, VA: The Mitchie Co.

Aptekar, R.G., Ford, F., & Bleck, E.E. (1976). Light patterns as a means of assessing and recording gait: 2. Results in children with cerebral palsy. *Developmental Medicine and Child Neurology, 18*, 37-40.

Arheim, D., & Sinclair, W. (1985). *Physical education for special populations.* Englewood Cliffs, NJ: Prentice-Hall.

Arieff, A.J., Pysik, S.W., Tigay, E.L., & Bernsohn, J. (1960). Some metabolic studies in quadraplegia following spinal cord injury [Abstract]. *Illinois Medical Journal, 117*, 219.

Armstrong, J.D. (1975). Evaluation of man-machine systems in the mobility of the visually handicapped. In R.M. Pickett & T.J. Triggs (Eds.), *Human factors in health care.* DC Heath, Lexington, MA: Lexington Books.

Arnhold, R.W., & McGrain, P. (1985). Selected kinematic patterns of visually impaired youth in sprint running. *Adapted Physical Activity Quarterly, 2*, 206-213.

Arnold, J.D., Shephard, R.J., & Kakis, G. (1985). Lipid profile, physical fitness, and job activity of Canadian postal workers. *Journal of Cardiopulmonary Rehabilitation, 5*, 373-337.

Arvidsson, S., Dencker, S.J., & Grimby, G. (1970). Fysisk traning pa mentalsjukhus [Physical education in mental hospitals]. *Lakartidningen, 67*, 58-64.

Asmussen, E. (1968). Correlation between various physiological test results in handicapped persons. *Communications of Testing and Observation Institute, 27*.

Asmussen, E., & Heebøll-Nielsen, K. (1956). The physical performance and growth in children, influence of sex, age and intelligence. *Journal of Applied Physiology, 8*, 371-380.

Asmussen, E., & Molbech, S.V. (1954). Methods and standards for evaluation of the physical working capacity of patients. *Communications of Testing and Observation Institute, 4*, 1-16.

Asmussen, E., & Poulsen, E. (1966). A battery of physiological tests applied to two different groups of handicapped persons. *Communications of Testing and Observation Institute, 13*, 1-13.

Asmussen, E., Poulsen, E., & Bøgh, H.E. (1964). Measurements of muscle strength necessary for driving a motor car. *Communications of Testing and Observation Institute, 19*, 1-12.

Åstrand, I. (1960). Aerobic work capacity in men and women with special reference to age. *Acta Physiologica Scandinavica,* **49**(Suppl. 169), 1-91.

Åstrand, I., Guharay, A., & Wahren, J. (1968). Circulatory responses to arm exercise with different arm positions. *Journal of Applied Physiology,* **25**, 528-532.

Åstrand, P.O., Ekblöm, B., Messin, R., Saltin, B., & Stenberg, J. (1965). Intra-arterial blood pressure during exercise with different muscle groups. *Journal of Applied Physiology,* **20**, 253-256.

Åstrand, P.O., Rodahl, K. (1977). *Textbook of work physiology* (2nd ed.). New York: McGraw-Hill.

Åstrand, P.O., & Saltin, B. (1961). Maximal oxygen uptake and heart rate in various types of muscular activity. *Journal of Applied Physiology,* **16**, 977-981.

Aufsesser, P.M. (1982). Comparison of the attitudes of physical education, recreation and special education majors toward the disabled. *American Corrective Therapy Journal,* **36**, 35-41.

Australian Council for Rehabilation of the Disabled. (1974). *Recreation for the handicapped.* Melbourne: Author.

Auxter, D. (1981). Equal educational opportunity for the handicapped through physical education. *Physical Educator,* **38**, 8-14.

Auxter, D. (1983). Generalization of motor skills from training to natural environments. In R.L. Eason, T.L. Smith, & F. Caron (Eds.), *Adapted physical education: From theory to application* (pp. 180-188). Champaign, IL: Human Kinetics.

Auxter, D., & Pyfer, J. (1985). *Principles of adapted physical education and recreation.* St. Louis: Times Mirror/Mosby.

Axelson, P. (1986). Facilitation of integrated recreation. In C.A. Sherrill (Ed.), *Sport and disabled athletes* (pp. 81-89). Champaign, IL: Human Kinetics.

Axelson, P., & McCormack, J. (1983). Mixing it up. *Sport 'N Spokes,* **9**(4), 16-17.

Badal, J. (1966). Preventive measures against cardiovascular disease in Czechoslovakia. In W. Raab (Ed.), *Prevention of ischemic heart disease: Principles and practice.* Springfield, IL: Charles C Thomas.

Bailey, D.A. (1974). Exercise, fitness and physical education for the growing child. In W.A.R. Orban (Ed.), *Proceedings of the national conference on fitness and health* (pp. 13-22). Ottawa, ON: Health & Welfare Canada.

Bailey, D.A., Shephard, R.J., & Mirwald, R.L. (1976). Validation of a self-administered home test of cardiorespiratory fitness. *Canadian Journal of Applied Sport Sciences,* **1**, 67-78.

Baka, R.S. (1986). Australian government involvement in sport: A delayed, eclectic approach. In G. Redmond (Ed.), *Sport and politics* (pp. 27-32). Champaign, IL: Human Kinetics.

Bandura, A. (1977). Self-efficacy: Towards a unifying theory of behavioral change. *Psychological Review,* **84**, 191-215.

Bard, G. (1963). Energy expenditure of hemiplegic subjects during walking. *Archives of Physical Medicine and Rehabilitation,* **44**, 368-370.

Bard, G., & Ralston, H.J. (1959). Measurement of energy expenditure during ambulation, with special reference to evaluation of assistive devices. *Archives of Physical Medicine and Rehabilitation,* **40**, 415-420.

Barker, R.G., Wright, B.A., & Gonick, H.R. (1983). Adjustment to physical handicap and illness: A survey of the social psychology of physique and disability. *Social Science Research Council Bulletin,* **55**(5), 5.

Bar-Or, O. (1981). Le test anaérobie de Wingate. Charactéristiques et applications [The Wingate anaerobic test. Characteristics and applications]. *Symbioses,* **13**, 157-171.

Bar-Or, O. (1983). *Pediatric sports medicine for the practitioner.* New York: Springer Verlag.

Bar-Or, O., & Inbar, O. (1978). Relationships among anaerobic capacity, sprint and middle-distance running of schoolchildren. In R.J. Shephard & H. Lavallée (Eds.), *Physical fitness assessment* (pp. 142-147). Springfield, IL: Charles C Thomas.

Bar-Or, O., Inbar, O., & Spira, R. (1976). Physiological effects of a sports rehabilitation program on cerebral palsied and post-poliomyelitic adolescents. *Medicine and Science in Sports and Exercise,* **8**, 157-161.

Bar-Or, O., Skinner, J.S., Bergsteinova, V., Shearburn, C., Royer, D., Bell, W., Haas, J., & Buskirk, E.R. (1971). Maximal aerobic capacity of 6-15 year old girls and boys with subnormal intelligence quotients. *Acta Paediatrica Scandinavica* (Suppl. 217), 108-113.

Bar-Or, O., & Zwiren, L.D. (1975). Maximal oxygen consumption test during arm exercise—reliability and validity. *Journal of Applied Physiology,* **38**, 424-426.

Beal, O.P., Glaser, R.M., Petrofsky, J.S., Smith, P.A., & Fox, E.L. (1981). Static components of handgrip muscles for various wheelchair propulsion methods. *Federation Proceedings,* **40**, 497.

Beasley, C.R. (1982). Effects of a jogging program on cardiovascular fitness and work performance of mentally retarded adults. *American Journal of Mental Deficiency,* **86**, 609-613.

Becker, M.H., & Maiman, L. (1975). Socio-behavioral determinants of compliance with health and medical care recommendations. *Medical Care,* **13**, 10-24.

Beckmann, P. (1966). Combined environmental-emotional and physical cardiac prevention programs in the West German reconditioning centres. In W. Raab (Ed.), *Prevention of ischemic heart disease: Principles and practice* (pp. 393-400). Springfield, IL: Charles C Thomas.

Bedbrook, G.M. (1974). Outdoor recreation and camping. In J. Yeo (Ed.), *Recreation for the handicapped* (pp. 65-68). Melbourne: Australian Council for Rehabilitation of Disabled.

Behnke, A.R. (1961). Quantitative assessment of body build. *Journal of Applied Physiology,* **16**, 960-986.

Ben Ari, E., Inbar, O., & Bar-Or, O. (1978). The aerobic capacity and maximal anaerobic power of 30- to 40-year old men and women. In F. Landry & W.A.R. Orban (Eds.), *Biomechanics of sport and kinanthropometry* (pp. 427-433). Miami, FL: Symposia Specialists.

Bennedik, J. (1985). Winter sports NHSRA style. *Palaestra,* **1**(3), 25-29.

Bennett, B.L. (1978). A history of comparative physical education and sport, or how a new discipline is born and grows. In U. Simri (Ed.), *Comparative physical education and sport* (pp. 14-32). Natanya, Israel: Wingate Institute.

Bennett, B.L., Howell, M.L., & Simri, U. (1983). *Comparative physical education and sport* (2nd ed., pp. 1-283). Philadelphia: Lea & Febiger.

Benson, T.B., & Williams, E. (1979). The younger disabled unit at Fazakerley Hospital. *British Medical Journal, 2,* 369-371.

Berg, K. (1970). Effect of physical training of school children with cerebral palsy. *Acta Paediatrica Scandinavica,* (Suppl. 204), 27-33.

Berg, K., & Bjure, J. (1970). Methods for evaluation of the physical working capacity of school children with cerebral palsy. *Acta Paediatrica Scandinavica,* (Suppl. 204), 15-26.

Berg, K., & Isaksson, B. (1970). Maximal oxygen uptake of cerebral palsied children in relation to body cell mass. In M. Maček (Ed.), *Proceedings of Second Pediatric Work Physiology Symposium* (pp. 89-90). Prague: Charles University.

Berg, K., & Olsson, T. (1970). Energy requirements of school children with cerebral palsy as determined from indirect calorimetry. *Acta Paediatrica Scandinavica,* (Suppl. 204), 71-80.

Bergh, U., Kanstrup, I.L., & Ekblöm, B. (1976). Maximal oxygen uptake during exercise with various combinations of arm and leg work. *Journal of Applied Physiology, 41,* 191-196.

Bergofsky, E.H., Turino, G.M., & Fishman, A.P. (1959). Cardiorespiratory failure in kyphoscoliosis. *Medicine, 38,* 263-317.

Berry, M.R., Baldes, E.J., Essex, H.F., & Wakim, K.G. (1948). A compensating plethysmokymograph for measuring blood flow in human extremities. *Journal of Laboratory and Clinical Medicine, 33,* 191-195.

Best, G. (1971). Treatment of children afflicted with C.P. through remedial physical exercises. In U. Simri (Ed.), *Sports as a means of rehabilitation* (pp. 12/1-12/7). Natanya, Israel: Wingate Institute.

Beuter, A.C. (1983). Effects of mainstreaming on motor performance of intellectually normal and trainable mentally retarded students. *American Corrective Therapy Journal, 37,* 48-52.

Beuter, A., & Garfinkel, A. (1985). Phase plane analysis of limb trajectories in non-handicapped and cerebral palsied subjects. *Adapted Physical Activity Quarterly, 2,* 214-227.

Bevegard, S., Freyschuss, U., & Strandell, T. (1966). Circulatory adaptation to arm and leg exercise in supine and sitting position. *Journal of Applied Physiology, 21,* 37-46.

Bhatt, D.R., Isabel-Jones, J.B., Villoria, G.J., Lendriem, B.L., & Harris, J.B. (1978). Accuracy of echocardiography in assessing left ventricular dimensions and volumes. *Circulation, 57,* 699-707.

Bicknell, J. (1972). Riding for the handicapped. *Outdoors, 3*(3), 33. (Available from the Physical Education Association of Great Britain and Northern Ireland).

Bieber, N. (1986). Characteristics of physically disabled riders in equestrian competition at the national level. In C. Sherrill (Ed.), *Sport and disabled athletes* (pp. 245-250). Champaign, IL: Human Kinetics.

Biering-Sorensen, F. (1980). Classification of paralyzed and amputee sportsmen. In H. Natvig (Ed.), *First International Medical Congress on Sports and the Disabled* (pp. 44-54). Oslo: Royal Ministry of Church and Education.

Biering-Sorensen, F. (1983). Problems of the ISOD classification system. In J.H. Hoeberigs & H. Vorsteveld (Eds.), *Proceedings of the Workshop on Disabled and Sports* (pp. 106-110). Amersfoort, Netherlands: Nederlandse Invaliden Sportbond.

Bird, P.J., & Gansneder, B.M. (1979). Preparation of physical education teachers as required under Public Law 94-142. *Exceptional Children,* **45**, 464-466.

Birrer, R.B. (1984). The Special Olympics: An injury overview. *The Physician and Sportsmedicine,* **12**, 95-97.

Bitcon, C. (1976). *The clinical and educational use of Orff-Schülwerk.* Santa Ana, CA: Rosha Press.

Björke, G., Hagen, R., Lie, H., & Klieve, I. (1978). Fysisk aktivisering av mentalt retarderte barn [Physical activation of mentally retarded children]. *Tidsskrift for den Norske Laegeforening,* **98**(3), 134-136.

Bjüre, J., Grimby, G., & Nachemson, A. (1969). The effect of physical training in girls with idiopathic scoliosis. *Acta Orthopaedica Scandinavica,* **40**, 325-333.

Black, B.C. (1983). The effect of an outdoor experiential adventure program on the development of dynamic balance and spatial veering for the visually impaired adolescent. *Therapeutic Recreation Journal,* **17**, 39-49.

Bleck, E., & Nagel, D. (Eds.) (1982). *Physically handicapped children: A medical atlas for teachers* (2nd ed.). New York: Grune & Stratton.

Blocker, W.P., Merrill, J.M., Krebs, M.A., Cardus, D.P., & Ostermann, H.J. (1983). An electrocardiographic survey of patients with chronic spinal cord injury. *American Corrective Therapy Journal,* **37**, 101-104.

Blohmke, M. (1966). Objective results of physical training therapy at rural reconditioning centers. In W. Raab (Ed.), *Prevention of ischemic heart disease. Principles and practice* (pp. 409-413). Springfield, IL: Charles C Thomas.

Bloomquist, L.E. (1986). Injuries to athletes with physical disabilities: Prevention implications. *The Physician and Sportsmedicine,* **14**, 97-105.

Bobath, B. (1971). Motor development: Its effect on general development and application to the treatment of cerebral palsy. *Physiotherapy,* **57**, 526-532.

Bobbert, A.C. (1960). Physiological comparison of three types of ergometry. *Journal of Applied Physiology,* **15**, 1007-1014.

Borg, G. (1971). The perception of physical performance. In R.J. Shephard (Ed.), *Frontiers of fitness* (pp. 280-294). Springfield, IL: Charles C Thomas.

Botvin Madorsky, J.G., & Curtis, K. (1984). Wheelchair sports medicine. *American Journal of Sports Medicine,* **12**, 128-132.

Bouchard, C., Godbout, P., Monder, J.-C., & LeBlanc, C. (1979). Specificity of maximal aerobic power. *European Journal of Applied Physiology,* **40**, 85-93.

Bouchard, C., Lesage, R., Lortie, G., Simoneau, J-S., Hamel, P., Boulay, M.R., Perusse, L., Theriault, G., & LeBlanc, C. (1986). Aerobic performance in brothers, dizygotic and monozygotic twins. *Medicine and Science in Sports and Exercise,* **18**, 639-646.

Bowker, J.H., & Halpin, P.J. (1978). Factors determining success in reambulation of the child with progressive muscular dystrophy. *Orthopedic Clinics of North America, 9*, 431-436.

Boyd, J. (1967). Comparison of motor behavior in deaf and hearing boys. *American Annals of the Deaf, 112*, 598-605.

Brabant, J. (1982). High level sailing. *Sports 'N Spokes, 8*(3), 11-12.

Brandmeyer, G.A., & McBee, G.F. (1986). Social status and athletic competition for the disabled athlete: The case of wheelchair roadracing. In C. Sherrill (Ed.), *Sport and disabled athletes* (pp. 181-188). Champaign, IL: Human Kinetics.

Brattgard, S., Grimby, G., & Hook, O. (1970). Energy expenditure and heart rate in driving a wheelchair ergometer. *Scandinavian Journal of Rehabilitation Medicine, 2*, 143-148.

Brattnas, B. (1974). International comparisons. In W.A.R. Orban (Ed.), *Proceedings of the National Conference on Fitness and Health* (pp. 101-103). Ottawa, ON: Health & Welfare Canada.

Brauer, R.L. (1972). *An ergonomic analysis of wheelchair wheeling*. Unpublished doctoral dissertation, University of Illinois, Champaign.

Braun, J.R., & LaForo, D. (1968). Fakability of the 16 PF questionnaire, Form C. *Journal of Psychology, 68*, 3-7.

Breithaupt, D.J., Jousse, A.T., & Wynne-Jones, M. (1961). Late causes of death and life expectancy in paraplegia. *Canadian Medical Association Journal, 85*, 73-77.

Briggs-Myers, I. (1986). *Introduction to type*. Palo Alto, CA: Consulting Psychologists Press.

Bright, R. (1974). Music—Its role in recreation. In J. Yeo (Ed.), *Recreation for the handicapped* (pp. 52-55). Melbourne: Australian Council for Rehabilitation of Disabled.

Brinkmann, J.R., & Hoskins, T.A. (1979). Physical conditioning and altered self-concept in rehabilitated hemiplegic patients. *Physical Therapy, 59*, 859-865.

Bromley, I. (1981). *Tetraplegia and paraplegia: A guide for physiotherapists*. Edinburgh: Churchill Livingstone.

Brooks, G.A., & Fahey, T.D. (1984). *Exercise physiology: Human bioenergetics and its applications*. Toronto: John Wiley.

Brouha, L., & Korbath, H. (1967). Continuous recording of cardiac and respiratory functions in normal and handicapped persons. *Human Factors, 9*, 567-571.

Brown, A. (1982). More than fun—The role of competitive sport for cerebral palsied children. In U. Simri (Ed.), *Social aspects of physical education and sport* (p. 124). Natanya, Israel: Wingate Institute.

Brown, J. (1967). Comparative performance of trainable mentally retarded on the Kraus-Weber test. *Research Quarterly, 38*, 348-351.

Brownell, K.D., & Smoller, J.W. (1985). Exercise in the clinical management of obesity. In P. Welsh & R.J. Shephard (Eds.), *Current therapy in sports medicine* (pp. 60-64). Burlington, ONT: B.C. Decker.

Brubaker, C. (1984). Determination of the effects of mechanical advantage on propulsion with hand rims. In N.G. Stamp & C. McLaurin (Eds.), *Wheelchair mobility 1982-3* (pp. 1-3). Richmond, VA: Rehabilitation Engineering Center, University of Virginia.

Brubaker, C., & McClay, I. (1983). Determination of the relationship of mechanical advantage with propulsion efficiency. In N.G. Stamp & C. McLaurin (Eds.), *Wheelchair mobility 1983-4* (pp. 1-7). Richmond, VA: Rehabilitation Engineering Center, University of Virginia.

Brubaker, C., & McLaurin, C. (1982). Ergonomics of wheelchair propulsion. In T.L. Golbranson & R.W. Wirta (Eds.), *Wheelchair III* (pp. 22-42). Bethesda, MD: Resna.

Bruderman, I., Najenson, T., Gelbard, C., Serepka, M., & Solsi, P. (1971). The cardio-pulmonary response following physical training in amputees with peripheral vascular disease. In U. Simri (Ed.), *Sports as a means of rehabilitation* (pp. 6/1-6/11). Natanya, Israel: Wingate Institute.

Bruin, M.I. de, & Binkhorst, R.A. (1984). Cardiac output of paraplegics during exercise. *International Journal of Sports Medicine, 5*, 175-176.

Bruininks, V.L. (1978). Peer status and personality characteristics of learning disabled and non-disabled students. *Journal of Learning Disabilities, 11*(18), 484-489.

Brunt, D., & Broadhead, G.D. (1982). Motor proficiency traits of deaf children. *Research Quarterly, 53*, 236-238.

Brunt, D., Layne, C.S., Cook, M., & Rowe, L. (1984). Automatic postural responses of deaf children from dynamic and static positions. *Adapted Physical Activity Quarterly, 1*, 247-252.

Bryan, E. (1976). Come on dummy: An observational study of children's communications. *Journal of Learning Disabilities, 9*(10), 66-69.

Buehl, A.N. (1979). The effects of creative dance movement on large muscle control and balance in congenitally blind children. *Journal of Visual Impairment and Blindness, 73*, 127-133.

Buell, C. (1979). Association for blind athletes as seen by a blind sportsman. *Journal of Visual Impairment and Blindness, 73*, 412-413.

Buell, C.E. (1982). *Physical education and recreation for the visually handicapped*. Washington, DC: American Alliance for Health, Physical Education, Recreation and Dance.

Buell, C.E. (1983). How to include blind children in vigorous public school physical education. In R.L. Eason, T.L. Smith, & F. Caron (Eds.), *Adapted physical activity; From theory to application* (pp. 89-92). Champaign, IL: Human Kinetics.

Buell, C.E. (1984). *Physical education for blind children* (2nd ed.). Springfield, IL: Charles C Thomas.

Buell, C.E. (1987). Blind athletes who compete in the mainstream. In M. Berridge & G. Ward (Eds.), *International perspectives in adapted physical activity* (pp. 173-178). Champaign, IL: Human Kinetics.

Bulbulian, R., Johnson, R., Bruber, J., & Darabos, B. (1987). Body composition in paraplegic male athletes. *Medicine and Science in Sports and Exercise, 19*, 195-210.

Bundschuh, E., & Cureton, K. (1982). Effect of bicycle ergometer conditioning on the physical work capacity of mentally retarded adolescents. *American Corrective Therapy Journal*, **36**, 159-163.

Burke, E.J., Auchinachie, J.A., Hayden, R., & Loftin, J.M. (1985). Energy cost of wheelchair basketball. *The Physician and Sportsmedicine*, **13**, 99-105.

Burkett, L.N., Chisum, J., Pierce, J., Pomeroy, K., Fisher, J., & Martin, M. (1988). Blood flow and lactic acid levels in exercising paralyzed wheelchair-bound individuals. *Adapted Physical Activity Quarterly*, **5**, 60-73.

Burkett, L.N., & Ewing, N. (1984). Max $\dot{V}O_2$ uptake on five trainable, mentally-retarded high school students. In W. Kroll (Ed.), *Abstracts of research papers presented at the Anaheim, CA, Convention of the American Alliance of Health, Physical Education, Recreation and Dance* (p. 73). Reston, VA: American Alliance for Health, Physical Education, Recreation and Dance.

Butterfield, S.A. (1986). Gross motor profiles of deaf children. *Perceptual and Motor Skills*, **62**, 68-70.

Butterfield, S.A. (1987). The influence of age, sex, hearing loss, etiology, and balance ability on the fundamental motor skills of deaf children. In M. Berridge & G. Ward (Eds.), *International perspectives in adapted physical activity* (pp. 43-51). Champaign, IL: Human Kinetics.

Butterfield, S.A., & Ersing, W.F. (1986). Influence of age, sex, etiology and hearing loss on balance performance by deaf children. *Perceptual and Motor Skills*, **62**, 659-663.

Cahill, T. (1982). Sculling for the disabled. *The Oarsman*, **13**(6), 22.

Caillet, R. (1980). Exercise in multiple sclerosis. In J.V. Basmajian (Ed.), *Therapeutic exercise* (3rd ed., pp. 375-388). Baltimore: Williams & Wilkins.

Caiozzo, V.J., Perrine, J.J., & Edgerton, V.R. (1981). Training induced alterations of the *in vivo* force velocity relationship of human muscle. *Journal of Applied Physiology, Respiratory, Environmental and Exercise Physiology*, **51**, 750-754.

Cameron, B.J., Ward, G.R., & Wicks, J.R. (1978). Relationship of type of training to maximum oxygen uptake and upper limb strength in male paraplegic athletes. *Medicine and Science in Sports and Exercise*, **9**, 58.

Campbell, J. (1972). Physical fitness and the MR: A review of research. *Mental Retardation*, **2**(5), 26-29.

Campbell, J. (1978). Evaluation of physical fitness programs for retarded boys. *Journal for Special Educators of the Mentally Retarded*, **14**, 78-83.

Campbell, S.C. (1986). Youth sport in the United Kingdom. In M.R. Weiss & D. Gould (Eds.), *Sport for children and youths* (pp. 21-26). Champaign, IL: Human Kinetics.

Canabal, M.Y., Sherrill, C., & Rainbolt, W.J. (1987). Psychological mood profiles of elite cerebral palsied athletes. In M. Berridge & G. Ward (Eds.), *International perspectives in adapted physical activity* (pp. 157-163). Champaign, IL: Human Kinetics.

Canada Fitness Survey. (1983). *Fitness and lifestyle in Canada*. Ottawa, ON: Directorate of Fitness and Amateur Sport.

Canada Fitness Survey. (1986). *Physical activity among activity-limited and disabled adults in Canada*. Ottawa, ON: Canada Fitness and Lifestyle Research Institute.

Carlson, R.B. (1972). Assessment of motor ability of selected deaf children in Kansas. *Perceptual and Motor Skills, 34*, 303-305.

Carroll, J.E., Hagberg, J.M., Brooke, M.H., & Shumate, J.B. (1979). Bicycle ergometry and gas exchange. Measurements in neuromuscular diseases. *Archives of Neurology, 36*, 457-461.

Cartmel, J.L., & Banister, E.W. (1968). The physical working capacity of blind and deaf schoolchildren. *Canadian Journal of Physiology and Pharmacology, 47*, 833-836.

Caspersen, C.J., Powell, K.E., & Christenson, G.M. (1985). Physical activity, exercise and physical fitness: Definitions and distinctions for health-related research. *Public Health Reports, 100*, 126-131.

Cauette, M., & Reid, G. (1985). Increasing the work output of severely retarded adults on a bicycle ergometer. *Education and Training of the Mentally Retarded, 20*, 296-304.

Cerebral Palsy International Sports and Recreation Association. (1983). *Classification and sport rules manual* (2nd ed.). Netherlands: Author.

Cermak, J., Kuta, I., & Pařízková, J. (1975). Some predispositions for top performance in speed canoeing and their changes during the whole year training programme. *Journal of Sports Medicine and Physical Fitness, 15*, 243-251.

Cerquiglini, S., Figura, F., Marchetti, M., & Ricci, B. (1981). Biomechanics of wheelchair propulsion. In A. Moreki, K. Fideles, K. Kedzior, & A.J. Wit (Eds.), *Biomechanics VIIA*. Baltimore: University Park Press.

Cerretelli, P., Pendergast, D., Paganelli, W.C., & Rennie, D.W. (1979). Effects of specific muscle training on $\dot{V}O_2$ response and early blood lactate. *Journal of Applied Physiology, 47*, 761-769.

Chasey, W.C. (1970). The effects of clinical physical education on the motor fitness of educable mentally retarded boys. *American Corrective Therapy Journal, 24*, 74-75.

Chasey, W.C., Swartz, J.D., & Chasey, C.G. (1974). Effect of motor development on body image scores for institutionalized mentally retarded children. *American Journal of Mental Deficiency, 78*, 440-445.

Chasey, W.C., Swartz, J.D., Chasey, C.G., Brogman, R., & Sandler, H. (1975). Attitude change following exposure to handicapped children in clinical physical education. *Therapeutic Recreation Journal, 9*, 68-74.

Chasey, W.C., & Wyrick, W. (1971). Effects of a physical developmental program on psychomotor ability of retarded children. *American Journal of Mental Deficiency, 75*, 566-570.

Chawla, J.C., Bar, C., Creber, I., Price, J., & Andrews, B. (1977). Techniques for improving the strength and fitness of spinal injured patients. *Paraplegia, 17*, 185-189.

Cheshire, D.J.E., & Coats, D.A. (1966). Respiratory and metabolic management in acute tetraplegia. *Paraplegia, 4*, 1-23.

Chrétien, R., Simard, C.P., & Dorion, A. (1987). Effects of relaxation on the peripheral chronaxie of persons having multiple sclerosis. In M. Berridge & G. Ward (Eds.), *International perspectives on adapted physical activity* (pp. 65-72). Champaign, IL: Human Kinetics.

Clark, B.A., Wade, M.G., Massey, B.H., & Van Dyke, R. (1973). Response of institutionalized geriatric mental patients to a twelve week program of regular physical activity. *Journal of Gerontology, 30*, 565-573.

Clark, G., French, R., & Henderson, H. (1985). Teaching techniques that develop positive attitudes. *Palaestra, 1*, 14-17.

Clark, M.W. (1980). Competitive sports for the disabled. *American Journal of Sports Medicine, 8*, 366-369.

Clark-Carter, D.D., Heyes, A.D., & Howarth, C.I. (1986a). The efficiency and walking speed of visually impaired people. *Ergonomics, 29*, 779-789.

Clark-Carter, D.D., Heyes, A.D., & Howarth, C.I. (1986b). The effect of non-visual preview upon the walking speed of visually impaired people. *Ergonomics, 29*, 1575-1581.

Clarke, D.H. (1973). Adaptations in strength and muscular endurance resulting from exercise. *Exercise and Sports Sciences Reviews, 1*, 74-102.

Clarke, H.H. (1966). *Muscular strength and endurance in man*. Englewood Cliffs, NJ: Prentice-Hall.

Claus-Walker, J., & Halstead, L. (1981). Metabolic and endocrine changes in spinal cord injury: 1. The nervous system before and after transection of the spinal cord. *Archives of Physical Medicine and Rehabilitation, 62*, 595-601.

Claus-Walker, J., & Halstead, L. (1982). Metabolic and endocrine changes in spinal cord injury: 4. Compounded neurological dysfunctions. *Archives of Physical Medicine and Rehabilitation, 63*, 632-638.

Claus-Walker, J., Halstead, L.S., & Carter, R.E., & Campos, R.J. (1974). Physiological responses to cold stress in healthy subjects and in subjects with cervical cord injuries. *Archives of Physical Medicine and Rehabilitation, 55*, 485-490.

Clausen, J.P. (1973). Muscle blood flow during exercise and its significance for maximal performance. In J. Keul (Ed.), *Limiting factors of physical performance* (pp. 253-266). Stuttgart: Thieme.

Clausen, J.P. (1977). Effects of physical training on cardiovascular adjustments to exercise in man. *Physiological Reviews, 57*, 779-815.

Clausen, J.P., Klausen, K., Rasmussen, B., & Trap-Jensen, J. (1973). Central and peripheral circulatory changes after training of the arms and legs. *American Journal of Physiology, 225*, 675-682.

Clausen, J.P., & Trap-Jensen, J. (1976). Heart rate and arterial blood pressure during exercise in patients with angina pectoris: Effect of training and of nitroglycerin. *Circulation, 53*, 436-442.

Clausen, J.P., Trap-Jensen, J., & Lassen, N.A. (1970). The effect of training on the heart rate during arm and leg exercise. *Scandinavian Journal of Clinical and Laboratory Investigation, 26*, 295-301.

Clinkingbeard, J.R., Gersten, J.W., & Hoehn, D. (1964). Energy cost of ambulation in traumatic paraplegic. *American Journal of Physical Medicine, 43*, 157-165.

Clumpner, R.A. (1986). Pragmatic coercion: The role of government in sport in the United States. In G. Redmond (Ed.), *Sport and politics* (pp. 5-12). Champaign, IL: Human Kinetics.

Cohen, S. (1977). *Special people*. Englewood Cliffs, NJ: Prentice-Hall.

Colantonio, A., Davis, G.M., Shephard, R.J., Simard, C., & Godin, G. (1986). Prediction of leisure time exercise behaviour among a group of lower-limb disabled adults. In M. Berridge & G. Ward (Eds.), *Proceedings of the International Conference on Adapted Physical Activity* (p. 15). Toronto: School of Physical and Health Education.

Coleman, A., Ayoub, M., & Friedrich, D. (1976). Assessment of the physical work capacity of institutionalized mentally retarded males. *American Journal of Mental Deficiency*, **80**, 629-635.

Coleman, M. (1973). *Serotonin in Down's syndrome*. New York: American Elsevier.

Coleman, R.S., & Whitman, T.L. (1984). Developing, generalizing and maintaining physical fitness in mentally retarded adults: Toward a self-directed program. *Analysis and Intervention in Developmental Disabilities*, **4**, 109-127.

Collier, D., & Reid, G. (1987). A comparison of two models designed to teach autistic children a motor task. *Adapted Physical Activity Quarterly*, **4**, 226-236.

Compton, D.M., Witt, P.A., & Ellis, G.D. (1983). Development and validation of a leisure diagnostic battery for handicapped children and youth. In R.L. Eason, T.L. Smith, & F. Caron (Eds.), *Adapted physical activity: From theory to application* (pp. 124-138). Champaign, IL: Human Kinetics.

Conine, T.A. (1969). Acceptance or rejection of disabled persons by teachers. *The Journal of School Health*, **39**, 278-281.

Connolly, B.H., & Michael, B.T. (1986). Performance of retarded children, with and without Down's Syndrome, on the Bruinincks Oseretsky test of motor proficiency. *Physical Therapy*, **66**, 344-348.

Cook, E.N. (1942). War injuries of urinary tract. *Proceedings of the Staff Meetings of the Mayo Clinic*, **17**, 561-565.

Cook, T.C., LaPorte, R.E., Washburn, D.E., Traven, N.D., Slemenda, C.W., & Metz, K.F. (1986). Chronic low level physical activity as a determinant of high density lipoprotein cholesterol and subfractions. *Medicine and Science in Sports and Exercise*, **18**, 653-657.

Cooke, R.E. (1984). Atlanto-axial instability in children with Down's syndrome. *Adapted Physical Activity Quarterly*, **1**, 194-195.

Cooper, I.S., Rynearson, E.H., MacCarty, C.S., & Power, M.H. (1950). Metabolic consequences of spinal cord injuries [Abstract]. *Endocrinology*, **10**, 858.

Cooper, K.H. (1968a). *Aerobics*. New York: Evans.

Cooper, K.H. (1968b). A means of assessing oxygen intake. *Journal of the American Medical Association*, **203**, 201-204.

Cooper, M., Sherrill, C., & Marshall, D. (1986). Attitudes toward physical activity of elite cerebral palsied athletes. *Adapted Physical Activity Quarterly*, **3**, 14-21.

Cooper, R.H., O'Rourke, R.A., Karliner, J.S., Peterson, K.L., & Leopold, G.R. (1972). Comparison of the ultra-sound and cineangiographic measurements of the mean rate of circumferential fiber shortening in man. *Circulation*, **46**, 914-923.

Corbett, J.L., Debarge, O., Frankel, H.L., & Mathias, C. (1975). Cardiovascular responses in tetraplegic man to muscle spasm, bladder percussion and head-up tilt. *Clinical and Experimental Pharmacology and Physiology*, (Suppl. 2), 189-193.

Corbett, J.L., Frankel, H.L., & Harris, P.J. (1971). Cardiovascular responses to tilting in tetraplegic man. *Journal of Physiology* (London), **215**, 411-413.

Corcoran, P.J. (1971). Energy expenditure during ambulation. In J.A. Downey & R.C. Darling (Eds.), *Physiological basis of rehabilitation medicine* (pp. 185-198). Philadelphia: W.B. Saunders.

Corcoran, P.J., Goldman, R.F., Hoerner, E.F., Kling, C., Knuttgen, H.G., Marquis, B., McCann, B.C., & Rossier, A.B. (1980). Sports medicine and the physiology of wheelchair marathon racing. *Orthopedic Clinics of North America*, **11**, 697-716.

Corcoran, P.J., Jebsen, R.H., Brengelmann, G.L., & Simons, B.C. (1970). Effects of plastic and metal leg braces on speed and energy cost of hemi-paretic ambulation. *Archives of Physical Medicine and Rehabilitation*, **51**, 69-77.

Corder, W.O. (1966). Effects of physical education on the intellectual, physical and social development of educable mentally retarded boys. *Exceptional Children*, **32**, 357-364.

Council of Europe. (1970). Sport for all—Five countries report. Strasbourg: Author.

Coutts, K.D. (1986). Physical and physiological characteristics of elite wheelchair marathoners. In C. Sherrill (Ed.), *Sport and disabled athletes* (pp. 157-161). Champaign, IL: Human Kinetics.

Coutts, K.D., Rhodes, E.C., & McKenzie, D.C. (1983). Maximal exercise responses of tetraplegics and paraplegics. *Journal of Applied Physiology*, **55**, 479-482.

Coutts, K.D., & Stogryn, J.L. (1987). Aerobic and anaerobic power of Canadian wheelchair athletes. *Medicine and Science in Sports and Exercise*, **19**, 62-65.

Cowell, L.L., Squires, W.G., & Raven, P.B. (1986). Benefits of aerobic exercise for the paraplegic: A brief review. *Medicine and Science in Sports and Exercise*, **18**, 501-508.

Cowin, L.W., O'Riain, M.D., Sibille, J., & Layeux, G. (1987). Motor soccer and the wheelchair bumper. In M. Berridge & G. Ward (Eds.), *International perspectives in adapted physical activity* (pp. 203-208). Champaign, IL: Human Kinetics.

Cratty, B.J. (1973). Physical activity and educational programs for the retarded. In O. Grüpe (Ed.), *Sport in the modern world—Chances and problems* (pp. 265-269). Berlin: Springer Verlag.

Cratty, B.J. (1980). *Adapted physical education for the handicapped and youth*. Denver: Love Publishing.

Cratty, B.J., Cratty, I.J., & Cornell, S. (1986). Motor planning abilities in deaf and hearing children. *American Annals of the Deaf*, **131**, 281-284.

Crews, D., Purkett, L., Wells, C.L., & McKeeman, V. (1982). Cardiovascular characteristics of wheelchair marathon racers compared with marathon runners [Abstract]. *International Journal of Sports Medicine*, **3**, 64.

Crews, T.R., & Roberts, J.A. (1976). Effects of interaction of frequency and intensity of training. *Research Quarterly, 47*, 48-55.

Croce, R.V. (1987). Motor skill training: A neurobehavioral approach. In M. Berridge & G. Ward (Eds.), *International perspectives in adapted physical activity* (pp. 35-41). Champaign, IL: Human Kinetics.

Croce, R.V., & Jacobson, W.H. (1986). Application of two-point cane technique for motor control and learning of visually impaired performers. *Journal of Visual Impairment and Blindness, 80*, 780-793.

Cross, D.R. (1980). The influence of physical fitness training as a rehabilitation tool. *International Journal of Rehabilitation Research, 3*, 163-175.

Croucher, N. (1976). Sports and disability. In J.G.P. Williams & P.N. Sperryn (Eds.), *Sports medicine* (pp. 523-538). London: Arnold.

Croucher, R.J. (1978). Outdoor activities. *Physiotherapy, 64*, 294-295.

Crowe, W.C., Auxter, D., & Pyfer, J. (1981). *Principles and methods of adapted physical education and recreation*. St. Louis: C.V. Mosby.

Cruts, H.E.P., Van Alste, J.A., de Vries, J., & Huisman, K. (1985). Cardiac loads during prosthetic training in leg amputees. In J.H. Hoeberigs & H. Vorsteveld (Eds.), *Proceedings of Workshop on Disabled and Sports* (pp. 60-78). Amersfoort: Nederlandse Invaliden Sportbond.

Cumming, G.R. (1971). Correlation of physical performance with laboratory measures of fitness. In R.J. Shephard (Ed.), *Frontiers of fitness* (pp. 265-279). Springfield, IL: Charles C Thomas.

Cumming, G.R., Goulding, D., & Baggley, G. (1971). Working capacity of deaf and visually and mentally handicapped children. *Archives of Disease in Childhood, 46*, 490-494.

Cumming, G.R., & Keynes, R. (1967). A fitness performance test for school children and its correlation with physical working capacity and maximal oxygen uptake. *Canadian Medical Association Journal, 96*, 1262-1269.

Cummins, R.D., & Gladden, L.B. (1983). Responses to submaximal and maximal arm cycling above, at and below heart level. *Medicine and Science in Sports and Exercise, 15*, 295-298.

Curtis, K.A. (1984). Wheelchair sportsmedicine: Part 4. Athletic injuries. *Sports 'N Spokes, 82*(7:January/February), 20-24.

Curtis, K.A., & Dillon, D.A. (1986). Survey of wheelchair athletic injuries— Common patterns and prevention. In C.A. Sherrill (Ed.), *Sport and disabled athletes* (pp. 211-216). Champaign, IL: Human Kinetics.

Dalton, R.B. (1980). *Effects of exercise and vitamin B-12 supplementation on the depression scale scores of a wheelchair-confined population*. Unpublished doctoral dissertation, University of Missouri, St. Louis.

Daniels, L., & Worthington, C. (1972). *Muscle testing*. (3rd ed.). Philadelphia: Saunders.

Danielson, R.R., & Danielson, K.F. (1979). On-going motivation in employee fitness programming. In R. Wanzel (Ed.), *Employee fitness: The how to . . .* (pp. 129-160). Toronto: Ministry of Culture and Recreation.

Davies, C.T.M., Few, J., Foster, K.G., & Sargeant, A.J. (1974). Plasma catecholamine concentration during dynamic exercise involving different muscle groups. *European Journal of Applied Physiology, 32*, 195-206.

Davies, C.T.M., & Knibbs, A.V. (1971). The training stimulus: The effect of intensity, duration and frequency of effort on maximum aerobic power output. *Internationale Zeitschrift für Angewandte Physiologie einschliesslich Arbeitsphysiologie, 29,* 299-305.

Davies, C.T.M., & Sargeant, A.J. (1974). Physiological responses to standardized arm work. *Ergonomics, 17,* 41-49.

Davies, C.T.M., & Sargeant, A.J. (1975). Effects of training on the responses to one- and two-leg work. *Journal of Applied Physiology, 38,* 377-381.

Davies, J.A. (1976). *The reins of life.* London: J.A. Allen.

Davis, G.M. (1985). *Cardiovascular fitness and muscle strength in lower limb disabled males.* Unpublished doctoral dissertation, University of Toronto.

Davis, G.M., Jackson, R.W., & Shephard, R.J. (1984a). Sports and recreation for the physically disabled. In R.H. Strauss (Ed.), *Sports medicine* (pp. 286-304). Philadelphia: W.B. Saunders.

Davis, G.M., Kofsky, P.R., Shephard, R.J., & Jackson, R.W. (1981). Classification of psycho-physiological variables in the lower-limb disabled. *Canadian Journal of Applied Sport Sciences, 6,* abstract.

Davis, G.M., Kofsky, P.R., Shephard, R.J., Keene, G., & Jackson, R.W. (1980). Fitness levels in the lower limb disabled. *Canadian Journal of Applied Sport Sciences, 5.*

Davis, G.M., & Shephard, R.J. (1988). Cardio-respiratory fitness in highly active versus less active paraplegics. *Medicine and Science in Sports and Exercise, 20,* 463-468.

Davis, G.M., Shephard, R.J., & Jackson, R.W. (1981). Cardiorespiratory fitness and muscular strength in the lower-limb disabled. *Canadian Journal of Applied Sport Sciences, 6,* 159-165.

Davis, G.M., Shephard, R.J., & Leenen, F.H.H. (1987). Cardiac effects of short-term arm crank training in paraplegics: Echocardiographic evidence. *European Journal of Applied Physiology, 56,* 90-96.

Davis, G.M., Shephard, R.J., & Ward, G.R. (1984b). Alteration of dynamic strength following forearm crank training of disabled subjects [Abstract]. *Medicine and Science in Sports and Exercise, 16,* 147.

Davis, G.M., Tupling, S.J., & Shephard, R.J. (1986). Dynamic strength and physical activity in wheelchair users. In C. Sherrill (Ed.), *Sport and disabled athletes* (pp. 139-146). Champaign, IL: Human Kinetics.

Davis, J.A., Vodak, P., Wilmore, J.H., Vodak, J., & Kurtz, P. (1976). Anaerobic threshold and maximal aerobic power for three modes of exercise. *Journal of Applied Physiology, 41,* 544-550.

Davis, R. (1985). *Backward wheelchair propulsion in sprint start by Class I cerebral palsied athletes.* Unpublished doctoral dissertation, Texas Women's University, Denton.

Davis, W.E. (1987). Evidence for muscle activation deficiency in mentally handicapping conditions. In M. Berridge & G. Ward (Eds.), *International perspectives in adapted physical activity* (pp. 53-64). Champaign, IL: Human Kinetics.

Dawson, M. (1981). A biomechanical analysis of gait patterns of the visually impaired. *American Corrective Therapy Journal, 35,* 66-71.

Day, H. (1984). Rehabilitation for leisure: Attitudes and opportunities. In L.M. Wells (Ed.), *Proceedings: The Integration of the Physically Disabled Into Community Living: A colloquium* (pp. 234-253). Toronto: University of Toronto School of Social Work.

DeBoer, L.B., Kallal, J.E., & Longo, R.M. (1982). Upper extremity prone position exercise as aerobic capacity indicator. *Archives of Physical Medicine and Rehabilitation, 63*, 467-471.

deBusk, R.F., Valdez, R., Houston, N., & Haskell, W.L. (1978). Cardiovascular responses to dynamic and static effort soon after myocardial infarction. *Circulation, 58*, 368-375.

Decker, R. (1973). Movement education with mentally retarded children: Introduction. In O. Grüpe (Ed.), *Sport in the modern world: Problems and chances* (pp. 263-265). Berlin: Springer Verlag.

Delateur, B., & Giaconi, R. (1979). Effect on maximal strength of submaximal exercise in Duchenne muscular dystrophy. *American Journal of Physical Medicine, 58*, 26-36.

Delforge, G.D. (1973). Attitudes of physically handicapped and non-handicapped college students towards physical activity. *Dissertation Abstracts International, 34*, 1116A.

DeMaria, A.N., Neumann, A., Lee, G., Fowler, W., & Mason, D.T. (1978). Alterations in ventricular mass and performance induced by exercise training in man evaluated by echocardiography. *Circulation, 57*, 237-244.

Dempsey, J. (1987). Exercise-induced imperfections in pulmonary gas exchange. *Canadian Journal of Sport Sciences, 12*(Suppl.), 66S-70S.

DeMyer, M.K. (1976). Motor, perceptual-motor, intellectual disabilities of autistic children. In L. Wing (Ed.), *Early childhood autism* (2nd ed.). New York: Pergamon Press.

Dendy, E. (1978). Recreation for disabled people—What do we mean? *Physiotherapy, 64*, 290-297.

DePauw, K.P. (1981). Physical education for the visually impaired: A review of the literature. *Journal of Visual Impairment and Blindness, 75*, 162-164.

DePauw, K.P. (1984). Total body mass centroid and segmental mass centroid locations found in Down's Syndrome individuals. *Adapted Physical Activity Quarterly, 1*, 221-229.

de Potter, J-C. (1981). Vigilance et rapidité motrice d'adolescents arrières mentaux [Vigilance and motor speed in mentally retarded adolescents]. In J-C. de Potter (Ed.), *Activités physiques adaptées* (pp. 43-50). Brussels: Editions de l'Université de Bruxelles.

de Potter, J-C. (1987). A trial evaluation of a motor aptitude scale for mentally deficient persons. In M. Berridge & G. Ward (Eds.), *International perspectives in adapted physical activity* (pp. 179-182). Champaign, IL: Human Kinetics.

Desoille, H., Scherrer, J., & Truhaut, R. (1984). *Précis de Medicine du Travail* [Abstracts of occupational medicine]. (4th ed.). Paris: Masson.

Dibner, S.S., & Dibner, A.S. (1973). *Integration or segregation for the physically handicapped child?* (pp. 1-201). Springfield, IL: Charles C Thomas.

DiCarlo, S.E., Supp, M.D., & Taylor, H.C. (1983). Effect of arm ergometry on physical work capacity of individuals with spinal cord injuries. *Physical Therapy, 63,* 1104-1107.

DiNatale, J.M., Lee, M., Ward, G., & Shephard, R.J. (1985). Loss of physical condition in sightless adolescents during a summer vacation. *Adapted Physical Activity Quarterly, 2,* 144-150.

DiNatale, J.M., Pierrynowski, M.R., Tupling, S.J., & Forsyth, R.D. (1984). Length and volume change in the spinal cord injured using photogrammetric anthropometry. In *Human Locomotion III.* Paper presented at Annual meeting of the Canadian Society of Biomechanics, Winnipeg.

DiRocco, P. (1986). Tethered swimming and the development of cardio-pulmonary fitness for non-ambulatory individuals. *American Corrective Therapy Journal, 40,* 43-47.

Dishman, R.K. (1985). Medical psychology in exercise and sport. *Medical Clinics of North America, 69,* 123-143.

Dishman, R.K. (1988). Exercise adherence: Its impact on public health. Champaign, IL: Human Kinetics.

Dishman, R.K., Sallis, J.F., & Orenstein, D.R. (1985). The determinants of physical activity and exercise. *Public Health Reports, 100,* 158-171.

Dobbins, D., Garron, R., & Rarick, G. (1981). The motor performance of EMR and intellectually normal boys after covariate control for differences in body size. *Research Quarterly for Exercise and Sport, 52*(1), 1-8.

Dodds, A.G., & Carter, D.D.C. (1983). Memory for movement in blind children: The role of previous visual experience. *Journal of Motor Behavior, 15,* 343-352.

Doll-Tepper, G.M. (1983). Physical education programs for mentally retarded children in Germany. In R.L. Eason, T.L. Smith, & F. Caron (Eds.), *Adapted physical education: From theory to application* (pp. 19-24). Champaign, IL: Human Kinetics.

Dordel, H-J. (1971). Physical education and sport for the visually handicapped and blind. In U. Simri (Ed.), *Sports as a means of rehabilitation* (pp. 9/1-9/10). Natanya, Israel: Wingate Institute.

Douglas, F.G.V., & Becklake, M.R. (1968). Effect of seasonal training on maximum cardiac output. *Journal of Applied Physiology, 25,* 600-605.

Downey, J.A., Darling, R.C., & Chiodi, H.P. (1967). The response of the tetraplegic patients to cold. *Archives of Physical Medicine and Rehabilitation, 48,* 645-649.

Drake, V., Jones, G., Brown, J.R., & Shephard, R.J. (1968). Fitness performance tests and their relationship to maximum oxygen uptake. *Canadian Medical Association Journal, 99,* 844-848.

Dransart, G. (1977). *Contribution à la connaissance du canoe kayak* [Contributions to knowledge about kayaking] Thesis for diploma, National Institute of Sports and Physical Education, Paris.

Dreisinger, T.E. (1978). *Wheelchair ergometry: A training study.* Unpublished doctoral dissertation, University of Missouri, Columbia.

Dreisinger, T.E., & Londeree, B.R. (1982). Wheelchair exercise: A review. *Paraplegia, 20,* 20-34.

Dresen, M.H.W. (1985). Physical training of handicapped children. In R.A. Binkhorst, H.C.G. Kemper, & W.H.M. Saris (Eds.), *Children and exercise XI* (pp. 203-209). Champaign, IL: Human Kinetics.

Dresen, M.H.W., Groot, G. de., Brandt Corstius, J.J., Krediet, G.H.B., & Meijer, M.J.H. (1982). Physical work capacity and daily activities of handicapped and non-handicapped children. *European Journal of Applied Physiology,* **48**, 241-251.

Dresen, M.H.W., Vermeulen, H., Netelenbos, B.J., & Krot, H. (1982). Physical work capacity and classroom attention of handicapped and non-handicapped children. *International Journal of Rehabilitation Research,* **5**, 5-12.

Drouin, D., Simard, C., & Cloutier, L. (1981). Analyse du quotient d'habilités motrices d'enfants normaux et de déficients mentaux légers [Analysis of motor ability quotients for normal and mildly retarded children]. In J-C. de Potter (Ed.), *Activités physiques adaptées* (pp. 11-20). Brussels: Editions de l'Université de Bruxelles.

DuBow, L.L., Witt, P.K., Kadaba, M.P., Reyes, R., & Cochrane, G.V.B. (1983). Oxygen consumption of elderly persons with bilateral below-knee amputations: Ambulation vs. wheelchair propulsion. *Archives of Physical Medicine and Rehabilitation,* **64**, 255-259.

Dummer, G.M., Ewing, M.E., Habeck, R.V., & Overton, S.R. (1987). Attributions of athletes with cerebral palsy. *Adapted Physical Activity Quarterly,* **4**, 278-292.

Dunn, D.J. (1969). *Adjustment to spinal cord injury in the rehabilitation hospital setting* (Doctoral dissertation, University of Maryland, College Park). *Dissertation Abstracts International,* **31**, 911B.

Dunn, J.M. (1983). Physical activity for the severely handicapped: Theoretical and practical considerations. In R.L. Eason, T.L. Smith, & F. Caron (Eds.), *Adapted physical activity: From theory to application* (pp. 63-73). Champaign, IL: Human Kinetics.

Durnin, J.V.G.A., & Passmore, R. (1967). *Energy, work, and leisure.* London: Heinemann.

Durnin, J.V.G.A., & Womersley, J.A. (1974). Body fat assessed from total body density and its estimation from skinfold thickness: Measurements on 481 men and women aged from 16 to 72 years. *British Journal of Nutrition,* **32**, 77-97.

Eason, B.L., Smith, T.L., & Stamps, L.E. (1981). Response time and heart rate differences between minimally retarded and gifted children: Part 2. In J-C. de Potter (Ed.), *Activités physiques adaptées* (pp. 37-42). Brussels: Editions de l'Université de Bruxelles.

Eberhart, H.D., Elftman, H., & Inman, V.T. (1954). The locomotor mechanism of the amputee. In P.E. Klopsteg & D.D. Wilson (Eds.), *Iluman limbs and their substitutes* (pp. 472-480). New York: McGraw-Hill.

Edgerton, V.R. (1978). Mammalian muscle fibre types and their adaptability. *American Zoological Journal,* **18**, 113-125.

Edstrom, L., & Ekblöm, B. (1972). Difference in size of red and white muscle fibres in vastus lateralis of musculus quadriceps femoris of normal individuals and athletes: Relation to physical performance. *Scandinavian Journal of Clinical and Laboratory Investigation,* **30**, 175-181.

Effgen, S.K. (1981). Effect of an exercise program on the static balance of deaf children. *Physical Therapy,* **61**, 873-877.

Ehsani, A.A., Health, G.W., Hagberg, G.M., & Schechtman, K. (1981). Noninvasive assessment of changes in left ventricular function induced by graded isometric exercise in healthy subjects. *Chest,* **80**, 51-55.

Eichstaedt, C.B., & Seiler, P.J. (1978). Signing. *Journal of Physical Education and Recreation,* **49**(5), 12-21.

Eickelberg, W., Less, M., & Engels, W. (1976). Respiratory, cardiac and learning changes in exercised muscular dystrophic children [Abstract]. *Perceptual and Motor Skills,* **43**, 66.

Eisenberg, M., Griggins, C., & Duval, R. (1982). *Disabled people as second class citizens.* New York: Springer Verlag.

Ekblöm, B., & Lundberg, A. (1968). Effect of physical training on adolescents with severe motor handicaps. *Acta Paediatrica Scandinavica,* **57**, 17-23.

Emes, C. (1978). Physical work capacity of wheelchair athletes. *Research Quarterly,* **48**, 209-212.

Emes, C. (July, 1984). *Modifying motor behavior of blind children for participation in sport and physical activity.* Paper presented at Olympic Sports Medicine Congress, Eugene, OR.

Engel, R., & Hildebrandt, G. (1971). Zur Arbeitsphysiologische Beurteilung verschiedenen handbetriebenen Krankenfahrstuehlen [On the work physiology of children and hand-driven wheelchairs]. *Zeitschrift für Physikalische Medizin,* **2**, 95-102.

Engel, R., & Hildebrandt, G. (1973). Long-term spiroergometric studies of paraplegics during the clinical period of rehabilitation. *Paraplegia,* **11**, 105-110.

Engel, R., & Hildebrandt, G. (1974). Wheelchair design: Technological and physiological aspects. *Proceedings of the Royal Society of Medicine,* **67**, 409-411.

Enoka, R.M., Miller, D.I., & Burgess, E.M. (1982). Below-knee amputee running gait. *American Journal of Physical Medicine,* **61**, 66-84.

Erdman, W.J., Hettinger, T., & Saez, F. (1960). Comparative work stress for above-knee amputees using artificial legs or crutches. *American Journal of Physical Medicine,* **39**, 225-232.

Fait, H. (1983). Evaluation of motor skills of the handicapped: Theory and practice. In R.L. Eason, T.L. Smith, & F. Caron (Eds.), *Adapted physical activity: From theory to application* (pp. 172-179). Champaign, IL: Human Kinetics.

Fait, H.F., & Dunn, J.M. (1984). *Special physical education: Adapted, individualized, developmental* (5th ed.). Philadelphia: Saunders.

Fardy, P.S., Webb, D.P., & Hellerstein, H.K. (1976). Cardiorespiratory adaptation to submaximal and maximal exercise [Abstract]. *Medicine and Science in Sports and Exercise,* **8**, 49.

Fardy, P.S., Webb, D.P., & Hellerstein, H.K. (1977). Benefits of arm exercise in cardiac rehabilitation. *The Physician and Sportsmedicine,* **5**, 30-41.

Fernhall, B., & Tymeson, G.T. (1988). Validation of cardiovascular fitness field tests for adults with mental retardation. *Adapted Physical Activity Quarterly,* **5**, 49-59.

Fernhall, B., Tymeson, G.T., & Webster, G.E. (1988). Cardiovascular fitness of mentally retarded individuals. *Adapted Physical Activity Quarterly, 5,* 12-28.

Field, T., Roseman, S., DeStefano, L., & Koewler, J.H. (1982). The play of handicapped preschool children with handicapped and non-handicapped peers in integrated and non-integrated situations. *Topics in Early Childhood Education, 2,* 28-38.

Findlay, H. (1981). Adaptation of the Canada Fitness Award for the trainable mentally handicapped. *Canadian Association for Health, Physical Education & Recreation Journal, 48*(1), 5-12.

Fishbein, M., & Ajzen, I. (1975). *Belief, attitude, intention and behavior: An introduction to theory and research.* Reading, MA: Addison-Wesley.

Fisher, P. (1980). How a creative movement education program will affect the body-image and self-concept of the learning disabled child. *Scottish Journal of Physical Education, 8,* 5-9.

Fisher, S.V., & Gullickson, G. (1978). Energy cost of ambulation in health and disability: A literature review. *Archives of Physical Medicine and Rehabilitation, 59,* 124-132.

Fitzgerald, P.I., Sedlock, D.A., Knowlton, R.G., & Schneider, D.A. (1982). Cardiovascular responses of spinal cord injured women to prolonged submaximal wheelchair activity [Abstract]. *Medicine and Science in Sports and Exercise, 14,* 166.

Flordmark, A. (1986). Augmented auditory feedback as an aid in gait training of the cerebral-palsied child. *Developmental Medicine and Child Neurology, 28,* 147-155.

Floyd, W.F., Guttmann, L., Noble, C.W., Parkes, K.R., & Ward, J. (1966). A study of the space requirements of wheelchair users. *Paraplegia, 4,* 24-37.

Flynn, R.J., & Salomone, P.R. (1977). Performance of the MMPI in predicting rehabilitation outcome: A discriminant analysis, double cross-validation assessment. *Rehabilitation Literature, 38,* 12-15.

Folsom-Meek, S.L. (1984). Parents: Forgotten teacher aids in adapted physical education. *Adapted Physical Activity Quarterly, 1,* 275-281.

Forest, M. (1984). Reflections on a new kind of school. In L.M. Wells (Ed.), *Proceedings: The integration of the physically disabled into community living: A colloquium* (pp. 169-190). Toronto: University of Toronto School of Social Work.

Fowler, W.M., & Gardner, G.W. (1967). Quantitative strength measurements in muscular dystrophy. *Archives of Physical Medicine and Rehabilitation, 48,* 629-644.

Fox, E.L. (1984). *Sports physiology.* New York: CBC College.

Fox, E.L., Bartels, R.L., Billings, C.E., O'Brien, R., Bason, R., & Mathews, D.K. (1975). Frequency and duration of interval training programs and changes in aerobic power. *Journal of Applied Physiology, 38,* 481-484.

Fox, M.J. (1974). Access for the handicapped. In J. Yeo (Ed.), *Recreation for the handicapped* (pp. 36-39). Melbourne: Australian Council for Rehabilitation of the Disabled.

Fox, R., & Rotatori, A.F. (1982). Prevalence of obesity among mentally retarded adults. *American Journal of Mental Deficiency, 87*, 228-230.

Fox, V.M., Lawlor, V.A., & Luttges, M.W. (1984). Pilot study of novel test instrumentation to evaluate therapeutic horseback riding. *Adapted Physical Activity Quarterly, 1*, 30-36.

Francis, R.J., & Rarick, G.L. (1959). Motor characteristics of the mentally retarded. *American Journal of Mental Deficiency, 63*, 792-811.

Francis, R.S., & Nelson, A.G. (1981). Physiological and performance profiles of a world-class wheelchair athlete [Abstract]. *Medicine and Science in Sports and Exercise, 13*, 132.

Franklin, B.A. (1985). Exercise testing, training and arm ergometry. *Sports Medicine, 2*, 100-119.

Franklin, B.A. (1988). Program factors that influence exercise adherence: Practical adherence skills for the clinical staff. In R.K. Dishman (Ed.), *Exercise adherence* (pp. 237-258). Champaign, IL: Human Kinetics.

Franklin, B.A., Vander, L., Wrisley, D., & Rubenfire, M. (1983). Aerobic requirements of arm ergometry: Implications for exercise testing and training. *The Physician and Sportsmedicine, 11*, 81-90.

Frazier, C.H. (1918). *Surgery of the spine and spinal cord.* New York: D. Appleton.

French, R.W., & Jansma, P. (1982). *Special physical education.* Columbus, OH: C.E. Merrill.

Frewin, D.B., Levitt, M., Myers, S.J., Co, C.C., & Downey, J.A. (1973). Catecholamine responses in paraplegia. *Paraplegia, 11*, 238-244.

Frick, M.H., Sjögren, A.L., Perasalo, J., & Pajunen, S. (1970). Cardiovascular dimensions and moderate physical training in young men. *Journal of Applied Physiology, 29*, 452-458.

Fried, T., & Shephard, R.J. (1970). Assessment of a lower extremity training programme. *Canadian Medical Association Journal, 103*, 260-266.

Friedmann, L.N. (1972). Amputations and prostheses in primitive culture. *Bulletin of Prosthetic Research, 10-17*(Spring), 105-138.

Frison, J.C., Sanchez Massa, L., Garmacho, H., & Gimeno, V. (1979). Heart rate variations in tetraplegic patients. *British Medical Journal, I*, 1353-1354.

Frith, V., & Hermelin, B. (1969). The role of visual and motor cues for normal, subnormal and autistic children. *Archives of General Psychiatry, 20*, 155-165.

Fugl-Meyer, A.R., Grimby, G. (1971). Effects of respiratory muscle paralysis in tetraplegic and paraplegic patients. *Scandinavian Journal of Rehabilitation Medicine, 3*, 141-150.

Funk, D.C. (1971). Effects of physical education on fitness and motor development of trainable mentally retarded children. *Research Quarterly, 42*, 30-34.

Gaesser, G.A., & Brooks, G.A. (1975). Muscular efficiency during steady-state exercise: Effects of speed and work-rate. *Journal of Applied Physiology, 38*, 1132-1139.

Gailani, S., Danowski, T.S., & Fisher, D.S. (1958). Muscular dystrophy: Catheterization studies indicating latent congestive heart failure. *Circulation, 17*, 585-588.

Gairdner, J. (1983). *Fitness for the disabled: Wheelchair users.* Toronto: Fitzhenry & Whiteside.

Gamerale, F. (1972). Perceived exertion, heart rate, oxygen uptake and blood lactate in different work operations. *Ergonomics, 15*, 545-554.

Gandee, R., Porterfield, J., Narraway, A., Winningham, M., Deitchman, R., Dodd, R., & Hollering, B. (1981). Somatotype and isokinetic strength profile of an elite wheelchair marathon racer [Abstract]. *Medicine and Science in Sports and Exercise, 13*, 132.

Gandee, R., Winningham, M., Deitchman, R., & Narraway, A. (1980). The aerobic capacity of an elite wheelchair marathon racer [Abstract]. *Medicine and Science in Sports and Exercise, 12*, 142.

Ganguli, S., Datta, S.R., Chatterjee, B.B., & Roy, B.N. (1973). Performance evaluation of amputee-prosthesis system in below-knee amputees. *Ergonomics, 16*, 797-810.

Ganguli, S., Datta, S.R., Chatterjee, B.B., & Roy, B.N. (1974a). Ergonomic evaluation of above-knee amputee prosthesis combinations. *Ergonomics, 17*, 199-210.

Ganguli, S., Datta, S.R., Chatterjee, B.B., & Roy, B.N. (1974b). Biomechanical approach to the functional assessment of the use of crutches for amputation. *Ergonomics, 17*, 365-374.

Ganguli, S., Datta, S.R., Chatterjee, B.B., & Roy, B.N. (1974c). Metabolic cost of walking at different speeds with patellar-tendon bearing prostheses. *Journal of Applied Physiology, 36*, 440-443.

Gargiulo, R.M., & Yonker, R.J. (1983). Assessing teachers' attitudes toward the handicapped: A methodological investigation. *Psychology in the Schools, 20*, 229-233.

Gass, C.G., & Camp, E.M. (1979). Physiological characteristics of trained paraplegic and tetraplegic subjects. *Medicine and Science in Sports and Exercise, 11*, 256-265.

Gass, C.G., & Camp, E.M. (1984). The maximum physiological responses during incremental wheelchair and arm cranking exercise in male paraplegics. *Medicine and Science in Sports and Exercise, 16*, 355-359.

Gass, C.G., Camp, E.M., Davis, H.A., Eager, B., & Grout, L. (1981). The effects of prolonged exercise on spinally-injured subjects. *Medicine and Science in Sports and Exercise, 13*, 277-283.

Gauthier, R., Massicotte, D., Hermiston, R., & MacNab, R. (1983). The physical work capacity of Canadian children, aged 7 to 17, in 1983: A comparison with 1968. *CAHPER Journal, 50*(2), 1-9.

Geddes, D. (1977). Motor development of autistic monozygotic twins: A case study. *Perceptual and Motor Skills, 45*, 179-186.

Gehlsen, G., Beekman, K., Assman, N., Winant, D., Seidle, M., & Carter, A. (1986). Gait characteristics in multiple sclerosis: Progressive changes and effects of exercise on parameters. *Archives of Physical Medicine and Rehabilitation, 67*, 536-539.

Gehlsen, G.M., Grigsby, S.A., & Winant, D.M. (1984). Effects of an aquatic fitness program on the muscular strength and endurance of patients with muscular sclerosis. *Physical Therapy, 64*, 653-657.

Geis, H.J. (1972). The problem of personal worth in the physically disabled patient. *Rehabilitation Literature, 33*, 34-39.

Geisler, W.O., Jousse, A.T., & Wynne-Jones, M. (1977). Survival in traumatic transverse myelitis. *Paraplegia, 14*, 262-275.

George, C., & Patton, R. (1975). Development of an aerobic program for the visually impaired. *Journal of Health, Physical Education and Recreation, 46*, 39-40.

Gersten, J., Brown, I., Speck, L., & Grueter, B. (1963). Comparison of tension development and circulation in bicep and tricep in man. *American Journal of Physical Medicine, 42*, 156-165.

Gessaroli, M.E., & Robertson, D.G.E. (1980). Comparison of two wheelchair sprint starts. *Canadian Journal of Applied Sport Sciences, 5*.

Getman, L., Greninger, L., & Molnar, S. (1968). Efficiency of wheeling after training [Abstract]. *Proceedings of the Annual Convention of the Southern District of the American Alliance for Health, Physical Education and Recreation, 7*, 83.

Ghosh, A.K. (1980). *Selection of clinically suitable tests/methods for ergonomic/ physiological evaluation of lower extremity handicapped persons*. Unpublished doctoral dissertation, University of Calcutta, India.

Ghosh, A.K., Tibarewala, D.N., Mukherjee, P., Chakraborty, S., & Ganguli, A. (1979). Preliminary study of static weight distribution under human foot as a measure of lower extremity disability. *Medical and Biological Engineering and Computing, 17*, 737-741.

Gilbert, C.A., Nutter, D.D., Felner, J.M., Perkins, J.V., Heymsfield, S.B., & Schlant, R.C. (1977). Echocardiographic study of cardiac dimensions and function in the endurance trained athlete. *American Journal of Cardiology, 40*, 528-533.

Giles, M.T. (1968). Classroom research leads to physical fitness for retarded youth. *Education and Training of the Mentally Retarded, 3*, 67-74.

Gipsman, S.C. (1981). Effect of visual condition on use of proprioceptive cues in performing a balance task. *Journal of Visual Impairment and Blindness, 75*, 50-54.

Glaser, R.M. (1987). Exercise and locomotion for the disabled. In M. Berridge & G. Ward (Eds.), *International perspectives in adapted physical activity*. Champaign, IL: Human Kinetics.

Glaser, R.M., & Collins, S.R. (1981). Validity of power output estimation for wheelchair locomotion. *American Journal of Physical Medicine, 60*, 180-189.

Glaser, R.M., Edwards, M., Barr, S.A., & Wilson, G.H. (1975). Energy cost and cardiorespiratory response to wheelchair ambulation and walking [Abstract]. *Federation Proceedings, 34*, 461.

Glaser, R.M., Fichtenbaum, B.M., Simsen-Harold, C.A., Petrofsky, J.S., & Surprayasad, A.G. (1982). Efficiency of young and geriatric individuals during wheelchair locomotion. *Federation Proceedings, 41*, 1675.

Glaser, R.M., Foley, D.M., Laubach, L.L., Sawka, M.N., & Surprayasad, A.G. (1978a). An exercise test to evaluate fitness for wheelchair activity. *Paraplegia, 16*, 341-349.

Glaser, R.M., Giner, J.F., & Laubach, L.L. (1977). Validity and reliability of wheelchair ergometry. *Physiologist, 20*, 34-37.

Glaser, R.M., Laubach, L.L., Sawka, M.N., & Surprayasad, A.G. (1978b). Exercise stress fitness evaluation and training of wheelchair users. In A.S. Leon & G.J. Amundson (Eds.), *Proceedings of First International Conference on Lifestyle and Health* (pp. 167-194). Minneapolis: University of Minnesota.

Glaser, R.M., Sawka, M.N., Brune, M.F., & Wilde, S.W. (1980a). Physiological responses to maximal effort wheelchair and arm crank ergometry. *Journal of Applied Physiology, Respiratory, Environmental and Exercise Physiology,* **48**, 1060-1064.

Glaser, R.M., Sawka, M.N., Durbin, R.J., Foley, D.M., & Surprayasad, A.G. (1980b). Exercise program for wheelchair activity. *American Journal of Physical Medicine,* **60**, 67-75.

Glaser, R.M., Sawka, M.N., Laubach, L.L., & Surprayasad, A.G. (1979). Metabolic and cardiopulmonary responses to wheelchair and bicycle ergometry. *Journal of Applied Physiology,* **46**, 1066-1070.

Glaser, R.M., Sawka, M.N., & Miles, D.S. (1984). Efficiency of wheelchair and low power bicycle ergometry. *Proceedings of the IEEE National Aerospace and Electronics Conference* (Vol. 2, pp. 946-953). New York: Institute of Electronics and Electronic Engineers.

Glaser, R.M., Sawka, M.N., Wilde, S., Woodrow, B. & Surprayasad, A.G. (1981). Energy cost and cardiopulmonary responses for wheelchair locomotion and walking on tile and carpet. *Paraplegia,* **19**, 220-226.

Glaser, R.M., Sawka, M.N., Young, R.E., & Surprayasad, A.G. (1980c). Applied physiology for wheelchair design. *Journal of Applied Physiology, Respiratory, Environmental and Exercise Physiology,* **48**, 41-44.

Glaser, R.M., Simsen-Harold, C.A., Petrofsky, J.S., Kahn, S.E., & Surprayasad, A.G. (1983). Metabolic and cardio-pulmonary responses of older wheelchair dependent and ambulatory patients during locomotion. *Ergonomics,* **26**, 687-697.

Glaser, R.M., Young, R.E., & Surprayasad, A.G. (1977). Reducing energy cost and cardiopulmonary stresses during wheelchair activity. *Federation Proceedings,* **36**, 580.

Glick, S.J. (1953). Emotional problems of 200 cerebral palsied adults. *Cerebral Palsy Review,* **14**, 3-7.

Godfrey, R. (1980). *Outward bound: Schools of the possible.* Garden City, NY: Anchor Press/Doubleday.

Godin, G., Colantonio, A., Davis, G.M., Shephard, R.J., & Simard, C. (1986). Prediction of leisure-time exercise behavior among a group of lower-limb disabled adults. *Journal of Clinical Psychology,* **42**, 272-279.

Godin, G., & Shephard, R.J. (1986). Importance of type of attitude to the study of exercise behavior. *Psychological Reports,* **58**, 991-1000.

Goffman, E. (1963). *Stigma: Notes on the management of spoiled identity.* Englewood Cliffs, NJ: Prentice-Hall.

Goldberg, G., & Shephard, R.J. (1982). Personality profiles of disabled individuals in relation to physical activity patterns. *Journal of Sports Medicine and Physical Fitness,* **22**, 477-484.

Goldspink, G. (1970). The proliferation of myofibrils during muscle fiber growth. *Journal of Cell Science,* **6**, 593-603.

Gollnick, P.D., Armstrong, R.B., Saubert, C.W., Piehl, K., & Saltin, B. (1972). Enzyme activity and fiber composition in skeletal muscle of untrained and trained men. *Journal of Applied Physiology, 33*, 312-319.

Gonyea, W.J. (1980). Rate of exercise in inducing increases of skeletal muscle fiber number. *Journal of Applied Physiology, 48*, 421-426.

Gonzalez, E.G., Corcoran, P.J., & Reyes, R.L. (1974). Energy expenditure in below-knee amputees: Correlation with stump length. *Archives of Physical Medicine and Rehabilitation, 55*, 111-119.

Goode, W. (1978). *The celebration of heroes: Prestige as a social control system.* Berkeley: University of California Press.

Gordon, E., & Vanderwalde, H. (1956). Energy requirements in paraplegic ambulation. *Archives of Physical Medicine and Rehabilitation, 37*, 285-289.

Gorton, B., & Gavron, S. (1987). A biomechanical analysis of the running pattern of blind athletes in the 100-m dash. *Adapted Physical Activity Quarterly, 4*, 192-203.

Goslin, B., & Graham, T.E. (1985). A comparison of "anaerobic" components of O_2 debt and the Wingate test. *Canadian Journal of Applied Sport Sciences, 10*, 134-140.

Goswami, A., Ghosh, A.L., Ganguli, S., & Banerjee, A.K. (1984). Aerobic capacity of severely disabled Indians. *Ergonomics, 27*, 1267-1269.

Gouldner, A. (1965). *Enter Plato: Classical Greece and the origins of social theory.* New York: Basic Books.

Gray, P.G., & Todd, J.E. (1967). *Mobility and reading habits of the blind* (Government Social Survey 386). London: Her Majesty's Stationery Office.

Greenway, R.M., Houser, H.B., Lindan, O., & Weir, D.R. (1970). Long term changes in gross body composition of paraplegic and quadriplegic patients. *Paraplegia, 7*, 310-318.

Greenway, R.M., Littell, A.S., Houser, H.B., Lindan, O., & Weir, D.R. (1965). An evaluation of the variability in measurement of some body composition parameters [Abstract]. *Proceedings of the Society for Experimental Biology and Medicine, 120*, 487.

Grimby, G. (1980). Aerobic capacity, muscle strength and fiber composition in young paraplegics. In H. Natvig (Ed.), *First International Medical Congress on Sports for the Disabled.* Oslo: Royal Ministry for Church and Education.

Grosfield, I.N. (1980). Classification of asymmetrical quads in swimming and track. In H. Natvig (Ed.), *The First International Medical Congress on Sports for the Disabled.* Oslo: Royal Ministry of Church and Education.

Grossman, H.J. (Ed.) (1984). *Manual on terminology and classification in mental retardation.* Washington, DC: American Association on Mental Deficiency.

Grundy, D.J., & Silver, J.R. (1983). Amputation for peripheral vascular disease in the paraplegic and tetraplegic. *Paraplegic, 21*, 305-311.

Gurlt, I. (1889). In Thorburn, W. (Ed.), *A contribution to the surgery of the spinal cord.* London: C. Griffin. (Original work published 1864)

Guttmann, L. (1946). Rehabilitation after injuries to the spinal cord and cauda equina. *British Journal of Physical Medicine, 9*, 130-137.

Guttmann, L. (1954). Statistical survey of one thousand paraplegics and initial treatment of traumatic paraplegia. *Proceedings of the Royal Society of Medicine, 47*, 1099.

Guttmann, L. (1973). Development of sport for the disabled. In O. Grüpe (Ed.), *Sport in the modern world* (pp. 254-256). Berlin: Springer Verlag.

Guttmann, L. (1976a). *Textbook of sport for the disabled*. Oxford: H.M. & M. Publishers.

Guttmann, L. (1976b). Reflection on the 1976 Toronto olympiad for the physically disabled. *Paraplegia, 14,* 225-226.

Guttmann, L., Munro, A.F., Robison, R., & Walsh, J.J. (1963). Effect of tilting on the cardiovascular responses and plasma catecholamine levels in spinal man. *Paraplegia, 1,* 4-18.

Guttmann, L., Whitteridge, D., & Jonason, P.H. (1947). The treatment and prognosis of traumatic paraplegia. *Proceedings of the Royal Society of Medicine, 40,* 219-232.

Hamill, J., Knutzen, K.M., & Bates, B.T. (1985). Ambulatory consistency of the visually impaired. In D.A. Winter, R.W. Norman, R.P. Wells, K.C. Hayes, & A.E. Patla (Eds.), *Biomechanics IXA* (pp. 570-574). Champaign, IL: Human Kinetics.

Hamilton, E.A., & Nichols, P.J.R. (1972). Rehabilitation of the lower-limb amputee. *British Medical Journal, 2,* 95-99.

Hamilton, E.J., & Anderson, S. (1983). Effects of leisure activities on attitudes toward people with disabilities. *Therapeutic Recreation Journal, 17*(3), 50-57.

Hannah, R.E., Morrison, J.B., & Chapman, A.E. (1984). Prosthesis alignment: Effect on gait of persons with below-knee amputations. *Archives of Physical Medicine and Rehabilitation, 65,* 159-162.

Harber, V.J., & Sutton, J. (1984). Endorphins and exercise. *Sports Medicine, 1,* 154-171.

Hardison, G.T., Israel, R.G., & Somes, G.W. (1987). Physiological responses to different cranking rates during submaximal arm ergometry in paraplegic males. *Adapted Physical Activity Quarterly, 4,* 94-105.

Hardy, R.E., & Cull, J.D. (1972). *Social and rehabilitation services for the blind.* Springfield, IL: Charles C Thomas.

Harper, D.C. (1978). Personality characteristics of physically impaired adolescents. *Journal of Clinical Psychology, 34,* 97-104.

Harper, D.C., & Richman, L.C. (1978). Personality profiles of physically impaired adolescents. *Journal of Clinical Psychology, 34,* 636-642.

Harper, D.C., & Richman, L.C. (1980). Personality profiles of physically impaired young adults. *Journal of Clinical Psychology, 36,* 668-671.

Hartley, X.Y. (1986). A summary of recent research into the development of children with Down's Syndrome. *Journal of Mental Deficiency Research, 30,* 1-14.

Hattin, H., Fraser, M., Ward, G., & Shephard, R.J. (1986). Are deaf children unusually fit? A comparison of fitness between deaf and blind children. *Adapted Physical Activity Quarterly, 3,* 268-275.

Hay, C. (1982). Wilderness travel on horseback. *Sports 'N Spokes, 7*(6), 6-8.

Hayden, F.J. (1962). *Physical activity for the severely retarded.* Paper presented at the annual meeting of the Canadian Association for the Mentally Retarded, Halifax, NS.

Hayden, F.J. (1968). The nature of physical performance in the trainable retarded. In G.A. Jervis (Ed.), *Expanding concepts in mental retardation*. Springfield, IL: Charles C Thomas.

Hayes, G.A., & Smith, D. (1973). Municipal recreation services for special populations in Texas. *Therapeutic Recreation Journal, 7*(1), 23-30.

Heigenhauser, G.F., Ruff, C.L., Miller, B., & Faulkner, J.A. (1976). Cardiovascular responses of paraplegics during graded arm ergometry [Abstract]. *Medicine and Science in Sports and Exercise, 8*, 68.

Hellerstein, H.K. (1977). Limits of marathon running in the rehabilitation of coronary patients: Anatomic and physiological determinants. *Annals of the New York Academy of Sciences, 301*, 484-494.

Hellerstein, H.K., & Franklin, B.A. (1984). Exercise testing and prescription. In N. Wenger & H.K. Hellerstein (Eds.), *Rehabilitation of the coronary patient* (2nd ed., pp. 197-284). New York: John Wiley.

Henriksson, K.G. (1980). Muscle histochemistry and muscle function. *Acta Paediatrica Scandinavica, 283*(Suppl.), 15-19.

Henriksson, J., & Reitman, J.S. (1977). Time course of changes in human skeletal muscle succinate dehydrogenase and cytochrome oxidase activities and maximal oxygen uptake with physical activity and inactivity. *Acta Physiologica Scandinavica, 99*, 91-97.

Henschen, K., Horvat, M., & French, R. (1984). A visual comparison of psychological profiles between able-bodied and wheelchair athletes. *Adapted Physical Activity Quarterly, 1*, 118-124.

Herzlich, C. (1973). *Health and illness*. London: Academic Press.

Hettinger, T.L. (1961). *Physiology of strength*. Springfield, IL: Charles C Thomas.

Heyes, A.D., Armstrong, J.D., & Willans, P.R. (1976). A comparison of heart rates during blind mobility and car driving. *Ergonomics, 19*, 489-497.

Hickson, R.C. (1980). Interference of strength development by simultaneous training for strength and endurance. *European Journal of Applied Physiology, 45*, 255-263.

Higgs, C. (1983). Analysis of racing wheelchairs used at the 1980 Olympic Games for the Disabled. *Research Quarterly, 54*, 229-233.

Higgs, C. (1986). Propulsion of racing wheelchairs. In C. Sherrill (Ed.), *Sport and disabled athletes* (pp. 165-172). Champaign, IL: Human Kinetics.

Higgs, C. (1987). Science, research, and special populations: The view from biomechanics. In M. Berridge & G. Ward (Eds.), *International perspectives in adapted physical activity* (pp. 193-201). Champaign, IL: Human Kinetics.

Hildebrandt, G., Voight, E., Bahn, D., Berendes, B., & Krager, J. (1970). Energy costs of propelling a wheelchair at various speeds: Cardiac responses and effect on steering accuracy. *Archives of Physical Medicine and Rehabilitation, 51*, 131-136.

Hill, F.T. (1974). Widening horizons in recreation for the handicapped. In J. Yeo (Ed.), *Recreation for the handicapped* (pp. 29-32). Melbourne: Australian Council for Rehabilitation of the Disabled.

Hjeltnes, N. (1977). Oxygen uptake and cardiac output in graded arm exercise in paraplegics with low level spinal lesions. *Scandinavian Journal of Rehabilitation Medicine*, **9**, 107-113.

Hjeltnes, N. (1980). Control of medical rehabilitation of para and tetraplegics. In H. Natvig (Ed.), *First International Medical Congress on Sports for the Disabled*. Oslo: Royal Ministry of Church and Education.

Hjeltnes, N. (1984). Control of medical rehabilitation of para- and tetraplegics by repeated evaluation of endurance capacity. *International Journal of Sports Medicine*, **5**, 171-174.

Hjeltnes, N., & Vokac, Z. (1979). Circulatory strain in everyday life of paraplegics. *Scandinavian Journal of Rehabilitation Medicine*, **11**, 67-73.

Ho, K.W., Roy, R.R., Tweedle, C.D., Heusner, W.W., Van Huss, W.D., & Carrow, R.E. (1980). Skeletal muscle fiber splitting with weight lifting in rats. *American Journal of Anatomy*, **157**, 433-440.

Hoeberigs, J.H. (1985). How big is the problem of "disabled and sports"? Presentation of some epidemiological data. In J.H. Hoeberigs & H. Vorsteveld (Eds.), *Proceedings of the Workshop on Disabled and Sports* (pp. 142-147). Amersfoort, Netherlands: Nederlandse Invaliden Sportbond.

Hoes, M., Binkhorst, R.A., Smeekes-Kuyl, A., & Vissurs, A.C. (1968). Measurement of forces exerted on a pedal crank during work on the bicycle ergometer at different loads. *Internationale Zeitschrift für Angewandte und Arbeitsphysiologie*, **26**, 33-42.

Hoffman, M.D. (1986). Cardiorespiratory fitness and training in quadriplegics and paraplegics. *Sports Medicine*, **3**, 312-330.

Hollmann, W., & Venrath, H. (1962). Experimentelle Untersuchungen zur Bedeutung eines Trainingsunterhalb und oberhalb der Dauerbelastungsgranze [Experimental investigations on the importance of training below and above the steady work limit]. In I. Korbs (Ed.), *Carl Diem Festschrift*. Frankfurt: W.U.A.

Holloszy, J.O., & Booth, F.W. (1976). Biochemical adaptations to endurance exercise in muscle. *Annual Review of Physiology*, **38**, 273-291.

Holm, G.A.L., & Krotkiewski, M.J. (1985). Exercise in the treatment of diabetes mellitus. In P. Welsh & R.J. Shephard (Eds.), *Current therapy in sports medicine* (pp. 105-106). Burlington: B.C. Decker.

Holmgren, A. (1967). Cardiorespiratory determinants of cardiovascular fitness. *Canadian Medical Association Journal*, **96**, 697-705.

Hook, O. (1971). Arm ergometer for patients with paraplegia. *Scandinavian Journal of Rehabilitation Medicine*, **3**, 77-79.

Hopkins, W.G., Gaeta, H., Thomas, A.C., & Hill, P.M. (1987). Physical fitness of blind and sighted children. *European Journal of Applied Physiology*, **56**, 69-73.

Hopper, C.A. (1986). Socialization of wheelchair athletes. In C. Sherrill (Ed.), *Sport and disabled athletes* (pp. 197-202). Champaign, IL: Human Kinetics.

Horvat, M.A. (1982). Effect of a home learning program on learning disabled children's balance. *Perceptual and Motor Skills*, **55**, 1158.

Horvat, M.A. (1987). Effects of a progressive resistance training program on an individual with spastic cerebral palsy. *American Corrective Therapy Journal*, **41**, 7-11.

Horvat, M.A., Golding, L.A., Beutel-Horvat, T., & McConnell, T.J. (1984). A treadmill modification for wheelchairs. *Research Quarterly, 55,* 297-301.

Hoskin, M., Erdman, W., Bream, J., & MacAvay, C. (1974). Therapeutic horseback riding for the handicapped. *Archives of Physical Medicine and Rehabilitation, 55,* 473-474.

Hosking, G.P., Bhat, U.S., Dubowitz, V., & Edwards, R.H.T. (1976). Measurements of muscle strength and performance in children with normal and diseased muscle. *Archives of Disease in Childhood, 51,* 957-963.

Hottinger, K. (1980). Downhill skiing: Schuss the slopes in a Smith sled. *Sports 'N Spokes, 6,* (November/December), 6-7.

Howald, H. (1975). Ultrastructural adaptation of skeletal muscle to prolonged physical exercise. In H. Howald & J.R. Poortmans (Eds.), *Metabolic adaptations to prolonged physical exercise* (pp. 372-383). Basel: Birkhauser Verlag.

Howe, C. (1959). A comparison of motor skills of mentally retarded and normal children. *Exceptional Children, 25,* 352-354.

Howell, M.L., & Macnab, R.J. (1968). *The physical capacity of Canadian children 7-17 years.* Ottawa: Canadian Association for Health, Physical Education and Recreation.

Howell, R. (1978). The western world and sport: National government programs. In U. Simri (Ed.), *Comparative physical education and sport* (pp. 176-188). Natanya, Israel: Wingate Institute.

Hrubec, Z., & Ryder, R.A. (1980). Traumatic limb amputations and subsequent mortality from cardiovascular disease and other causes. *Journal of Chronic Diseases, 33,* 239-250.

Huang, C.T., McEachran, A.B., Kuhlmeier, K.V., DeVivo, M.J., & Fine, P.R. (1983). Prescriptive arm ergometry to optimize muscular endurance in acutely injured paraplegic patients. *Archives of Physical Medicine and Rehabilitation, 64,* 578-582.

Huberman, G. (1971). Wheelchair sports: Historical notes. In U. Simri (Ed.), *Sport as a means of rehabilitation* (pp. 15-1 to 15-17). Natanya, Israel: Wingate Institute.

Huberman, G. (1976). Organized sports activities with cerebral palsied adolescents. *Rehabilitation Literature, 37,* 103-107.

Hullemann, K-O., List, M., Matthes, D., Wiese, G., & Zika, D. (1975). Spiroergometric and telemetric investigations during the XXI International Stoke Mandeville Games, 1972, in Heidelberg. *Paraplegia, 13,* 109-123.

Hunt, P. (1966). *Stigma: The experience of disability.* London: Chapman.

Hutchison, P. (1980). Perceptions of disabled persons regarding barriers to community involvement. *Journal of Leisurability, 7,* 4-16.

Ikai, M., & Fukunaga, T. (1968). Calculation of muscle strength per unit cross-sectional area of human muscle by means of ultrasonic measurement. *Internationale Zeitschrift für Angewandte und Arbeitsphysiologie, 26,* 26-32.

Inkley, S.R., Oldenburg, F.C., & Vignos, P.J. (1974). Pulmonary function in Duchenne muscular dystrophy related to stages of the disease. *American Journal of Medicine, 56,* 297-306.

Inman, V.T., Barnes, G.H., Levy, S.W., Loon, H.E., & Ralston, H.J. (1961). Medical problems of amputees. *California Medicine, 94,* 132-138.

Inman, V.T., & Ralston, H.J. (1962). *Energy expenditure in certain types of disability.* (final project report). Washington, DC: Veterans' Administration Research & Development Division, Prosthetic and Sensory Aids Service.

Institute for Personality and Ability Testing. (1972). *IPAT Staff Administrator's manual for 16 PF and tabular supplement.* Champaign, IL: Author.

International Sports Organization for the Disabled. (1981). *Les autres classification: ISOD handbook* (SHIF, Idrottens Hus, S-123 87). Farsta, Sweden: ISOD Secretary General.

International Stoke Mandeville Games Federation. (1982). *ISMGF guide for doctors.* Aylesbury, England: Author.

Irmischer, T. (1980). *Motopadagogik bei geistig behinderten* [Motor learning in moderately retarded]. Schorndorf, West Germany: Hofmann Verlag.

Ispa, J. (1981). Social interaction among teachers, handicapped children and non-handicapped children in a mainstreamed preschool. *Journal of Applied Developmental Psychology,* **1**, 131-150.

Jackson, R.W., Davis, G.M., Kofsky, P.R., Shephard, R.J., & Keene, G.C.R. (1981). Fitness levels in the lower limb disabled [Abstract]. *Transactions of the 27th Annual Meeting, Orthopedics Research Society,* **6**.

Jackson, R.W., & Frederickson, A. (1979). Sports for the physically disabled: The 1976 Olympiad (Toronto). *American Journal of Sports Medicine,* **7**, 293-296.

James, U. (1973). Oxygen uptake and heart rate during prosthetic walking in healthy male unilateral above-knee amputees. *Scandinavian Journal of Rehabilitation Medicine,* **5**, 71-80.

Jankowski, L.W., & Evans, J.K. (1981). The exercise capacity of blind children. *Journal of Visual Impairment and Blindness,* **75**, 248-251.

Jansma, P., & Schultz, B. (1982). Validation and use of a mainstreaming attitude inventory with physical educators. *American Corrective Therapy Journal,* **36**, 150-158.

Jayasuriya, A. (1974). *Traditional curative methods in Sri Lanka and their popularity today.* Colombo, Sri Lanka: Ministry of Health.

Jefferies, S.C. (1986a). Youth sport in the Soviet Union. In M.R. Weiss & D. Gould (Eds.), *Sport for children and youths* (pp. 35-40). Champaign, IL: Human Kinetics.

Jefferies, S.C. (1986b). An analysis of the organizational structure of the Soviet Youth Sports System. In G. Redmond (Ed.), *Sport and politics* (pp. 51-57). Champaign, IL: Human Kinetics.

Jochheim, K.A. (1971). Physical education of the mentally retarded. In U. Simri (Ed.), *Sports as a means of rehabilitation* (pp. 1/1-1/7). Natanya, Israel: Wingate Institute.

Jochheim, K.A., & Strohkendl, H. (1973). The value of particular sports of the wheelchair disabled in maintaining health of the paraplegic. *Paraplegic,* **11**, 173-178.

Johnson, L., & Londeree, B. (1976). *Motor fitness testing manual for the moderately mentally retarded.* Washington, DC: American Alliance for Health, Physical Education and Recreation.

Johnson, M.A., Polgar, J., Weightman, D., & Appleton, D. (1973). Data on the distribution of fibre types in thirty six human muscles: An autopsy study. *Journal of Neurological Science, 18,* 111-129.

Johnson, R.H., & Park, D.M. (1973). Effect of change of posture on blood pressure and plasma renin concentration in men with spinal transections. *Clinical Science, 44,* 539-546.

Jokl, E. (1958). *The clinical physiology of physical fitness and rehabilitation.* Springfield, IL: Charles C Thomas.

Jokl, E. (1980). Sir Ludwig Guttmann—A personal tribute. *Internal Journal of Sports Medicine, 1,* 144-145.

Jones, J.A. (1984). *Training guide to cerebral palsy sports* (2nd ed.). Champaign, IL: Human Kinetics.

Jones, N., & Campbell, E.J.M. (1982). *Clinical exercise testing.* Toronto: W.B. Saunders.

Josef, K. (1967). *Musik als Hilfe in der Erziehung geistig Behinderter* [Music as an aid to training the moderately retarded]. Berlin: Marhold.

Jousse, A.T., Wynne-Jones, M., & Breithaupt, D.J. (1968). A follow-up study of life-expectancy and mortality in traumatic transverse myelitis. *Canadian Medical Association Journal, 98,* 427-435.

Kabsch, A. (1973). The ski camp as a rehabilitative aspect in the training of the gait of above-knee amputees with a prosthesis. In O. Grüpe (Ed.), *Sport in the modern world* (pp. 260-261). Berlin: Springer Verlag.

Kallio, V. (1982). Medical and social problems of the disabled. *EURO Reports and Studies (WHO), 73,* 1-35.

Kamenetz, H.L. (1969). *The wheelchair book.* Springfield, IL: Charles C Thomas.

Kanehisa, H., & Miyashita, M. (1983a). Effects of isometric and isokinetic muscle training on static strength and dynamic power. *European Journal of Applied Physiology, 50,* 365-371.

Kanehisa, H., & Miyashita, M. (1983b). Specificity of velocity in strength training. *European Journal of Applied Physiology, 52,* 104-106.

Kanner, L. (1943). Autistic disturbance of affective contact. *The Nervous Child,* 43(4), 80-81.

Kaplan, P.E., Gandhavadi, B., Richards, L., & Goldschmidt, J. (1978). Calcium balance in paraplegic patients, influence of injury duration and ambulation. *Archives of Physical Medicine and Rehabilitation, 59,* 447-450.

Karper, W.B., & Martinek, T.J. (1985). Teachers' expectations in a mainstreamed physical activity program. *Palaestra, 1*(3), 19-21, 41.

Karrer, R. (1985). Input, central and motor segments of response time in mentally retarded and normal children. In M.C. Wade (Ed.), *Motor skill acquisition of the mentally handicapped.* Amsterdam: North Holland.

Karvonen, M., Kentala, K., & Mustala, O. (1957). The effects of training on heart rate: A longitudinal study. *Annales Medicinae Experimentalis et Biologiae Fenniae, 35,* 307-315.

Kasch, F.W., & Zasueta, S.A. (1971). Physical capacities of mentally retarded children. *Acta Paediatrica Scandinavica,* (Suppl. 217), 114-117.

Katz, R.C., & Singh, N.N. (1986). Increasing recreational behavior in mentally retarded children. *Behavior Modification, 10,* 508-519.

Katz, S., Shurks, E., & Florian, V. (1978). The relationship between physical disability, social perception and psychological stress. *Scandinavian Journal of Rehabilitation Medicine,* **10,** 109-113.

Kavanagh, T. (1980). *The healthy heart programme.* Toronto: Van Nostrand.

Kavanagh, T., & Shephard, R.J. (1973). The application of exercise testing to the elderly amputee. *Canadian Medical Association Journal,* **108,** 314-317.

Kay, C., & Shephard, R.J. (1969). On muscle strength and the threshold of anaerobic work. *International Zeitschrift für Angewandte Physiologie,* **27,** 311-328.

Kay, L. (1973). Sonic glasses for the blind: A progress report. *American Foundation for the Blind Research Bulletin,* **25,** 25-58.

Keene, G.C.R., Davis, G.M., Jackson, R.W., & Shephard, R.J. (1979). The physically disabled—Exercise testing. *Proceedings, Canadian Orthopaedic Association Annual Meeting.*

Kegel, B., Burgess, E.M., Starr, T.W., & Daly, W.K. (1981). Effects of isometric muscle training on residual limb volume, strength, and gait of below-knee amputees. *Physical Therapy,* **61,** 1419-1426.

Kelly, L.E., Rimmer, J.H., & Ness, R.A. (1986). Obesity levels in institutionalized mentally retarded adults. *Adapted Physical Activity Quarterly,* **3,** 167-176.

Kennedy, A.B., & Thurman, S.K. (1982). Inclinations of non-handicapped children to help their handicapped peers. *Journal of Special Education,* **16**(3), 319-327.

Kennedy, M. (1980). Sport role socialization and attitudes toward physical activity. Unpublished master's thesis, Eugene, OR.

Kenyon, G.S. (1968a). A conceptual model for characterising physical activity. *Research Quarterly,* **39,** 96-105.

Kenyon, G.S. (1968b). Six scales for assessing attitudes towards physical activity. *Research Quarterly,* **39,** 566-574.

Kenyon, G.S. (1970). Attitude toward sport and physical activity among adolescents from four English-speaking countries. In G. Lüschen (Ed.), *The cross-cultural analysis of sport and games* (pp. 138-155). Champaign, IL: Stipes.

Keogh, J.F., & Oliver, J.N. (1968). Physical performance of retarded children: Diagnosis and prescription. In G.A. Jervis (Ed.), *Expanding concepts in mental retardation.* Springfield, IL: Charles C Thomas.

Kerr, R., & Blais, C. (1985). Motor skill acquisition by individuals with Down's Syndrome. *American Journal of Mental Deficiency,* **90,** 313-318.

Kerr, R., & Hughes, K. (1987). Movement difficulty and learning disabled children. *Adapted Physical Activity Quarterly,* **4,** 72-79.

Kessler, H.H. (1970). *Disability—Determination and evaluation.* Philadelphia: Lea & Febiger.

Keys, A, Aravanis, C., Blackburn, H., Van Buchem, F.S.P., Buzina, R., Djordjevic, B.S., Fidanza, F., Karvonen, M.J., Menotti, A., Puddu, V., & Taylor, H.L. (1972). Coronary heart disease: Overweight and obesity. *Annals of Internal Medicine,* **77,** 15-27.

Kilburn, J. (1984). Changing attitudes. *Teaching Exceptional Children,* **16**(2), 124-127.

Killian, K.J., Joyce-Petrovich, R.A., Menna, L., & Arena, S.A. (1984). Measuring water orientation and beginner swim skills of autistic individuals. *Adapted Physical Activity Quarterly*, **1**, 287-295.

Kindermann, V.W., Keul, J., & Lehmann, M. (1975). Anaerobe Kapazität bei Kindern und Jugendlichen in Beziehung zum Erwachsenen [Anaerobic capacity of children and adolescents in relation to growth]. *Sportarzt und Sportmedizin*, **6**, 112-115.

Kinney, W.B. (1979). Relationship of body image and perceptual motor performance of trainable mental retardates in a therapeutic recreational setting. *International Journal of Rehabilitation Research*, **2**, 215-224.

Kiphard, E.J. (1973). Sensory-motor training with mentally retarded children. In O. Grüpe (Ed.), *Sport in the modern world—Problems and chances* (pp. 269-271). Berlin: Springer Verlag.

Kiphard, E.J. (1979). *Motopadagogik* [Motor Learning]. Dortmund, West Germany: Verlag Modernes Lernen.

Kiphard, E.J. (1983). Adapted physical education in Germany. In R.L. Eason, T.L. Smith, & F. Caron (Eds.), *Adapted physical activity: From theory to application* (pp. 25-32). Champaign, IL: Human Kinetics.

Kiphard, E.J., & Leger, A. (1975). *Psychomotorische Elementarerziehung: Ein Bildband* [Elementary psychomotor education: An illustrated manual]. Gutersloh, West Germany: Flottmann Verlag.

Kirchhoff, H.W. (1966). Cardiovascular function before and after reconditioning periods in a mountainous terrain. In W. Raab (Ed.), *Prevention of ischemic heart disease: Principles and practice* (pp. 401-408). Springfield, IL: Charles C Thomas.

Kirillyuk, V. (1981). *Sport: The Soviet Union today and tomorrow*. Moscow: Novosti Press Agency.

Kisabeth, K.L., & Richardson, D.B. (1985). Changing attitudes toward disabled individuals: The effect of one disabled person. *Therapeutic Recreation Journal*, **19**(2), 24-33.

Klausen, K., Rasmussen, B., Clausen, J.P., & Trap-Jensen, J. (1974). Blood lactate from exercising extremities before and after arm or leg training. *American Journal of Physiology*, **227**, 67-72.

Klemz, A. (1977). *Blindness and partial sight*. Cambridge: Woodhead-Falkner.

Knowles, C.J. (1983). Individualized instruction for special students: A challenge for change in physical education. In R.L. Eason, T.L. Smith, & F. Caron (Eds.), *Adapted physical activity: From theory to practice* (pp. 53-62). Champaign, IL: Human Kinetics.

Knowlton, R.G., Fitzgerald, P.I., & Sedlock, D.A. (1981). The mechanical efficiency of wheelchair dependent women during wheelchair ergometry. *Canadian Journal of Applied Sport Sciences*, **6**, 187-190.

Knutsson, E., Lewenhaupt-Olsson, E., & Thorsen, M. (1973). Physical work capacity and physical conditioning in paraplegic patients. *Paraplegia*, **11**, 205-216.

Kofsky, P.R., Davis, G.M., Jackson, R.W., Keene, G.C.R., & Shephard, R.J. (1983a). Field-testing—Assessment of physical fitness of disabled adults. *European Journal of Applied Physiology*, **51**, 109-120.

Kofsky, P.R., Davis, G.M., & Shephard, R.J. (1983b). Muscle strength and aerobic power of the lower-limb disabled. *Annali del I.S.E.F.*, **2**, 201-208.

Kofsky, P.R., Davis, G.M., Shephard, R.J., Keene, G.C.R., & Jackson, R.W. (1980). Cardio-respiratory fitness in the lower-limb disabled [Abstract]. *Canadian Journal of Applied Sport Sciences,* **5**.

Kofsky, P.R., Davis, G.M., Shephard, R.J., Keene, G.C.R., & Jackson, R.W. (1982). Strength and aerobic power in the wheelchair bound [Abstract]. *Canadian Journal of Applied Sport Sciences,* **7**.

Kofsky, P.R., & Shephard, R.J. (1985). *Factors influencing fitness and life adjustment of disabled individuals* (final report to Grant 6605-1915-46). Ottawa, ON: Health & Welfare Canada.

Kofsky, P.R., Shephard, R.J., Davis, G.M., & Jackson, R.W. (1986). Fitness classification tables for lower-limb disabled individuals. In C. Sherrill (Ed.), *Sport and disabled athletes* (pp. 147-156). Champaign, IL: Human Kinetics.

Kolko, D.J., Anderson, L., & Campbell, M. (1980). Sensory preference and over-selective responding in autistic children. *Journal of Autism and Developmental Disorders,* **10**, 259-271.

Kraus, H. (1963). *Therapeutic exercise* (2nd ed., pp. 1-249). Springfield, IL: Charles C Thomas.

Krause, R. (1981). Two dimensional echocardiography. In A.S. Abbasi (Ed.), *Echocardiographic interpretation* (pp. 430-455). Springfield, IL: Charles C Thomas.

Kreze, A., Zelinda, M., Julias, J., & Gargara, M. (1974). Relationship between intelligence and relative prevalence of obesity. *Human Biology,* **46**, 109-113.

Krotkiewski, M., Björntorp, P., Sjöstrom, L., & Smith, U. (1983). Impact of obesity on metabolism in men and women: Importance of regional adipose tissue distribution. *Journal of Clinical Investigation,* **72**, 1150-1162.

Kruimer, A. (1985). The classification system of CP-ISRA and its possible problems. In J.H. Hoeberigs & H. Vorsteveld (Eds.), *Proceedings of the Workshop on Disabled and Sports* (pp. 111-117). Amersfoort, Netherlands: Nederlandse Invaliden Sportbond.

Lagerstom, D. (1980). Sports for the deaf. In H. Natvig (Ed.), *First International Medical Congress on Sports for the Disabled* (pp. 100-105). Oslo: Royal Ministry of Church and Education.

Lais, G., & Schurke, P. (1982). Canoeing in the boundary waters: Wilderness inquiry II. *Sports 'N Spokes,* **8**(3).

Lakomy, H.K.A., Campbell, I., & Williams, C. (1987). Treadmill performance and selected physiological characteristics of wheelchair athletes. *British Journal of Sports Medicine,* **21**, 130-133.

LaMere, T., & Labonowich, S. (1984a). The history of sport wheelchairs: 1. Background of the basketball wheelchair. *Sports 'N Spokes,* **9**(6), 6-11.

LaMere, T., & Labonowich, S. (1984b). The history of sport wheelchairs: 2. The racing wheelchair. *Sports 'N Spokes,* **10**(2), 12-16.

Landin, S., Hagenfeldt, L., Saltin, B., & Wahren, J. (1977). Muscle metabolism during exercise in hemiparetic patients. *Clinical Science and Molecular Medicine,* **53**, 257-269.

Langsner, S., & Anderson, S. (1987). Outdoor challenge education and self-esteem and locus of control in children with behavior disorders. *Adapted Physical Activity Quarterly,* **4**, 237-246.

LaPorte, R.E., Brenes, G., Dearwater, S., Murphy, M.A., Cauley, J.A., Dietrick, R., & Robertson, R. (1983). HDL cholesterol across a spectrum of physical activity from quadriplegia to marathon running. *Lancet,* **1**, 1212-1213.

Laughlin, S. (1975). A walking-jogging program for blind persons. *New Outlook for the Blind,* **69**, 312-313.

Lavay, B., Giese, M., Bussen, M., & Dart, S. (1987). Comparison of three measures of predictor VO₂ maximum test protocols of adults with mental retardation: A pilot study. *Mental Retardation,* **25**, 39-42.

Lawrence, G. (1981). *Aquafitness for women.* Toronto: Personal Library.

Lazar, A.L., Demos, G.D., Gaines, L., Rogers, D., & Stirnkorb, M. (1978). Attitudes of handicapped and non-handicapped university students on three attitude scales. *Rehabilitation Literature,* **38**, 49-52.

Lazarus, B., Cullinane, E., & Thompson, P.D. (1981). Comparison of the results and reproducibility of arm and leg exercise tests in men with angina pectoris. *American Journal of Cardiology,* **47**, 1075-1079.

Leatt, P., Shephard, R.J., & Plyley, M. (1987). Specific muscular development in under 18 soccer players. *Journal of Sport Sciences.* **5**, 165-175.

Lebow, F. (1983). Guest spot: Wheelchairs are welcome everywhere, but do they belong in races? *Runners' World,* **18**, 178.

Lee, M., Ward, G., & Shephard, R.J. (1985). Physical capacities of sightless adolescents. *Developmental Medicine and Child Neurology,* **27**, 767-774.

Lehmann, J.F., DeLateur, B.J., Warren, C.G., Simons, B.C., & Guy, A.W. (1969). Biomechanical evaluation of braces for paraplegics. *Archives of Physical Medicine and Rehabilitation,* **50**, 179-188.

Leonard, J.A., (1969). Static and mobile balancing performance of blind adolescent grammar school children. *The New Outlook for the Blind,* **63**, 65-72.

Levarlet-Joye, H. (1978). The development of motor competency in normal and slightly mentally handicapped children. *Padiatrie und Padogologie,* **13**, 357-364.

Levarlet-Joye, H., & Ribauville, A. (1981). Les aptitudes sportives et les possibilités motrices des handicapés mentaux de 12 à 13 ans [Athletic ability and psychomotor potential of mentally handicapped aged 12-13 years]. In J-C. de Potter (Ed.), *Activités physiques adaptées* (pp. 51-57). Bruxelles: Université de Bruxelles.

Levine, H., & Langness, L. (1983). Context, ability and performance: Comparison of competitive athletics among mildly mentally retarded and non-retarded adults. *American Journal of Mental Deficiency,* **87**, 528-538.

Lewallen, R., Quanbury, A.O., Ross, K., & Letts, R.M. (1985). A biomechanical study of normal and amputee gait. In D.A. Winter, R.W. Norman, R.P. Wells, K.C. Hayes, & A.E. Patla (Eds.), *Biomechanics IXA* (pp. 587-591). Champaign, IL: Human Kinetics.

Lewis, S., Higham, L., & Cherry, D. (1985). Development of an exercise program to improve the static and dynamic balance of profoundly hearing impaired children. *American Annals of the Deaf, 130*(4), 278-283.

Lewis, S., Thompson, P., Areskog, N.H., Vodak, P., Marconyak, M., DeBusk, R., Mellan, S., & Haskell, W. (1980). Transfer effects of endurance training to exercise with untrained limbs. *European Journal of Applied Physiology, 44*, 25-34.

Lewko, J.H. (1981). Social and psychological considerations in physical recreation and sport for the disabled. In J.R. Richardson (Ed.), *Report of the Research Priority Development Conference, March 17th and 18th, 1981* (pp. 23-28). Ottawa: Fitness & Amateur Sport.

Lillis, K.M. (1977). *Assessment of needs in physical education and sport in Africa: Report to ICSPE*. Paris: United Nations Educational, Scientific, and Cultural Organisation.

Lindh, M. (1978). Energy expenditure during walking in patients with scoliosis: The effect of surgical correction. *Spine, 3*, 122-134.

Lindsey, D., & O'Neal, J. (1976). Static and dynamic balance skills of eight year old deaf and hearing children. *American Annals of the Deaf, 121*, 49-55.

Lindstrom, H. (1984). Sports for disabled alive and well. *Rehabilitation World, 8*, 12-16.

Lindstrom, H. (1986). Sports classification for locomotor disabilities. In C. Sherrill (Ed.), *Sport and disabled athletes* (pp. 131-136). Champaign, IL: Human Kinetics.

Lipton, B.H. (1970). Role of wheelchair sports in rehabilitation. *International Rehabilitation Review, 21*, 25-27.

Liska, J.S. (1974). Discovering & developing recreation for visually impaired people. In J. Yeo (Ed.), *Recreation for the handicapped* (pp. 80-82). Melbourne: Australian Council for Rehabilitation of Disabled.

Loetze, R. (1981). Judo mit Sherbehinderten und Blinden Kindern [Judo for visually impaired and blind children]. *Praxis der Psychomotorik, 6*, 108-113.

Logan, M., Rubal, B., Raven, P., English, W., & Walters, N. (1981). Heart structure and function of females with multiple sclerosis: A deconditioned population [Abstract]. *Medicine and Science in Sports and Exercise, 13*, 133.

Londeree, B., & Johnson, L. (1974). Motor fitness of TMR vs. EMR and normal children. *Medicine and Science in Sports, 6*, 247-252.

Long, C., & Lawton, E.B. (1955). Functional significance of spinal cord lesion level. *Archives of Physical Medicine and Rehabilitation, 36*, 249-255.

Lorenzen, H. (1961). *Lehrbuch des Versehrtensports* [Textbook of sport for the visually impaired]. Stuttgart: Ferdinand Enke Verlag.

Lotter, V. (1966). Services for a group of autistic children in Middlesex. In J.K. Wing (Ed.). *Early childhood autism* (pp. 241-255). London: Pergamon Press.

Loy, J.W., & Ingham, A. (1973). Play, games and sport in the psychological development of child and youth. In G.L. Rarick (Ed.), *Physical activity: Human growth and development* (pp. 257-302). New York: Academic Press.

Lundberg, A. (1973). Changes in the working pulse during the school year in adolescents with cerebral palsy. *Scandinavian Journal of Rehabilitation Medicine, 5*, 12-17.

Lundberg, A. (1975). Mechanical efficiency in bicycle ergometer work of young adults with cerebral palsy. *Developmental Medicine and Child Neurology,* **17**, 434-439.

Lundberg, A. (1976). Oxygen consumption in relation to workload in students with cerebral palsy. *Journal of Applied Physiology,* **40**, 873-875.

Lundberg, A. (1978). Maximal aerobic capacity of young people with spastic cerebral palsy. *Developmental Medicine and Child Neurology,* **20**, 205-210.

Lundberg, A. (1980). Wheelchair driving: Evaluation of a new training outfit. *Scandinavian Journal of Rehabilitation Medicine,* **12**, 67-72.

Lundberg, A., Ovenfors, C.O., & Saltin, B. (1967). Effect of physical training on schoolchildren with cerebral palsy. *Acta Paediatrica Scandinavica,* **56**, 182-188.

Lundberg, A., & Pernow, B. (1970). The effect of physical training on oxygen utilization and lactate formation in the exercising muscle of adolescents with motor handicaps. *Scandinavian Journal of Clinical and Laboratory Investigation,* **26**, 89-96.

Lundberg, O. (1973). Methods of estimating morbidity and prevalence of disablement by use of mortality statistics. *Acta Psychiatrica Scandinavica,* **49**, 324-331.

Lüschen, G. (1970). The interdependence of sport and culture. In G. Lüschen (Ed.), *The cross-cultural analysis of sport and games* (pp. 85-99). Champaign, IL: Stipes.

Lussier, L., Knight, J., Bell, G., Lohman, T., & Morris, A.F. (1983). Body composition comparison in two elite female wheelchair athletes. *Paraplegia,* **21**, 16-22.

Luyben, P.D., Funk, D.M., Morgan, J.K., Clark, K.A., & Delulio, D.W. (1986). Team sports for the severely retarded: Training a side of the foot soccer pass using a maximum-to-minimum prompt reduction strategy. *Journal of Applied Behavior Analysis,* **19**, 431-436.

Lynch, F.W., & Stein, R. (1982). Perspectives on parent participation in special education. *Special Education,* **3**, 56-63.

MacGowan, H.E. (1983). The kinematic analysis of the walking gait of congenitally blind and sighted children: Ages 6-10 years. *Dissertation Abstracts International,* **44**, 703A.

MacGowan, H.E. (1985). Kinematic analysis of the walking gait of sighted and congenitally blind children: Ages 6-10 years. In D.A. Winter, R.W. Norman, R.P. Wells, K.C. Hayes, & A.E. Patla (Eds.), *Biomechanics IXA* (pp. 575-580). Champaign, IL: Human Kinetics.

MacGregor, D. (1980). Classification system for cerebral palsy competitive sport. In H. Natvig (Ed.), *First International Medical Congress on Sports for the Disabled.* Oslo: Royal Ministry of Church and Education.

MacIntosh, D., Franks, C.E.S., & Bedecki, T. (1986). Canadian government involvement in sport: Some consequences and issues. In G. Redmond (Ed.), *Sport and politics* (pp. 21-26). Champaign, IL: Human Kinetics.

Magel, J.R., Foglia, G.F., McArdle, W.D., Gutlin, B., Pechar, G.S., & Katch, F.I. (1975). Specificity of swim training on maximum oxygen uptake. *Journal of Applied Physiology,* **38**, 151-155.

Magel, J.R., McArdle, W.D., Toner, M., & Delio, D.J. (1978). Metabolic and cardiovascular adjustments to arm training. *Journal of Applied Physiology,* **45**, 75-79.

Maki, B.E., Rosen, J.H., & Simon, R. (1985). Modification of spastic gait through mechanical damping. *Journal of Biomechanics,* **18**, 431-443.

Maksud, M.G., & Hamilton, L.H. (1974). Physiological responses of EMR children to strenuous exercise. *American Journal of Mental Deficiency,* **79**, 32-38.

Malkia, E.A., Joukamaa, M., Maatela, J., Aromaa, A., & Heliovaara, M. (1987). The physical activity of mentally disturbed Finnish adults. In M. Berridge & G. Ward (Eds.), *International perspectives in adapted physical activity* (pp. 149-156). Champaign, IL: Human Kinetics.

Mangum, M., Ribisl, P.M., & Miller, H.S. (1983). The prediction of oxygen consumption during arm work ergometry. *Journal of Sports Sciences,* **1**, 121-130.

Margaria, R. (1966). An outline for setting significant tests of muscular performance. In H. Yoshimura & J.S. Weiner (Eds.), *Human adaptability and its methodology* (pp. 205-211). Tokyo: Society for the Promotion of Sciences.

Marincek, C.R.T. (1980). Exercise testing of paraplegic sportsmen. In H. Natvig (Ed.), *First International Medical Congress on Sports for the Disabled.* Oslo: Royal Ministry of Church and Education.

Marincek, C.R.T., & Valencic, V. (1978). Arm cyclo-ergometry and kinetics of oxygen consumption in paraplegics. *Paraplegia,* **15**, 178-185.

Marr, S. (1987). *Socialization into sport of persons with spina bifida.* Unpublished master's thesis, Texas Women's University, Denton.

Marshall, T. (1982). Marathons and road racing. *Sports 'N Spokes,* **8**, 27.

Martens, R. (1974). Arousal and motor performance. *Exercise and Sport Sciences Review,* **2**, 155-188.

Martens, R. (1986). Youth sport in the USA. In M.R. Weiss & D. Gould (Eds.), *Sport for Children and Youth* (pp. 27-33). Champaign, IL: Human Kinetics.

Martinek, T.J., & Karper, W.B. (1981). Teachers' expectations for handicapped and non-handicapped children in mainstreamed physical education classes. *Perceptual and Motor Skills,* **53**, 327-330.

Marwick, C. (1984). Wheelchair calisthenics keeps patients fit [Letter]. *Journal of the American Medical Association,* **251**, 303.

Massie, J.M., & Shephard, R.J. (1971). Physiological and psychological effects of training. *Medicine and Science in Sports,* **3**, 110-117.

Mastro, J.V., & French, R. (1986). Sport anxiety and blind athletes. In C. Sherrill (Ed.), *Sport and disabled athletes* (pp. 203-208). Champaign, IL: Human Kinetics.

Mastro, J., French, R., Henschen, K., & Horvat, M. (1986). Selected psychological characteristics of blind golfers and their coaches. *American Corrective Therapy Journal,* **40**, 111-114.

Mastro, J., Sherrill, C., Gench, B., & French, R. (1987). Psychological characteristics of elite visually impaired athletes: The iceberg profile. *Journal of Sport Behavior,* **10**, 39-46.

Mathias, C.J., Christensen, N.J., Corbett, J.L., Frankel, H.L., & Spalding, J.M.K. (1976a). Plasma catecholamines during paroxysmal neurogenic hypertension in quadriplegic man. *Circulation Research*, **39**, 204-208.

Mathias, C.J., Frankel, H.L., Christensen, N.J., & Spalding, J. (1976b). Enhanced pressor response to noradrenaline in patients with cervical spinal cord transection. *Brain*, **99**, 757-770.

Mathias, C.J., Hillier, K., Frankel, H.L., & Spalding, J.M.K. (1975). Plasma prostaglandin E during neurogenic hypertension in tetraplegic man. *Clinical Science and Molecular Medicine*, **49**, 625-628.

Maughan, R.J., Watson, J.S., & Weir, J. (1983). Relationship between muscle strength and muscle cross-sectional area in male sprinters and endurance runners. *European Journal of Applied Physiology*, **50**, 309-318.

McBeath, A.A., Bahrke, M., & Balke, B. (1974). Efficiency of assisted ambulation determined by oxygen consumption measurement. *Journal of Bone and Joint Surgery* (America), **56**, 994-1000.

McCafferty, W.R., & Horvath, S.M. (1977). Specificity of exercise and specificity of training: A sub-cellular response. *Research Quarterly*, **48**, 358-371.

McCann, B.C. (1979a). Wheelchair medical classification system. In R.D. Steadward (Ed.), *Proceedings of First International Conference on Sport and Training of the Physically Disabled Athlete* (pp. 1-24). Edmonton: University of Alberta.

McCann, B.C. (1979b). Problems and future trends in classifying disabled athletes. In R.D. Steadward (Ed.), *Proceedings of First International Conference on Sport and Training of the Physically Disabled Athlete* (pp. 25-35). Edmonton: University of Alberta.

McCann, B.C. (1984). Classification of the locomotor disabled for competitive sports: Theory and practice. *International Journal of Sports Medicine*, **5**(Suppl.), 167-170.

McCann, B.C. (1985). I.S.M.G.F. classification problems. In J.H. Hoeberigs & H. Vorsteveld (Eds.), *Proceedings of the Workshop on Disabled and Sports* (pp. 90-96). Amersfoort, Netherlands: Nederlandse Invaliden Sportbond.

McCann, B.C. (1987). The structure and future of sport for the disabled: The Arnhem seminar. *Palaestra*, **3**(4), 9-11, 40.

McCormick, D.P. (1984). Handicapped skiing: An overview. In R.C. Cantu (Ed.), *Clinical sports medicine* (pp. 63-70). Lexington: Collamore Press.

McCormick, D.P. (1985). Injuries in handicapped Alpine ski racers. *The Physician and Sportsmedicine*, **13**, 93-97.

McCubbin, J.A., & Jansma, P. (1987). The effects of training selected psychomotor skills and the relationship to adaptive behavior. In M.E. Berridge & G. Ward (Eds.), *International perspectives in adapted physical activity* (pp. 119-126). Champaign, IL: Human Kinetics.

McCubbin, J.A., & Shasby, G.B. (1985). Effects of isokinetic exercise on adolescents with cerebral palsy. *Adapted Physical Activity Quarterly*, **2**, 56-64.

McDonald, J.J., & Chusid, J.G. (1952). *Correlative anatomy and functional neurology*. Los Airos, CA: Lange Medical.

McDonell, E., Brassard, L., & Taylor, A.W. (1980). Effects of an arm ergometer training program on wheelchair subjects [Abstract]. *Canadian Journal of Applied Sport Sciences, 5*.

McFayden, G.M., & Stoner, D.L. (1980). Polyurethane foam wheelchair cushions: Retention of supportive properties. *Archives of Physical Medicine and Rehabilitation, 61*, 234-237.

McGill, S.M., & Dainty, D.A. (1984). Computer analysis of energy transfer in children walking with crutches. *Archives of Physical Medicine and Rehabilitation, 65*, 115-120.

McIntosh, P.C. (1980). *"Sport for all" programmes throughout the world* (UNESCO Contract 207604). Paris: United Nations Educational, Scientific and Cultural Organisation.

McKenzie, D.C., Fox, E.L., & Cohen, K. (1978). Specificity of metabolic and circulatory responses to arm or leg interval training. *European Journal of Applied Physiology, 39*, 241-248.

McLeish, E. (1983). In-service training in physical education for teachers in inner London schools for the educationally subnormal. In R.L. Eason, T.L. Smith, & F. Caron (Eds.), *Adapted physical activity: From theory to application* (pp. 13-18). Champaign, IL: Human Kinetics.

Menon, P.G. (1970). The handicapped as people. *Journal of Rehabilitation in Asia, 11*, 5-7.

Merkel, K.D., Miller, N.E., Westbrook, P.R., & Merritt, J.L. (1984). Energy expenditure of paraplegic patients standing and walking with two knee-ankle-foot orthoses. *Archives of Physical Medicine and Rehabilitation, 65*, 121-124.

Michael, J. (1986). Prosthetic feet for the amputee athlete. *Palaestra, 2*(3), 37-41.

Miles, D.S., Sawka, M.N., Glaser, R.M., Wilde, S.W., Doerr, B.M., & Frey, M.A.B. (1984). Central hemodynamics during progressive upper- and lower-body exercise and recovery. *Journal of Applied Physiology, 57*, 366-370.

Miles, D.S., Sawka, M.N., Wilde, S.W., Durbin, R.J., Gotshall, R.W., & Glaser, R.M. (1982). Pulmonary function changes in wheelchair athletes subsequent to exercise training. *Ergonomics, 25*, 239-246.

Millar, A.L. (1984). *The effect of endurance running on $\dot{V}O_2$max of Down's syndrome adolescents and young adults*. Unpublished doctoral dissertation, Arizona State University, Tempe.

Miller, D.I. (1981). Minireview: Biomechanical considerations in lower extremity amputee running and sports performance. *Australian Journal of Sports Medicine, 13*, 55-67.

Miller, E. (1958). Cerebral palsy children and their parents: A study in parent-child relationships. *Exceptional Child, 24*, 298-302.

Miller, N.E., Merritt, J.L., Merkel, K.D., & Westbrook, P.R. (1984). Paraplegic energy expenditure during negotiation of architectural barriers. *Archives of Physical Medicine and Rehabilitation, 65*, 778-779.

Molbech, S. (1966). Energy cost in level walking in subjects with an abnormal gait. In K. Evang & K.L. Andersen (Eds.), *Physical activity in health and disease* (pp. 146-155). Baltimore: Williams & Wilkins.

Molén, N.H. (1973). Energy/speed relation of below-knee amputees walking on motor-driven treadmill. *Internationale Zeitschrift für Angewandte Physiologie,* **31,** 173-185.

Moller, M.H.L., Oberg, B.E., & Gillquist, J. (1985). Stretching exercise and soccer: Effect of stretching on range of motion in the lower extremity in connection with soccer training. *International Journal of Sports Medicine,* **6,** 50-52.

Mollinger, L.A., Spurr, G.B., El Ghatit, A.Z., Barboriak, J.J., Rooney, C.B., Davidoff, D.D., & Bongard, R.D. (1985). Daily energy expenditure and basal metabolic rates of patients with spinal cord injury. *Archives of Physical Medicine and Rehabilitation,* **66,** 420-426.

Monnazzi, G. (1982). Paraplegics and sports: A psychological survey. *International Journal of Sports Psychology,* **13,** 85-95.

Montgomery, D.L., Reid, G., & Seidl, C. (in press). The effects of a physical fitness program on CSTF results by mentally retarded adults. *Canadian Journal of Applied Sport Sciences.*

Moon, M.S., & Renzaglia, K. (1982). Physical fitness and the mentally retarded: A critical review of the literature. *Journal of Special Education,* **16,** 268-287.

Moran, J.M., & Kalakian, L.H. (1977). *Movement experiences for the mentally retarded or emotionally disturbed child.* Minneapolis: Burgess.

Morgan, W.P. (1974). Exercise and mental disorders. In A.J. Ryan & F.L. Allman (Eds.), *Sports medicine.* New York: Academic Press.

Morgan, W.P. (1982). Psychological effects of exercise. *Behavioral Medicine Update,* **4,** 25-30.

Morganroth, J., Maron, B.J., Henry, W.L., & Epstein, S.E. (1975). Comparative left ventricular dimensions in trained athletes. *Annals of Internal Medicine,* **82,** 521-524.

Morisbak, I. (1980). Sports for the blind and partially sighted. In H. Natvig (Ed.), *First International Medical Congress on Sports for the Disabled* (pp. 93-99). Oslo: Royal Ministry of Church and Education.

Morton, H.W. (1963). *Soviet sport.* New York: Collier.

Mueller, A.D. (1962). Psychological factors in the rehabilitation of the paraplegic patients. *Archives of Physical Medicine and Rehabilitation,* **43,** 151-159.

Mulholland, R., & McNeill, A.W. (1985). Cardiovascular responses of three profoundly retarded, multiply handicapped children during selected motor activities. *Adapted Physical Activity Quarterly,* **2,** 151-160.

Muller, E.A., & Hettinger, T. (1953). Der Einfluss der Gehgeschwindigkeit auf den Energie-umsatz beim Gehen und das Gangbild des Kunstbeträgers [Effect of the speed of gait on the energy transformation in walking with artificial legs]. *Zeitschrift für Orthopädie und ihre Grenzgebiete,* **83,** 620-627.

Munaf, M., & Boenik, U. (1984). Verbesserter Pruef—Und Bewertungmethoden fuer Rollstuehle. In R. Scheunemann & F. Unz (Eds.), *Rollstühlentwicklung Deutsch-britische Statuskolloquium 1984* [German/British Colloquium 1984 on wheelchair design] (pp. 115-129). Bonn: Reha Verlag.

Munro, A.F., & Robinson, R. (1960). The catecholamine content of peripheral plasma in human subjects with complete transverse lesion of the spinal cord. *Journal of Physiology* (London), **154**, 244-253.

Murray, M.P., Mollinger, L.A., Sepic, S.B., Gardner, G.M., & Linder, M.T. (1983). Gait patterns in above-knee amputee patients: Hydraulic swing control vs constant friction knee components. *Archives of Physical Medicine and Rehabilitation,* **64**, 339-345.

Mushier, C.L. (1972). Personality and selected women athletes: A cross-sectional study. *International Journal of Sports Psychology,* **3**, 25-31.

Myklebust, H.R. (1964). *The psychology of deafness.* New York: Grune & Stratton.

Naftachi, N.E., Vian, A.T., Sell, G.H., & Lowman, E.W. (1980). Mineral metabolism in spinal cord injury. *Archives of Physical Medicine and Rehabilitation,* **61**, 139-142.

Nag, P.K., Panikar, J.T., Malvankar, M.G., Pradhan, C.K., & Chatterjee, S.K. (1982). Performance evaluation of lower extremity disabled people with reference to handcranked tricycle propulsion. *Applied Ergonomics,* **13**, 171-176.

Najenson, T., & Levy, M. (1971). Rehabilitation of amputees due to progressive vascular disease. In U. Simri (Ed.), *Sports as a means of rehabilitation* (pp. 5/1-5/15). Natanya, Israel: Wingate Institute.

Nakamura, Y. (1973). Working ability of the paraplegics. *Paraplegia,* **11**, 182-193.

Naor, M., & Milgram, R.A. (1980). Two pre-service strategies for preparing regular class teachers for mainstreaming. *Exceptional Children,* **47**, 126-129.

Natvig, H., Biering-Sorensen, F., & Jorgensen, P. (1980). Proposal for classification of athletes with "other locomotor disabilities." In H. Natvig (Ed.), *First International Medical Congress on Sports for the Disabled.* Oslo: Royal Ministry of Church and Education.

Nelipovich, M. (1983). Alcoholism and the visually impaired client. *Journal of Visual Impairment and Blindness,* **77**, 345-347.

Nelipovich, M., & Parker, R. (1981). The visually impaired substance abuser. *Journal of Visual Impairment and Blindness,* **75**, 305.

Nelson, R.R., Gobel, F.L., Jorgensen, C.R., Wang, K., Wang, Y., & Taylor, H.L. (1974). Hemodynamic predictors of myocardial oxygen consumption during static and dynamic exercise. *Circulation,* **50**, 1179-1189.

Nesbitt, J.A. (1983). Recreation for handicapped in the United States: A historical perspective. In R.L. Eason, T.L. Smith, & F. Caron (Eds.), *Adapted physical activity: From theory to application* (pp. 95-110). Champaign, IL: Human Kinetics.

Nichols, P.J. (1979). Wheelchair users' shoulder. *Scandinavian Journal of Rehabilitation Medicine,* **11**, 9-32.

Nilsson, S., Staff, D., & Pruett, E. (1975). Physical work capacity and the effect of training on subjects with long standing paraplegia. *Scandinavian Journal of Rehabilitation Medicine,* **7**, 51-56.

Nixon, H.L. (1988). Getting over the worry hurdle: Parental encouragement and the sports involvement of visually impaired children and youths. *Adapted Physical Activity Quarterly, 5,* 29-43.

Nordgren, B. (1970). Physical capabilities in a group of mentally retarded adults. *Scandinavian Journal of Rehabilitation Medicine, 2,* 125-132.

Nordgren, B. (1971). Physical capacity and training in a group of young adult mentally retarded persons. *Acta Paediatrica Scandinavica* (Suppl. 217), 119-121.

Nordgren, B. (1972). Physiological aspects of the rehabilitation of young mentally retarded persons. *Europa Medicophysica, 8,* 1-4.

Nordgren, B., & Backstrom, L. (1971). Correlations between muscular strength and industrial work performance in mentally retarded persons. *Acta Paediatrica Scandinavica,* (Suppl. 217), 122-126.

Nowicki, S., & Strickland, B.R. (1973). A locus of control scale for children. *Journal of Consulting and Clinical Psychology, 40,* 148-154.

Oberg, B.E., Moller, M., Ekstrand, J., & Gillquist, J. (1984). Muscle strength and flexibility in different positions of soccer players. *International Journal of Sports Medicine, 5,* 213-216.

Odeen, I. (1972). *Training of physical work capacity in wheelchair patients.* Sollentuna, Sweden: Rehabforlaget.

Ohry, A., Molho, M., & Rozin, R. (1975). Alterations of pulmonary function in spinal cord injured patients. *Paraplegia, 13,* 101-108.

Ornitz, E.M., Guthrie, D., & Farley, A.J. (1977). The early development of autistic children. *Journal of Autism and Childhood Schizophrenia, 7,* 208-229.

Ornstein, L.J., Skrinar, G.S., & Garrett, G.G. (1983). Physiological effects of swimming training in physically disabled individuals [Abstract]. *Medicine and Science in Sports and Exercise, 15,* 110.

Owens, N.F. (1968). *A study of personality changes in males with severe facial deformity during the first six months of adjustment after radical surgery for cancer* (Doctoral dissertation, New York University, 1968). *Dissertation Abstracts International, 30,* 722B.

Pachalski, A., & Mekarski, T. (1980). Effect of swimming on increasing of cardiorespiratory capacity of paraplegics. *Paraplegia, 18,* 190-196.

Padden, D.A. (1959). Ability of deaf swimmers to orient themselves when submerged in water. *Research Quarterly, 30,* 214-226.

Pandolf, K.B., Billings, D.S., Drolet, L.L., Pimental, N.A., & Sawka, M.N. (1984). Differentiated ratings of perceived exertion and various physiological responses during prolonged upper and lower body exercise. *European Journal of Applied Physiology, 53,* 5-11.

Parker, A.W., Bronks, R., & Snyder, C.W. (1986). Walking patterns in Down's syndrome. *Journal of Mental Deficiency Research, 30,* 317-330.

Pascoe, C. (1971, September). Towards a brighter tomorrow. *Canadian Doctor,* pp. 41-46.

Patrick, G.D. (1986). The effects of wheelchair competition on self-concept and acceptance of disability in novice athletes. *Therapeutic Recreation Journal, 20*(4), 61-71.

Patrick, G.D. (1987). Improving attitudes towards disabled persons. *Adapted Physical Activity Quarterly, 4,* 316-325.

Patton, J.F., & Duggan, A. (1985). Upper and lower body anaerobic power in elite biathletes [Abstract]. *Medicine and Science in Sports and Exercise, 17,* 247.

Pavlov, S. (1980). Physical culture and sport in socialist society. *Social Sciences, 2,* 13.

Peake, P., & Leonard, J.A. (1971). The use of heart rate as an index of stress in blind pedestrians. *Ergonomics, 14,* 189-204.

Peizer, E. (1961). On the energy requirements for prosthesis use by geriatric amputees. In *Conference on the Geriatric Amputee* (pp. 146-150, Publication No. 919). Washington, DC: National Academy of Sciences, National Research Council.

Peizer, E., Wright, D., & Freiberger, H. (1964). Bioengineering methods of wheelchair evaluation. *Bulletin of Prosthetics Research, 10,* 77-100.

Pender, R.H., & Patterson, P.E. (1982). A comparison of selected motor fitness items between congenitally deaf and hearing children. *Journal for Special Educators* (Valley Cottage, NY), **18**(4), 71-75.

Pendergast, S., Cerretelli, P., & Rennie, D.W. (1979). Aerobic and glycolytic metabolism in arm exercise. *Journal of Applied Physiology, 47,* 754-760.

Pennella, L. (1979). Motor ability and the deaf: Research implications. *American Annals of the Deaf, 124,* 366-372.

Perrault, H., Perronet, F., Cleroux, J., Cousineau, D., Nadeau, R., Pham-Huy, H., & Tremblay, G. (1978). Electro- and echocardiographic assessment of left ventricle before and after training in man [Abstract]. *Canadian Journal of Applied Sports Sciences, 3,* 180.

Persyn, U., & Hoeven, R. (1981). The balance problem in the crawlstroke of paralyzed swimmers. In J-C. de Potter (Ed.), *Activités physiques adaptées* (pp. 301-310). Brussels: Université de Bruxelles.

Persyn, U., Surmont, R.E., Wouters, L., & De Maeyer, J. (1975). Analysis of techniques used by swimmers in the Para-Olympic Games. In L. Lewillie & J.P. Clarys (Eds.), *Swimming II* (pp. 276-281). Baltimore: University Park Press.

Petrofsky, J.S. (1986). *Demonstration of electrical stimulation.* Paper presented at the Conference of International Committee on Physical Fitness Research, Jerusalem.

Petrofsky, J.S., Phillips, C.A., Sawka, M.N., Hanpeter, D., & Stafford, D. (1981). Blood flow and metabolism during isometric contractions in cat skeletal muscle. *Journal of Applied Psychology, 50,* 493-502.

Pilonchery, G., Minaire, P., Milan, J.J., & Revol, A. (1983). Urinary elimination of glycosaminoglycans during the immobilization osteoporosis of spinal cord injury patients. *Clinical Orthopedics and Related Research, 174,* 230-235.

Pimental, N.A., Sawka, M.N., Billings, D.S., & Trad, L.A. (1984). Physiological responses to prolonged upper body exercise. *Medicine and Science in Sports and Exercise, 16,* 360-365.

Polednak, A.P., & Auliffe, J. (1976). Obesity in institutionalized adult mentally retarded populations. *Journal of Mental Deficiency Research, 20,* 9-15.

Pollock, M.L. (1973). The quantification of endurance training programs. *Exercise and Sports Science Reviews,* **1,** 155-188.

Pollock, M.L., Miller, H., Linnerud, A., Laughridge, E., Coleman, E., & Alexander, E. (1974). Arm pedalling as an endurance training regimen for the disabled. *Archives of Physical Medicine and Rehabilitation,* **55,** 418-423.

Pomeroy, J. (1983). Recreation unlimited: Responding to persons with severe disabilities. In R.L. Eason, T.L. Smith, & F. Caron (Eds.), *Adapted physical activity: From theory to application* (pp. 111-123). Champaign, IL: Human Kinetics.

Pooley, J.C. (1978). Quantitative and qualitative analysis in comparative physical education and sport. In U. Simri (Ed.), *Comparative physical education and sport* (pp. 83-93). Natanya, Israel: Wingate Institute.

Pope, C.J. (1985). Sprint running in elite cerebral-palsied athletes: A kinematic analysis. Unpublished doctoral dissertation, Texas Women's University, Denton.

Pope, C.J. (1986, April). *A comparison of biomechanical characteristics based on limb involvement of elite cerebral palsied athletes performing a sprint run.* Paper presented at the American Alliance for Health, Physical Education, Recreation and Dance, Cincinnati, OH.

Pope, C.J., McGrain, P., & Arnhold, R.W. (1986). Running gait of the blind: A kinematic analysis. In C. Sherrill (Ed.), *Sport and disabled athletes* (pp. 173-177). Champaign, IL: Human Kinetics.

Pope, C.J., & Wilkerson, J. (1986, July). *A comparison of kinematic characteristics of elite cerebral palsied and able-bodied athletes performing a sprint run: Implications for improving performance.* Paper presented at International Sports Biomechanics Society, Halifax.

Potter, C.N., & Silverman, L.N. (1984). Characteristics of vestibular function and static balance skills in deaf children. *Journal of the American Physical Therapy Association,* **64,** 1071-1075.

Powers, S.K., Beadle, R.E., & Mangum, M. (1984). Exercise efficiency during arm ergometry: Effects of speed and work rate. *Journal of Applied Physiology,* **56,** 495-499.

President's Council on Physical Fitness and Sports. (1985). *National school population fitness survey.* Washington, DC: Author.

Price, R.J. (1986). The status of international activity in recreation, sports, and cultural activities with disabled persons. *Palaestra,* **3**(1), 32-37.

Price, R.J. (1987). Spinal cord injury, life stage and leisure satisfaction. In M. Berridge & G. Ward (Eds.), *International perspectives on adapted physical activity* (pp. 14). Champaign, IL: Human Kinetics.

Prior, M.R., & Chen, C.S. (1975). Learning set acquisition in autistic children. *Journal of Abnormal Psychology,* **84,** 701-708.

Pueschel, S.M. (1984). *The young child with Down's syndrome.* New York: Human Sciences Press.

Quintner, J. (1974). Recreation in the rehabilitation centre. In J. Yeo (Ed.), *Recreation for the handicapped* (pp. 48-51). Melbourne: Australian Council for Rehabilitation of Disabled.

Ragnarsson, K.T., Sell, H.G., McGarrity, M., & Reuven, O. (1975). Pneumatic orthosis for paraplegic patients: Functional evaluation and prescription considerations. *Archives of Physical Medicine and Rehabilitation,* **56**, 479-493.

Rainbolt, W., & Sherrill, C. (1987). Characteristics of blind athletes, competition experience and training practices. In M. Berridge & G. Ward (Eds.), *International perspectives on adapted physical activity* (pp. 165-171). Champaign, IL: Human Kinetics.

Ralston, H.J. (1965). Effects of immobilization of various body segments on the energy cost of human locomotion. In *Proceedings of the Second International Ergonomics Association Congress, Dortmund, 1964.* (Supplement to *Ergonomics,* **7**, 53-60).

Rappoport, A. (1982). Sledge hockey: Alternative to ice hockey for the disabled. *Sports 'N Spokes,* **8**(4), 24-25.

Rarick, G.L. (1971). *Special Olympics: Survey of adult reactions in two metropolitan areas.* Berkeley: University of California.

Rarick, G.L. (1980a). The factor structure of the motor domain of mentally retarded children and adolescents. In M. Ostyn, G. Beunen, & J. Simons (Eds.), *Kinanthropometry II* (pp. 149-160). Baltimore: University Park Press.

Rarick, G.L. (1980b). Cognitive-motor relationships in the growing years. *Research Quarterly for Exercise and Sport,* **51**, 174-192.

Rarick, G.L., & Beuter, A.C. (1985). The effect of mainstreaming on the motor performance of mentally retarded and non-handicapped students. *Adapted Physical Activity Quarterly,* **2**, 272-282.

Rarick, G.L., Dobbins, D.A., & Broadhead, G.D. (1976). *The motor domain and its correlates in educationally handicapped children.* Englewood Cliffs, NJ: Prentice-Hall.

Rarick, G.L., Widdop, J., & Broadhead, G.D. (1970). *The physical fitness and motor performance of educable mentally retarded children. Exceptional Children,* **36**, 509-512.

Rasmussen, B., Klausen, K., Clausen, J.P., & Trap-Jensen, J. (1975). Pulmonary ventilation, blood gases, and blood pH after training of the arms or the legs. *Journal of Applied Physiology,* **38**, 250-256.

Rathbone, J.L., & Lucas, C. (1970). *Recreation in total rehabilitation.* Springfield, IL: Charles C Thomas.

Reichenbach, M. (1973). Riding as a therapy. In O. Grüpe (Ed.), *Sport in the modern world* (pp. 261-262). Berlin: Springer Verlag.

Reid, G., Collier, D., & Morin, B. (1983). The motor performance of autistic individuals. In R.L. Eason, T.L. Smith, & F. Caron (Eds.), *Adapted physical activity: From theory to application* (pp. 201-218). Champaign, IL: Human Kinetics.

Reid, G., Montgomery, D.L., & Seidl, C. (1985). Performance of mentally retarded adults on the Canadian Standardized Test of Fitness. *Canadian Journal of Public Health,* **76**, 187-190.

Reybrouck, T., Heigenhauser, G.F., & Faulkner, J.A. (1975). Limitations to maximal oxygen uptake in arm, leg and combined arm-leg ergometry. *Journal of Applied Physiology,* **38**, 774-779.

Rhodes, E.C., McKenzie, D.C., Coutts, K.D., & Rogers, A.R. (1981). A field test for the prediction of aerobic capacity in male paraplegics and quadraplegics. *Canadian Journal of Applied Sport Sciences,* **6**, 182-186.

Ribadi, H., Rider, R.A., & Toole, T. (1987). A comparison of static and dynamic balance in congenitally blind, sighted and sighted blindfolded adolescents. *Adapted Physical Activity Quarterly,* **4**, 220-225.

Richardson, S.A., & Green, A. (1971). When is black beautiful: Colored and white children's reaction to skin color. *British Journal of Educational Psychology,* **41**(1), 62-69.

Riches, E.W. (1943). The methods and results of treatment in cases of paralysis of the bladder following spinal injury. *British Journal of Surgery,* **31**, 135-139.

Riddle, P.K. (1980). Attitudes, beliefs, behavioural intentions and behaviors of women and men toward regular jogging. *Research Quarterly,* **51**, 663-674.

Ridgway, M., Hamilton, N., Hendrick, B., Nirse, M., & Adrian, M. (1987, October 22-24). *Comparison of two wheelchair propulsion strokes during acceleration.* Paper presented at the Conference on Physical Activity for the Exceptional Individual, Fresno, CA.

Ridgway, M., Morse, M., Hendrick, B., Adrian, M., & Hamilton, N. (1987, October 22-24). *3-D hand patterns during wheelchair propulsion.* Paper presented at the Conference on Physical Activity for the Exceptional Individual, Fresno, CA.

Riechert, H., Bruhn, L., Schwalm, U., & Schnizer, W. (1977). Ein Ausdauerstraining im Rahmen des Schulsports bei vorwiegend spastisch gelähmten Kindern [Endurance training in physical education lessons for spastic handicapped children]. *Medizinische Welt,* **28**, 1694-1701.

Rimland, B. (1964). *Infantile autism: The syndrome and its implications for a neural theory of behavior.* New York: Appleton-Century Croft.

Rincover, A., Cook, R., Peoples, A., & Packard, D. (1979). Using sensory extinction and sensory reinforcement principles for programming multiple adaptive behavior change. *Journal of Applied Behavior Analysis,* **12**, 221-233.

Rizzo, T.L. (1984). Attitudes of physical educators toward teaching handicapped pupils. *Adapted Physical Activity Quarterly,* **1**, 267-274.

Roberts, K. (1974). Sports for the disabled. *Physiotherapy,* **60**, 271-274.

Robertson, B.L. (1977). A therapeutic program for muscular dystrophy. *American Corrective Therapy Journal,* **31**, 70-74.

Robertson, B.L. (1980). A therapeutic program for the spastic child. *American Corrective Therapy Journal,* **34**, 102-104.

Robertson, I. (1986). Youth sport in Australia. In M.R. Weiss & D. Gould (Eds.), *Sport for children and youths* (pp. 3-10). Champaign, IL: Human Kinetics.

Robin, G.C., Span, Y., Steinberg, R., Makin, M., & Menczel, J. (1982). Scoliosis in the elderly: A follow-up study. *Spine,* **7**, 355-368.

Robson, P. (1968). The prevalence of scoliosis in adolescents and young adults with cerebral palsy. *Developmental Medicine and Child Neurology,* **10**, 417-452.

Rocha-Ferreira, M.B. (1986). Youth sport in Brazil. In M.R. Weiss & D. Gould (Eds.), *Sport for children and youths* (pp. 11-15). Champaign, IL: Human Kinetics.

Roeren, F.R. (1987). Sport for all: Sailing is fun. In M. Berridge & G. Ward (Eds.), *International perspectives on adapted physical activity* (pp. 209-211). Champaign, IL: Human Kinetics.

Rosen, N.B. (1973). The role of sports in rehabilitation of the handicapped. *Maryland State Medical Journal,* **22,** 35-39.

Rosenzweig, M. (1987). Horseback riding: The therapeutic sport. in M. Berridge & G. Ward (Eds.), *International perspectives on adapted physical activity* (pp. 213-219). Champaign, IL: Human Kinetics.

Rosman, N., & Spira, E. (1974). Paraplegic use of walking braces: A survey. *Archives of Physical Medicine and Rehabilitation,* **55,** 310-314.

Ross, C.D. (1983). Leisure in the deinstitutionalization process: A vehicle for change. *Journal of Leisurability,* **10,** 13-19.

Roswall, G.M., Roswall, P.M., & Dunleavy, A.O. (1986). Normative health related fitness data for special Olympians. In C. Sherrill (Ed.), *Sport and disabled athletes* (pp. 231-238). Champaign, IL: Human Kinetics.

Rotter, J.B. (1975). Some problems and misconceptions related to the construct validity of internal versus external control of reinforcement. *Journal of Consulting and Clinical Psychology,* **43,** 56-67.

Rotzinger, H., & Stoboy, H. (1974). Comparison between clinical judgment and electromyographic investigations of the effect of a special training program for CP-children. *Acta Paediatrica Belgica,* **28**(Suppl.), 121-128.

Rowe, J., & Stutts, R.M. (1987). Effects of practica type, experience and gender on attitudes of undergraduate physical education majors toward disabled persons. *Adapted Physical Activity Quarterly,* **4,** 268-277.

Rowell, L.B. (1974). Human cardiovascular adjustments to exercise and thermal stress. *Physiology Reviews,* **54,** 75-159.

Royce, J. (1959). Isometric fatigue curves in human muscle with normal and occluded circulation. *Research Quarterly,* **29,** 204-212.

Ruch, T., & Patton, H. (1966). *Physiology and biophysics.* Philadelphia: W.B. Saunders.

Rusch, H. (1981). Reflections on holiday camps for physically handicapped boys and girls. In U. Simri (Ed.), *Social aspects of physical education and sport* (p. 118). Natanya, Israel: Wingate Institute.

Ruschhaupt, D.G., Sodt, P.C., Hutcheon, N.A., & Arcilla, R.A. (1983). Estimation circumferential fiber shortening velocity by echocardiography. *Journal of Clinical Cardiology,* **2,** 77-84.

Russell, R.W. (1976). *Multiple sclerosis: Control of the disease.* New York: Pergamon Press.

Salend, S.J., & John, J. (1983). A tale of two teachers: Changing teacher commitment to mainstreaming. *Teaching Exceptional Children,* **15**(2), 82-85.

Salisbury, L.L., & Colman, A. (1969). A prosthetic device with automatic proportional control of grasp. In D. Bootzin & H.C. Muffley (Eds.), *Biomechanics* (pp. 27-38). New York: Plenum Press.

Saltin, B., Nazar, K., Costill, D.L., Stein, E., Jansson, E., Essén, B., & Gollnick, P.D. (1976). The nature of the training response: Peripheral and central adaptations to one-legged exercise. *Acta Physiologica Scandinavica,* **96,** 298-305.

Sanderson, D.J., & Sommer, H.J. (1985). Kinematic features of wheelchair propulsion. *Journal of Biomechanics, 18*, 423-429.

Sandler, A., & McLain, S. (1987). Sensory reinforcement: Effects of response contingent vestibular stimulation on multiply handicapped children. *American Journal of Mental Deficiency, 91*, 373-378.

Sanjak, M., Paulson, D., Sufit, R., Reddan, W., Beaulieu, D., Erickson, L., Shug, A., & Brooks, B.R. (1987). Physiologic and metabolic response to progressive and prolonged exercise in amyotrophic lateral sclerosis. *Neurology, 37*, 1217-1220.

Sapega, A.A., Nicholas, J.A., Sokolow, D., & Sarantini, A. (1982). The nature of torque overshoot in Cybex isokinetic dynamometry. *Medicine and Science in Sports and Exercise, 14*, 368-375.

Saunders, J.B., Inman, V.T., & Eberhart, H.D. (1953). The major determinants in normal and pathological gait. *Journal of Bone and Joint Surgery, 35A*, 543-558.

Sawka, M.N. (1986). Physiology of upper body exercise. *Exercise and Sport Science Reviews, 14*, 175-211.

Sawka, M.N., Foley, M.E., Pimental, N.E., & Pandolf, K.B. (1983b). Physiological factors affecting upper body exercise. *Ergonomics, 26*, 639-646.

Sawka, M.N., Foley, M.E., Pimental, N.E., Toner, M.M., & Pandolf, K.B. (1982a). Arm crank protocols for determination of maximal aerobic power [Abstract]. *Medicine and Science in Sports and Exercise, 14*, 168.

Sawka, M.N., Foley, M.E., Pimental, N.E., Toner, M.M., & Pandolf, K.B. (1983a). Determination of maximal aerobic power during upper body exercise. *Journal of Applied Physiology, 54*, 113-117.

Sawka, M.N., Glaser, R.M., Laubach, L.L., Al-Samkari, O., & Surprayasad, A.G. (1981). Wheelchair exercise performance in the young, middle-aged and elderly. *Journal of Applied Physiology, 50*, 824-828.

Sawka, M.N., Glaser, R.M., Wilde, S.W., & Von Luhrte, T.C. (1980). Metabolic and circulatory responses to wheelchair and arm crank exercise. *Journal of Applied Physiology, 49*, 784-788.

Sawka, M.N., Miles, D.S., Petrofsky, J.S., Wilde, S.W., & Glaser, R.M. (1982b). Ventilation and acid-base equilibrium for upper body and lower body exercise. *Aviation, Space and Environmental Medicine, 53*, 354-359.

Sawka, M.N., Pimental, D.A., & Pandolf, K.B. (1984). Thermoregulatory responses to upper body exercise. *European Journal of Applied Physiology, 52*, 230-234.

Schmidt, S., & Dunn, J. (1980). Physical education for the hearing impaired: A system of movement symbols. *Teaching Exceptional Children, 12*, 99-102.

Schover, L.R., & Newson, C.D. (1976). Over-selectivity, developmental level and over-training in autistic and normal children. *Journal of Abnormal Child Psychology, 4*, 289-298.

Schuman, S. (1979). Wheelchair frame modifications. *Sports 'N Spokes, 4*(5), 5-6.

Schurrer, R., Weltman, A., & Brammerl, H. (1985). Effects of physical training on cardiovascular fitness and behavior patterns of mentally retarded adults. *American Journal of Mental Deficiency, 90*, 167-170.

Schwade, J., Blomquist, C.G., & Shapiro, W. (1977). A comparison of the response to arm and leg work in patients with ischemic heart disease. *American Heart Journal,* **94,** 203-208.

Scott, N. (1974). Riding for the handicapped. In J. Yeo (Ed.), *Recreation for the handicapped* (pp. 69-71). Melbourne: Australian Council for Recreation of Disabled.

Scruton, J. (1979). Sir Ludwig Guttmann: Creator of a world sports movement for the paralysed and other disabled. *Paraplegia,* **17,** 52-55.

Seals, D.R., & Mullin, J.P. (1982). V̇O₂max in variable type exercise among well-trained upper body athletes. *Research Quarterly,* **53,** 58-63.

Secher, N.H., Ruberg-Larsen, N., Binkhorst, R.A., & Bonde-Petersen, F. (1974). Maximal oxygen uptake during arm cranking and combined arm plus leg exercise. *Journal of Applied Physiology,* **36,** 515-518.

Seeger, B.R., & Caudrey, D.J. (1983). Biofeedback therapy to achieve symmetrical gait in children with hemiplegic cerebral palsy: Long-term efficacy. *Archives of Physical Medicine and Rehabilitation,* **64,** 160-162.

Seelye, W. (1983). Physical fitness of blind and visually impaired Detroit public school children. *Journal of Visual Impairment and Blindness,* **77**(3), 117-118.

Seidl, C., Reid, G., & Montgomery, D.L. (1987). A critique of cardiovascular fitness testing with mentally retarded persons. *Adapted Physical Activity Quarterly,* **4,** 106-116.

Sengstock, W.L. (1966). Physical fitness of mentally retarded boys. *Research Quarterly,* **37,** 113-120.

Seymour, R.J., & Lacefield, W.E. (1985). Wheelchair cushion effect on pressure and skin temperature. *Archives of Physical Medicine and Rehabilitation,* **66,** 103-108.

Shasby, G., & Lyttle, J. (1981). Row, row, row your boat. *Sports 'N Spokes,* **7**(2), 5-7.

Shatin, L. (1970). The situational attitudes schedule: A morale scale for the chronic medical patient. *American Corrective Therapy Journal,* **24,** 137-140.

Shaw, D.J., Crawford, M.H., Karliner, J.S., Didonna, G., Carleton, R.M., Ross, J., & O'Rourke, R.A. (1974). Arm crank ergometry: A new method for the evaluation of coronary artery disease. *American Journal of Cardiology,* **33,** 801-805.

Shephard, R.J. (1966). Oxygen cost of breathing during vigorous exercise. *Quarterly Journal of Experimental Physiology,* **51,** 336-350.

Shephard, R.J. (1968). *Rapporteur: Meeting of investigators on exercise tests in relation to cardiovascular function* (World Health Organization Technical Report No. 388), Geneva: World Health Organization, pp. 1-30.

Shephard, R.J. (1969a). Learning, habituation and training. *Internationale Zeitschrift für Angewandte Physiologie,* **28,** 38-48.

Shephard, R.J. (1969b). Intensity, duration and frequency of exercise as determinants of the response to a training regime. *Internationale Zeitschrift für Angewandte Physiologie,* **26,** 272-278.

Shephard, R.J. (1974). *Men at work: Applications of ergonomics to performance and design.* Springfield, IL: Charles C Thomas.

Shephard, R.J. (1975). Future research on the quantifying of endurance training. *Journal of Human Ergology, 3*, 163-181.

Shephard, R.J. (1977). *Endurance fitness* (2nd ed.). Toronto: University of Toronto Press.

Shephard, R.J. (1978a). *Human physiological work capacity*. London: Cambridge University Press.

Shephard, R.J. (1978b). *The fit athlete*. Toronto: University of Toronto Press.

Shephard, R.J. (1980). Current status of the Canadian Home Fitness Test. *British Journal of Sports Medicine, 14*, 114-125.

Shephard, R.J. (1981). *Ischemic heart disease and exercise*. London: Croom-Helm.

Shephard, R.J. (1982a). *Physical activity and growth*. Chicago: Year Book Publishers.

Shephard, R.J. (1982b). *Physiology and biochemistry of exercise*. New York: Praeger.

Shephard, R.J. (1985a). Factors influencing the exercise behaviour of patients. *Sports Medicine, 2*, 348-366.

Shephard, R.J. (1985b). Motivation: The key to fitness compliance. *The Physician and Sportsmedicine, 13*, 88-101.

Shephard, R.J. (1985c). The value of physical fitness in preventive medicine. In D. Evered & J. Whelan (Eds.), *The value of preventive medicine* (pp. 164-174). London: CIBA Foundation.

Shephard, R.J. (1986a). *Economic benefits of enhanced endurance fitness*. Champaign, IL: Human Kinetics.

Shephard, R.J. (1986b). *Fitness of a nation: Lessons from the Canada Fitness Survey*. Basel, Switzerland: Karger.

Shephard, R.J. (1987). *Physical activity and aging* (2nd ed.). London: Croom-Helm.

Shephard, R.J., Davis, G.M., Kofsky, P.R., & Sutherland, S. (1983). Interactions between attitudes, personality and physical activity in the lower limb disabled [Abstract]. *Canadian Journal of Applied Sport Sciences, 8*, 173.

Shephard, R.J., Vandewalle, H., Bouhlel, E., & Monod, H. (1988). Muscle mass as a factor limiting physical work. *Journal of Applied Physiology, 64*, 1472-1479.

Shephard, R.J., Ward, G.R., & Lee, M. (1987). Physical ability of deaf and blind children. In J. Rutenfranz, R., Mocellin, & F. Klimt (Eds.), *Children and exercise XII* (pp. 355-362). Champaign, IL: Human Kinetics.

Sherrill, C. (1981). *Adapted physical education—A multidisciplinary approach* (2nd ed.). Dubuque, IA: Wm. C. Brown.

Sherrill, C. (1983). Pedagogy in the psychomotor domain for the severely handicapped. In R.L. Eason, T.L. Smith, & F. Caron (Eds.), *Adapted physical activity: From theory to application* (pp. 74-88). Champaign, IL: Human Kinetics.

Sherrill, C. (1986a). *Sport and disabled athletes*. Champaign, IL: Human Kinetics.

Sherrill, C. (1986b). Social and psychological dimensions. In C. Sherrill (Ed.), *Sport and disabled athletes* (pp. 21-23). Champaign, IL: Human Kinetics.

Sherrill, C. (1986c). *Adapted physical education and recreation*. Dubuque, IA: Wm. C. Brown.

Sherrill, C., Adams-Mushett, C., & Jones, J.A. (1986). Classification and other issues in sports for blind, cerebral palsied, les autres and amputee athletes. In C. Sherrill (Ed.), *Sport and disabled athletes* (pp. 113-130). Champaign, IL: Human Kinetics.

Sherrill, C., Pope, C., & Arnhold, R. (1986). Sport socialization of blind athletes. *Journal of Visual Impairment and Blindness, 80*, 740-744.

Sherrill, C., & Rainbolt, W.J. (1986). Sociological perspectives of cerebral palsy sports. *Palaestra, 2*(4), 21-26, 50.

Sherrill, C., & Rainbolt, W. (1987, June), *Self-actualization of adult cerebral palsied athletes: Gender and skill level differences*. Paper presented at the International Federation of Adapted Physical Activity, Brisbane, Australia.

Sherrill, C., Rainbolt, W., & Ervin, S. (1984). Attitudes of blind persons toward physical education and recreation. *Adapted Physical Activity Quarterly, 1*, 3-11.

Sherrill, C., Rainbolt, W., Montelione, T., & Pope, C. (1986). Sport socialization of blind and cerebral palsied elite athletes. In C. Sherrill (Ed.), *Sport and disabled athletes* (pp. 189-196). Champaign, IL: Human Kinetics.

Shingledecker, C.A. (1978). The effects of anticipation on performance and processing load in blind mobility. *Ergonomics, 21*, 355-371.

Shizume, K., Shishuba, Y., Sakuma, M., Yamauchi, H., Nakao, K., & Okinaka, S. (1966). Studies on the electrolyte metabolism in idiopathic and thyrotoxic periodic paralysis: 2. Total exchangeable sodium and potassium. *Metabolism, 15*, 145-149.

Shneerson, J.M. (1978). Pulmonary artery pressure in thoracic scoliosis during and after exercise while breathing air and pure oxygen. *Thorax, 33*, 747-754.

Shneerson, J.M., & Edgar, M.A. (1979). Cardiac and respiratory function before and after spinal fusion in adolescent idiopathic scoliosis. *Thorax, 34*, 658-661.

Shneerson, J.M., & Madgwick, R. (1979). The effect of physical training on exercise ability in adolescent idiopathic scoliosis. *Acta Orthopedica Scandinavica, 50*, 303-306.

Shneidman, N.N. (1978). *The Soviet road to Olympus—Theory and practice of Soviet physical culture and sport*. Toronto: Ontario Institute for Studies in Education.

Shontz, F.C. (1978). Psychological adjustment to physical disability: Trends in theories. *Archives of Physical Medicine and Rehabilitation, 59*, 251-254.

Short, F.X., & Winnick, J.P. (1986). The performance of adolescents with cerebral palsy on measures of physical fitness. In C. Sherrill (Ed.), *Sport and disabled athletes* (pp. 239-244). Champaign, IL: Human Kinetics.

Shriver, E.K. (1983). Keynote address, Third International Symposium on Adapted Physical Activity. In R.L. Eason, T.L. Smith, & F. Caron (Eds.), *Adapted physical activity: From theory to application* (pp. 3-9). Champaign, IL: Human Kinetics.

Sidney, K.H., & Shephard, R.J. (1978). Frequency and intensity of exercise training for elderly subjects. *Medicine and Science in Sports, 10*, 125-131.

Siefert, J., Lob, G., Stoephasium, E., Probst, J., & Brendel, W. (1972). Blood flow in muscles of paraplegic patients under various conditions measured by a double isotope technique. *Paraplegia, 10*, 185-191.

Siller, J.S. (1960). Psychological concomitants of amputation in children. *Child Development, 31*, 109-120.

Siller, J.S. (1982). Continuing research findings: Attitudes toward people with disabilities. *Rehabilitation Brief, 10*, 1-4.

Siller, J.S., & Peizer, E. (1957). Some problems of the amputee child in school. *Education, 78*(3), 141.

Silva, J., & Weinberg, R. (Eds.), (1984). *Psychological foundations of sport.* Champaign, IL: Human Kinetics.

Silver, J.R. (1963). The oxygen cost of breathing in tetraplegic patients. *Paraplegia, 1*, 204-209.

Simmons, R., & Shephard, R.J. (1971a). Effects of physical conditioning upon the central and peripheral response to arm work. *Internationale Zeitschrift für Angewandte Physiologie, 30*, 73-79.

Simmons, R., & Shephard, R.J. (1971b). Measurement of cardiac output in maximum exercise: Application of an acetylene rebreathing method to arm and leg exercise. *Internationale Zeitschrift für Angewandte Physiologie, 29*, 159-172.

Simon, J.I. (1971). Emotional aspects of physical disability. *American Journal of Occupational Therapy, 25*, 408-410.

Singh, B., & Chhina, G.S. (1974). Some reflections on ancient Indian physiology. In N.H. Keswani (Ed.), *The science of medicine and physiological concepts in ancient and medieval India.* New Delhi: All-India Institute of Physiological Sciences.

Siri, W.E. (1956). The gross composition of the body. *Advances in Biological and Medical Physics, 4*, 239-280.

Sjöstrand, T. (1967). Exercise tests. In T. Sjöstrand (Ed.), *Clinical physiology.* Stockholm: Svenska Bokfotlaget.

Skrinar, G.S., Evans, W.J., Ornstein, L.J., & Brown, D.A. (1982). Glycogen utilization in wheelchair dependent athletes. *International Journal of Sports Medicine, 3*, 215-219.

Skrobak-Kaczynski, J., & Vavik, T. (1980). Physical fitness and trainability of young male patients with Down's syndrome. In K. Berg & B.O. Ericksson (Eds.), *Children and exercise IX* (pp. 300-316). Baltimore: University Park Press.

Skrotsky, K. (1983). Gait analysis in cerebral palsied and non-handicapped children. *Archives of Physical Medicine and Rehabilitation, 64*, 291-295.

Slagle, D.K. (1982). ATVs, three-wheelers, and other alternative modes of transportation. *Sports 'N Spokes, 7*(6), 12-19.

Sloan, W. (1951). Motor proficiency and intelligence. *American Journal of Mental Deficiency, 55*, 394-406.

Smith, M.J., & Melton, P. (1981). Isokinetic versus isotonic variable resistance training. *American Journal of Sports Medicine, 9*, 275-279.

Smith, P.A., Glaser, R.M., Petrofsky, J.S., Underwood, P., Gibson, G., & Richard, J. (1983). Arm crank vs. hand rim wheelchair propulsion: Metabolic and cardio-respiratory responses. *Archives of Physical Medicine and Rehabilitation,* **64**, 249-254.

Snaith, I.C. (1974). Agency responsibility for the recreation of the handicapped. In J. Yeo (Ed.), *Recreation for the handicapped* (pp. 43-47). Melbourne: Australian Council for Recreation of Disabled.

Society of Actuaries (1959). *Build and blood pressure study.* Chicago: Author.

Sockolov, R., Irwin, B., Dressendorfer, R.H., & Bernauer, E.M. (1977). Exercise performance in 6 to 11 year old boys with Duchenne muscular dystrophy. *Archives of Physical Medicine and Rehabilitation,* **58**, 195-201.

Sommer, M. (1971). Improvements of motor skills and adaptations of the circulatory system in wheelchair bound children in cerebral palsy. In U. Simri (Ed.), *Sports as a means of rehabilitation* (pp. 11/1-11/11). Natanya, Israel: Wingate Institute.

Sommer, M. (1973). Training of the organs with cerebral-paretic children in the wheelchair. In O. Grüpe (Ed.), *Sport in the modern world—Problems and chances* (pp. 282-283). Berlin: Springer Verlag.

Songster, T.B. (1986). The special Olympics sport program: An international sport program for mentally retarded athletes. In C. Sherrill (Ed.), *Sport and disabled athletes* (pp. 73-80). Champaign, IL: Human Kinetics.

Sonka, J.J., & Bina, M.J. (1978). Cross country running for visually impaired young adults. *Journal of Visual Impairment and Blindness,* **72**, 212-214.

Sorenson, L., & Ulrich, P. (1977). *Ambulation guide for nurses.* Minneapolis: Sister Kenny Institute.

Speakman, H.G.B. (1977). The measurement of motor fitness in trainable mentally retarded children. *Canadian Association for Health, Physical Education and Recreation Journal,* **43**, 30-35.

Spielberger, C., Gorsuch, R., & Lushene, R. (1970). *STAI manual.* Palo Alto, CA: Consulting Psychologists Press.

Spira, R. (1967a). An investigation into the influence of sports activities on some physical aspects of post-poliomyelitis paralytic subjects. In R. Spira (Ed.), *Influence of sports activities on rehabilitation of paralytic subjects.* Natanya, Israel: Wingate Institute.

Spira, R. (1967b). Physical impact of sport activities in a group of post-poliomyelitic paralytic subjects. In U. Simri (Ed.), *Sports as a means of rehabilitation* (pp. 3/1-3/11). Natanya, Israel: Wingate Institute.

Spira, R. (1974). Contribution of the H-reflex to the study of spasticity in adolescents. *Developmental Medicine and Child Neurology,* **16**, 150-157.

Spooren, P. (1981). The technical characteristics of wheelchair racing. *Sports 'N Spokes,* November/December, 1981.

Stafford, G. (1939). *Sports for handicapped.* New York: Prentice-Hall.

Stamford, B.A. (1973). Effects of chronic institutionalization on the physical working capacity and trainability of geriatric men. *Journal of Gerontology,* **28**, 441-446.

Stamford, B.A. (1975). Cardiovascular endurance training for blind persons. *The New Outlook,* **33**, 308-311.

Stamford, B.A., Cuddihee, R.W., Moffatt, R.J., & Rowland, R. (1978). Task specific changes in maximal oxygen uptake resulting from arm versus leg training. *Ergonomics, 21,* 1-19.

Stamps, L.E., Eason, B.L., & Smith, T.L. (1983). Discriminatory response time and heart rate differences between gifted and learning disabled children. In R.L. Eason, T.L. Smith, & F. Caron (Eds.), *Adapted physical activity: From theory to application* (pp. 226-229). Champaign, IL: Human Kinetics.

Stanley, S.M., & Kindig, L.E. (1986). Improvisations for blind bowlers. *Palaestra, 2,* 38-39.

Staros, A. (1981). Testing manually propelled wheelchairs. *Prosthetics and Orthotics International, 5,* 75-84.

Steadward, R.D. (1979). Research on classifying wheelchair athletes. In R.D. Steadward (Ed.), *Proceedings, First International Conference on Sport and Training of the Physically Disabled Athlete* (pp. 36-40). Edmonton: University of Alberta.

Steadward, R.D. (1980). Analysis of wheelchair sports events. In H. Natvig (Ed.), *First International Medical Congress on Sports for the Disabled.* Oslo: Royal Ministry of Church and Education.

Steadward, R.D., & Walsh, C. (1986). Training and fitness programs for disabled athletes: Past, present and future. In C. Sherrill (Ed.), *Sport and disabled athletes* (pp. 3-19), Champaign, IL: Human Kinetics.

Stein, J.U. (1965). Physical fitness of mentally retarded relative to national age norms. *Rehabilitation Literature, 26,* 205-208.

Stein, J.U. (1975). *Testing for impaired, disabled, and handicapped individuals.* Washington, DC: American Alliance for Health, Physical Education and Recreation.

Stein, J.U. (1986). International perspectives: Physical education and sport for participants with handicapping conditions. In C. Sherrill (Ed.), *Sport and disabled athletes* (pp. 51-64), Champaign, IL: Human Kinetics.

Stein, J.U., & Gepford, G. (1982). *International survey on development of physical education and sport for the physically and mentally handicapped* (UNESCO Contract No. 516291 with ICHPER). Washington, DC: International Council for Health, Physical Education and Recreation.

Stein, R.A., Michielli, D., Fox., E.L., & Krasnow, N. (1978). Continuous ventricular dimensions in man during supine exercise and recovery: An echocardiographic study. *American Journal of Cardiology, 41,* 655-660.

Steinberg, U., Sunwoo, I., & Roettger, R.F. (1985). Prosthetic rehabilitation of geriatric amputee patients: A follow-up study. *Archives of Physical Medicine and Rehabilitation, 66,* 742-745.

Stenberg, J., Åstrand, P.O., Ekblöm, B., Royce, J., & Saltin, B. (1967). Hemodynamic response to work with different muscle groups sitting and supine. *Journal of Applied Physiology, 22,* 61-70.

Stewart, C.C. (1988). Modification of student attitudes toward disabled peers. *Adapted Physical Activity Quarterly, 5,* 44-48.

Stewart, D. (1986). Deaf sport in the community. *Journal of Community Psychology, 14,* 16-21.

Stewart, N. (1981). Value of sport in the rehabilitation of the physically disabled. *Canadian Journal of Applied Sport Sciences, 6*, 166-167.

Stewart, S.F., Palmieri, V., & Cochran, G.V. (1980). Wheelchair cushion effect on skin temperature, heat flux and relative humidity. *Archives of Physical Medicine and Rehabilitation, 61*, 229-233.

Stoboy, H. (1978). Pulmonary function and spiroergometric criteria in scoliotic patients before and after Harrington Rod surgery and physical exercise. In J. Borms & M. Hebbelinck (Eds.), *Pediatric work physiology* (pp. 72-81). Basel, Switzerland: Karger.

Stoboy, H. (1985). Effort tolerance in scoliosis. In P. Welsh & R.J. Shephard (Eds.), *Current therapy in sports medicine 1985-6* (pp. 114-116). Burlington, ON: Decker.

Stoboy, H., & Speierer, B. (1968). Lungenfunktionswerte und spiroergometrische Parameter wahrend der Rehabilitation von Patienten mit idiopathischer Skoliose [Lung function values and spiroergometric parameters during the rehabilitation of patients with idiopathic scoliosis]. *Archiv für Orthopaedische und Unfall-Chirurgie, 81*, 247-254.

Stoboy, J., Rich, B.W., & Lee, M. (1971). Workload and energy expenditure during wheelchair propelling. *Paraplegia, 8*, 223-230.

Stoboy, H., & Wilson-Rich, B. (1971). Muscle strength and electrical activity, heart rate and energy cost during isometric contractions in disabled and non-disabled. *Paraplegia, 8*, 217-222.

Stone, B., Beeckman, C., Hall, V., Guess, V., & Brooks, H.L. (1979). The effects of an exercise program on change in curve in adolescents with minimal idiopathic scoliosis: A preliminary study. *Physical Therapy, 59*, 759-763.

Stott, J.R.R., Hutton, W.C., & Stokes, I.A.F. (1973). Forces under the foot. *Journal of Bone and Joint Surgery, 55B*, 335-344.

Strauss, R.H., Haynes, R.L., Ingram, R.H., & McFadden, E.R. (1977). Comparison of arm versus leg work in induction of acute episodes of asthma. *Journal of Applied Physiology, 42*, 565-570.

Strohkendl, H. (1985). Classification system for wheelchair basketball. In J.H. Hoeberigs & H. Varsteveld (Eds.), *Workshop on disabled and sports* (pp. 124-134). Amersfoort, Netherlands: Nederlandse Invaliden Sportbond.

Strohkendl, H. (1986). The new classification system for wheelchair basketball. In C. Sherrill (Ed.), *Sport and disabled athletes* (pp. 101-112), Champaign, IL: Human Kinetics.

Sündberg, S. (1982). Maximal oxygen uptake in relation to age in blind and normal boys and girls. *Acta Paediatrica Scandinavica, 71*, 603-608.

Sündberg, S. (1983). Lung volume and exercise ventilation in blind and normal boys and girls. *Respiration, 44*, 444-449.

Susheela, A.K., & Walton, J.N. (1969). Note on the distribution of histochemical fiber types in some normal human muscles: A study on autopsy material. *Journal of Neurological Science, 8*, 201-207.

Suzuki, K., Takahama, M., Mizutani, Y., Arai, M., & Iwai, A. (1983). Locomotive mechanics of normal adults and amputees. In H. Matsui & K. Kobayashi (Eds.), *Biomechanics VIIIA & B: Proceedings of the Eighth International Congress of Biomechanics, Nagoya* (pp. 380-385). Champaign, IL: Human Kinetics.

Szyman, R.J. (1980). The effect of participation in wheelchair sports. *Dissertation Abstracts International,* **41**, 804A-805A.

Tahamont, M.V., & Knowlton, R.G. (1981). Effects of wheelchair exercise on able-bodied and wheelchair confined women [Abstract]. *Medicine and Science in Sports and Exercise,* **13**, 132.

Tahamont, M.V., Knowlton, R.G., Sawka, M.N., & Miles, D.S. (1986). Metabolic responses of women to exercise attributable to long term use of a manual wheelchair. *Paraplegia,* **24**, 311-317.

Tauscher, H. (1969). Rhythmische-musikalische Arbeit mit dem behinderten Kind [Rhythmic musical activity with the retarded child]. *Das Behinderte Kind,* **6**, 4-5.

Taylor, A.W. (1981). Physical activity for the disabled. In J.R. Richardson (Ed.), *Report of the research priority development conference, March 17th and 18th, 1981* (pp. 15-21). Ottawa: Fitness & Amateur Sport.

Taylor, A.W., McDonnell, E., & Brassard, L. (1986). The effect of an arm ergometer training programme on wheelchair subjects. *Paraplegia,* **24**, 105-114.

Taylor, A.W., McDonnell, E., Royer, D., Loiselle, R., Lush, N., & Steadward, R.D. (1979). Skeletal muscle analysis of wheelchair athletes. *Paraplegia,* **17**, 456-460.

Taylor, P. (1983). Pete Axelson: Building a better ski-sled is only part of the story. *Sports 'N Spokes,* **8**(6), 28-30.

Tesch, P.A., & Karlsson, J. (1983). Muscle fiber type characteristics of M. Deltoideus in wheelchair athletes: Comparison with other trained athletes. *American Journal of Physical Medicine,* **62**, 239-243.

Tesch, P.A., Piehl, K., Wilson, G., & Karlsson, J. (1984). Bases physiologiques du canoe-kayak [Physiological basis of kayaking]. In M. Robin & G. Peres (Trans.) & J.R. LaCour (Ed.). St. Etienne, France: University of St. Etienne.

Thacker, J.G., O'Reagan, J.R., Aylor, J.H., & Brubacker, C. (1980). Wheelchair dynamometer. In T.E. Shoup & J.G. Thacker (Eds.), *Proceedings of International Conference on Medical Devices and Sports Equipment* (pp. 107-112). New York: American Society of Mechanical Engineers.

Thorpe-Tracey, R. (1976). *Integrating the disabled: Report of the Snowdon Working Party* (p. 66). Horsham, England: National Fund for Research Into Crippling Diseases.

Thorstensson, A., Larsson, L., Tesch, P.A., & Karlsson, J. (1977). Muscle strength and fiber composition in athletes and sedentary men. *Medicine and Science in Sports and Exercise,* **9**, 26-30.

Tilley, A.D., Mosher, R.E., & Sinclair, G.D. (1987). A physical fitness assessment of British Columbia Special Olympic Athletes. In M. Berridge & G. Ward (Eds.), *International perspectives on adapted physical activity* (pp. 183-190). Champaign, IL: Human Kinetics.

Titlow, L., & Ishee, J.H. (1980). Cardiovascular testing on individuals who are visually impaired. *Journal of Visual Impairment and Blindness,* **80**, 726-728.

Titus, J.A., & Watkinson, J.E. (1987). Effects of segregated and integrated programs on the participation and social interaction of moderately mentally handicapped children in play. *Adapted Physical Activity Quarterly,* **4**, 204-219.

Tomporowski, P.D., & Ellis, N.R. (1984). Effects of exercise on the physical fitness, intelligence and adaptive behavior of institutionalized mentally retarded adults. *Applied Research in Mental Retardation, 5*, 329-337.

Tomporowski, P.D., & Ellis, N.R. (1985). The effects of exercise on the health, intelligence and adaptive behavior of institutionalized severely and profoundly retarded adults: A systematic replication. *Applied Research in Mental Retardation, 6*, 465-473.

Tomporowski, P.D., & Jameson, L.D. (1985). Effects of a physical fitness training program on the exercise behavior of institutionalized mentally retarded adults. *Adapted Physical Activity Quarterly, 2*, 197-205.

Topsfield, R.J. (1974). Recreation in special education. In J. Yeo (Ed.), *Recreation for the disabled* (pp. 33-35). Melbourne: Australian Council for Rehabilitation of Disabled.

Totel, G.R. (1974). Physiological responses to heat of resting man with impaired sweating capacity. *Journal of Applied Physiology, 37*, 346-352.

Totel, G.L., Johnson, R.E., Fay, R.A., Goldstein, J.A., & Schick, J.A. (1971). Experimental hyperthermia in traumatic quadraplegia. *International Journal of Biometeorology, 15*, 346-355.

Traugh, G.H., Corcoran, P.J., & Reyes, R.L. (1975). Energy expenditure of ambulation in patients with above-knee amputations. *Archives of Physical Medicine and Rehabilitation, 56*, 67-71.

Triandis, H. (1971). *Attitude and attitude change.* New York: Wiley.

Tringo, J. (1970). The hierarchy of preference towards disability groups. *Journal of Special Education, 4*(3), 295-305.

Trowbridge, R. (1974). Outdoor recreation and camping. In J. Yeo (Ed.), *Recreation for the disabled* (pp. 65-68). Melbourne: Australian Council for Rehabilitation of Disabled.

Tucker, W. (1968). *Investigation of the feasibility of using 16PF to identify personality traits of physically handicapped college students* (Doctoral dissertation, University of South Dakota). *Dissertation Abstracts International, 29*, 157A.

Tupling, S.J., Davis, G.M., Pierrynowski, M.R., & Shephard, R.J. (1986). Arm strength and impulse generation: Initiation of wheelchair movement by the physically disabled. *Ergonomics, 29*, 303-312.

Tupling, S.J., Davis, G.M., & Shephard, R.J. (1983). Arm strength and impulse generation in the physically disabled [Abstract]. *Canadian Journal of Applied Sport Sciences, 9*, 148.

Ulrich, D.A. (1983). A comparison of the qualitative motor performance of normal, educable and trainable mentally retarded students. In R.L. Eason, T.L. Smith, & F. Caron (Eds.), *Adapted physical activity: From theory to application* (pp. 219-225). Champaign, IL: Human Kinetics.

United Nations Educational, Scientific and Cultural Organization, International Council of Sport and Physical Education. (1964). *Declaration on Sport.* Paris: Author.

United Nations Educational, Scientific and Cultural Organization. (1982). *International Symposium on Physical Education and Sport Programs for the Physically and Mentally Handicapped* (UNESCO Contract No. 518.015 with the U.S. National Commission for UNESCO). Paris: Author.

U.S. Office of Education. (1977, Aug. 23). Education of handicapped children: Implementation of Part B of Education of the Handicapped Children Act. *Federal Register, Part II.*

U.S. President's Council on Physical Fitness. (1963). *Adult physical fitness.* Washington, DC: U.S. Government Printing Office.

VA Technical Bulletin on Spinal Injuries. (1948). Washington, DC: U.S. Veteran's Administration.

Vaccaro, P., Clarke, D.H., Morris, A.F., & Gray, P.R. (1984). Physiological characteristics of the world champion whitewater slalom team. In N. Bachl, L. Prokop, & R. Suckert (Eds.), *Current topics in sports medicine* (pp. 637-647). Vienna: Urban & Schwarzenburg.

Van Alste, J.A., Cruts, H.E.P., Huisman, L., & de Vries, J., (1985b). Exercise electrocardiography in leg amputees. In J.H. Hoeberigs & H. Varsteveld (Eds.), *Workshop on disabled and sports* (pp. 44-49). Amersfoort, Netherlands: Nederlandse Invaliden Sportbond.

Van Alste, J.A., la Haye, M.W., Huisman, L., de Vries, J., & Boom, H.B.K. (1985a). Exercise electrocardiography using rowing ergometer suitable for leg amputees. *International Journal of Rehabilitation Medicine, 7,* 1-5.

Van der Woude, L.H.V., de Groot, G., Hollander, A.P., Van Ingen Schenau, G.J., & Rozendal, R.H. (1986). Wheelchair ergonomics and physiological testing of prototypes. *Ergonomics, 29,* 1561-1573.

Vander, L.B., Franklin, B.A., Wrisley, D., & Rubenfire, M. (1984). Cardio-respiratory responses to arm and leg ergometry in women. *The Physician and Sportsmedicine, 12,* 101-106.

Van Hal, L., Rarick, G.L., & Vermeer, A. (1984). Sport for the mentally handicapped: Mentally handicapped sport symposium of the Netherlands—SA Bicentennial, September 20-25, 1982. Haarlem, Netherlands: Uitgeverij de Vrieseborch.

Vanlerberghe, J.O.C., & Slock, K. (1987). A study of wheelchair basketball skills. In M. Berridge & G. Ward (Eds.), *International perspectives on adapted physical activity* (pp. 221-232). Champaign, IL: Human Kinetics.

Van Loan, M.D., McCluer, S., Loftin, J.M., & Boileau, R.A. (1987). Comparison of physiological responses to maximal arm exercise among able-bodied, paraplegics and quadriplegics. *Paraplegia, 25,* 397-405.

Vargo, J.W. (1978). Some psychological effects of physical disability. *American Journal of Occupational Therapy, 32,* 31-34.

Venediktov, D.D. (1966). Prophylaxis of cardiovascular diseases in the Soviet Union. In W. Raab (Ed.), *Prevention of ischemic heart disease: Principles and practice* (pp. 377-387). Springfield, IL: Charles C Thomas.

Verbeek, L.A.M. (1984). Prevalence of some motoric handicaps in community. *International Journal of Sports Medicine, 5*(Suppl.), 165-166.

Vignos, P., & Watkins, N. (1966). The effect of exercise in muscular dystrophy. *Journal of the American Medical Association, 197,* 843-848.

Voight, E.D., & Bahn, D. (1969). Metabolism and pulse rate in physically handicapped when propelling a wheelchair up an incline. *Scandinavian Journal of Rehabilitation Medicine, 1,* 101-106.

Vokac, Z., Bell, H., Bautz-Holter, E., & Rodahl, K. (1975). Oxygen uptake/heart rate relationship in leg and arm exercise, sitting and standing. *Journal of Applied Physiology, 39*, 54-59.

Vorsteveld, H. (1985). The classification system of I.S.M.G.F. In J.H. Hoeberigs & H. Vorsteveld (Eds.), *Proceedings of the workshop on disabled and sports* (pp. 84-89). Amersfoort, Netherlands: Nederlandse Invaliden Sportbond.

Vrijens, J., Hoestra, P., Bouckaert, J., & Uytvanck, P. Van (1975). Effects of training on maximal working capacity and haemodynamic response during arm and leg exercise in a group of paddlers. *European Journal of Applied Physiology, 36*, 113-119.

Wahren, J., & Bygdeman, S. (1971). Onset of angina pectoris in relation to circulatory adaptation during arm and leg exercise. *Circulation, 44*, 432-441.

Wakim, K.G., Elkins, E.C., Worden, R.E., & Polley, H.F. (1949). The effect of therapeutic exercise on the peripheral circulation of normal and paraplegic individuals. *Archives of Physical Medicine, 30*, 86-94.

Walsh, C.M., Marchiori, G.E., & Steadward, R.D. (1986). Effect of seat position on maximal linear velocity in wheelchair sprinting. *Canadian Journal of Applied Sport Sciences, 11*, 186-190.

Walsh, C.M., & Steadward, R.D. (1984). *Get fit: Muscular fitness exercises for the wheelchair user*. Edmonton: University of Alberta.

Ward, G.R. (1985). Exercise and sensory disability. In P. Welsh & R.J. Shephard (Eds.), *Current therapy in sports medicine 1985-1986* (pp. 111-113). Burlington, ON: Decker.

Ward, G.R., & Fraser, L.N. (1984). Fitness characteristics of Canadian National wheelchair athletes [Abstract]. *Medicine and Science in Sports and Exercise, 16*, 142.

Ware, M. (1982). Canoe racing. *Sports 'N Spokes, 8*(3), 4-18.

Washburn, R.A., & Seals, D.R. (1983). Comparison of continuous and discontinuous protocols for the determination of peak oxygen uptake in arm cranking. *European Journal of Applied Physiology, 51*, 3-6.

Waters, R.L., Perry, J., Antonelli, D., & Hislop, H. (1976). Energy cost of walking of amputees: Influence of level of amputation. *Journal of Bone and Joint Surgery* (America), *58*, 42-46.

Watkinson, E.J., & Titus, J.A. (1985). Integrating the mentally handicapped in physical activity: A review and discussion. *Canadian Journal for Exceptional Children, 2*, 48-53.

Weege, R.D. (1985). Technische Voraussetzungen fuer den Aktivsport in Rollstühl [Technical specification for active wheelchair sports]. *Orthopaedie Technik, 36*, 395-402.

Weiss, J.L. (1980). Evaluation of the left ventricle by two dimensional echocardiography. In J.A. Kisslo (Ed.), *Two dimensional echocardiography* (pp. 93-107). New York: Churchill-Livingstone.

Weiss, M. (1971). Sports with paraplegics. In U. Simri (Ed.), *Sports as a means of rehabilitation* (pp. 14/1-14/12). Natanya, Israel: Wingate Institute.

Weiss, M., & Beck, J. (1973). Sports as a part of therapy and rehabilitation of paraplegics. *Paraplegia, 11*, 166-172.

Weiss, M., & Curtis, K.A. (1986). Controversies in medical classification of wheelchair athletes. In C. Sherrill (Ed.), *Sport and disabled athletes* (pp. 93-100), Champaign, IL: Human Kinetics.

Welford, A.T. (1962). Arousal, channel capacity and decision. *Nature, 194*(4826), 365-366.

Wells, K.F., & Luttgens, K. (1976). *Kinesiology: Scientific basis of human motion* (6th ed.). Philadelphia: Saunders.

Wendt, I.R., & Gibbs, C.L. (1973). Energy production of rat extensor digitorum longus muscle. *American Journal of Physiology, 224*, 1081-1086.

Werder, J.K., & Kalakian, L.H. (1985). *Assessment in adapted physical education*. Minneapolis: Burgess.

Wessel, J.A. (1983). Quality programming in physical education and recreation for all handicapped persons. In R.L. Eason, T.L. Smith, & F. Caron (Eds.), *Adapted physical activity: From theory to application* (pp. 35-52). Champaign, IL: Human Kinetics.

Whipp, B.J., & Wasserman, K. (1969). Efficiency of muscular work. *Journal of Applied Physiology, 26*, 644-648.

Whiting, R.B., Dreisinger, T.E., & Abbott, C. (1983a). Clinical value of exercise testing in handicapped subjects. *Southern Medical Journal, 76*, 1225-1227.

Whiting, R.B., Dreisinger, T.E., Dalton, R.B., & Londeree, B. (1983). Improved physical fitness and work capacity in quadriplegics by wheelchair exercise. *Journal of Cardiac Rehabilitation, 3*, 251-255.

Whiting, R.B., Dreisinger, T.E., & Hayden, T. (1984). Wheelchair exercise testing: A comparison of continuous and discontinuous exercise. *Paraplegia, 22*, 92-98.

Whitt, F.R., & Wilson, G.R. (1979). *Bicycle science, ergonomics and mechanics*. London: M.I.T. Press.

Wicks, J., Lymburner, K., Dinsdale, S., & Jones, N. (1977). The use of multistage exercise testing with wheelchair ergometry and arm cranking in subjects with spinal cord lesions. *Paraplegia, 15*, 252-261.

Wicks, J., Oldridge, N.B., Cameron, N.B., & Jones, N.L. (1983). Arm-cranking and wheelchair ergometry in elite spinal cord injured athletes. *Medicine and Science in Sports and Exercise, 5*, 224-231.

Wilcox, E.N., Stauffer, E.S., & Nickel, V.L. (1968). A statistical analysis of 423 consecutive patients admitted to the spinal cord injury center, Rancho Los Amigos Hospital, January 1st 1964 to December 31st 1967. *Paraplegia, 14*, 27-35.

Wilde, S.W., Miles, D.S., Durbin, R.J., Sawka, M.N., Surprayasad, A.G., Gotshall, R.W., & Glaser, R.M. (1981). Evaluation of myocardial performance during wheelchair ergometer exercise. *American Journal of Physical Medicine, 60*, 277-291.

Wiles, C.M., & Karni, Y. (1983). The measurement of muscle strength in patients with peripheral neuromuscular disorders. *Journal of Neurology, Neurosurgery and Psychiatry, 46*, 1006-1013.

Wilkinson, K. (1982). Skiing on water. *Sports 'N Spokes, 8*(2), 17.

Wilkinson, P.F. (1984). Providing integrated play environments for disabled children. In L.M. Wells (Ed.), *Proceedings: The integration of the physically disabled into community living. A colloquium* (pp. 133-145). Toronto: University of Toronto School of Social Work.

Williams, J., Cottrell, E., Powers, S.K., & McKnight, T. (1983). Arm ergometry: A review of published protocols and the introduction of a new weight-adjusted protocol. *Journal of Sports Medicine and Physical Fitness, 23,* 107-112.

Wing, J.K. (1966). *Early childhood autism.* London: Pergamon Press.

Wing, L. (1976). Diagnosis, clinical description and prognosis. In L. Wing (Ed.) *Early childhood autism* (2nd ed.). New York: Pergamon Press.

Winnick, J.P. (1984). Recent advances related to special physical education and sport. *Adapted Physical Activity Quarterly, 1,* 197-206.

Winnick, J.P. (1985). Performance of visually impaired youngsters in physical education activities: Implications for mainstreaming. *Adapted Physical Activity Quarterly, 2,* 292-299.

Winnick, J.P. (1987). An integration continuum for sport participation. *Adapted Physical Activity Quarterly, 4,* 157-161.

Winnick, J.P., Huxter, D., Jansma, P., Sculli, J., Stein, J., & Weiss, R.A. (1980). Implications of Section 504 of the Rehabilitation Act as related to physical education instructional, personnel preparation, intramural, and inter-scholastic/intercollegiate sport programs. *Practical Pointers, 3*(11), 1-20.

Winnick, J.P., & Short, F.X. (1984). The physical fitness of youngsters with spinal neuromuscular conditions. *Adapted Physical Activity Quarterly, 1,* 37-51.

Winnick, J.P., & Short, F.X. (1985). *Physical fitness testing of the disabled: Project Unique.* Champaign, IL: Human Kinetics.

Winnick, J.P., & Short, F.X. (1986). *Physical fitness of adolescents with auditory impairments. Adapted Physical Activity Quarterly, 3,* 58-66.

Winter, D.A., Wells, R.P., & Orr, G.W. (1981). Errors in the use of isokinetic dynamometers. *European Journal of Applied Physiology, 46,* 397-408.

Witman, J.P. (1987). The efficacy of adventure programming in the development of cooperation and trust with adolescents in treatment. *Therapeutic Recreation Journal, 21*(3), 22-29.

Witt, A.N. (1973). Sport for the disabled. In O. Grüpe (Ed.), *Sport in the modern world* (pp. 256-260). Berlin: Springer Verlag.

Witt, P.A. (1977). *Community leisure services and disabled individuals.* Ottawa, ON: Leisurability Publications.

Wolf, E., & Magora, A. (1976). Orthostatic and ergometric evaluation of cord injured patients. *Scandinavian Journal of Rehabilitation Medicine, 8,* 93-96.

Wolfe, G.A. (1978). Influence of floor surface on the energy cost of wheelchair propulsion. *Orthopedic Clinics of North America, 9,* 370-372.

Wolfe, G.A., Waters, R., & Hislop, H.J. (1977). Influence of floor surface on the energy cost of wheelchair propulsion. *Physical Therapy, 57,* 1022-1027.

Wolfe, L.A., Cunningham, D.A., Rechnitzer, P.A., & Nichol, P.M. (1979). Effects of endurance training on left ventricular dimensions in healthy men. *Journal of Applied Physiology, Respiratory, Environmental and Exercise Physiology, 47,* 207-212.

Wood, P.D., Haskell, W., & Blair, S.N. (1983). Increased exercise level and plasma lipoprotein concentrations: A one-year randomized controlled trial in sedentary middle-aged men. *Metabolism, 32,* 31-39.

World Health Organization. (1969). Research in health education. *Technical Report, 432,* 1-30.

World Health Organization. (1974). Health education: A programme review. *WHO Offset Publications, 7,* 1-78.

Wright, B.A. (1983). *Physical disability: A psycho-social approach.* New York: Harper & Row.

Wright, G.B. (1986). The evolution and role of the Sports Councils in Britain. In G. Redmond (Ed.), *Sport and politics* (pp. 59-66). Champaign, IL: Human Kinetics.

Wright, J., & Cowden, J.E. (1986). Changes in self-concept and cardiovascular endurance of mentally retarded youths in a special Olympics swim training program. *Adapted Physical Activity Quarterly, 3,* 177-183.

Wycherly, R.S., & Nicklin, B.H. (1970). The heart rate of blind and sighted pedestrians on a town route. *Ergonomics, 13,* 181-192.

Wylie, R. (1961). *The self concept—A critical survey of pertinent research literature.* Lincoln, NE: University of Nebraska Press.

Yale, M. (1982). Leisure time—Benefit or cop-out? *Journal of Leisure, 9,* 4-7.

Yeo, J. (1974). *Recreation for the handicapped.* Melbourne: Australian Council for Rehabilitation of the Disabled.

Yoshizawa, S., Ishizaki, T., & Honda, H. (1975). Aerobic capacity of mentally retarded boys and girls in junior high schools. *Journal of Human Ergology, 4,* 15-26.

Zankel, H.T. (1971). *Stroke rehabilitation.* Springfield, IL: Charles C Thomas.

Zasueta, A.S., & Kasch, F.W. (1973). Physical performance changes in educable mentally retarded children over two years. In O. Bar-Or (Ed.), *Pediatric work physiology* (pp. 303-314). Natanya, Israel: Wingate Institute.

Zeppilli, P., Sandric, S., Cecchetti, F., Spataro, A., & Fanelli, R. (1980). Echocardiographic assessments of cardiac arrangements in different sports activities. In T. Lubich & A. Venerando, *Sports cardiology* (pp. 723-734). Bologna: Aulo Gaggi.

Zhuo, D. (1985). *The Chinese exercise book: From ancient and modern China—Exercises for well-being and the treatment of illnesses.* Vancouver: Hartley & Marks.

Ziegler, E. (1976). Canada at the cross-roads in international sport. In P.J. Graham & H. Veberhorst (Eds.), *The modern Olympics* (pp. 209-225). West Point, NY: Leisure Press.

Zoneraich, S., Rhee, J.J., Zoneraich, O., Jordan, D., & Appel, J. (1977). Assessment of cardiac function in marathon runners by graphic noninvasive techniques. *Annals of New York Academy of Sciences, 301,* 900-917.

Zwiren, L., & Bar-Or, O. (1975). Responses to exercise of paraplegics who differ in conditioning level. *Medicine and Science in Sports and Exercise, 7,* 94-98.

Zwiren, L.D., Huberman, G., & Bar-Or, O. (1973). Cardio-pulmonary functions of sedentary and highly active paraplegics. *Medicine and Science in Sports, 5,* 63.

Index